OTHER MONOGRAPHS IN THE SERIES,
MAJOR PROBLEMS IN PATHOLOGY

Published

Evans and Cruickshank: *Epithelial Tumours of the Salivary Glands*

Mottet: *Histopathologic Spectrum of Regional Enteritis and Ulcerative Colitis*

Whitehead: *Mucosal Biopsy of the Gastrointestinal Tract, 2nd ed.*

Hughes: *Pathology of Muscle*

Thurlbeck: *Chronic Airflow Obstruction in Lung Disease*

Hughes: *Pathology of the Spinal Cord*

Fox: *Pathology of the Placenta*

Striker, Quadracci and Cutler: *Use and Interpretation of Renal Biopsy*

Asbury and Johnson: *Pathology of Peripheral Nerve*

Morson: *The Pathogenesis of Colorectal Cancer*

Azzopardi: *Problems in Breast Pathology*

Hendrickson and Kempson: *Surgical Pathology of the Uterine Corpus*

Katzenstein and Askin: *Surgical Pathology of Non-Neoplastic Lung Disease*

Forthcoming

Burke: *Surgical Pathology of the Spleen*

Jaffe: *Surgical Pathology of Lymph Nodes and Related Organs*

LiVolsi: *Pathology of the Thyroid*

Lukeman and Mackay: *Tumors of the Lung*

Mackay, Evans and Ayala: *Soft Tissue Tumors*

Mottet & Norris: *Histopathology of Inflammatory Bowel Disease, 2nd ed.*

Panke and McLeod: *Pathology of Burn Injury*

Phillips: *Pathology of the Liver*

Reagan and Fu: *Pathology of the Uterine Cervix, Vagina and Vulva*

Taylor, Chandor and Nakamura: *Immunomicroscopy*

Wigglesworth: *Perinatal Pathology*

WILLIAM J. FRABLE, M.D.

Director, Section of Surgical and Cytopathology
and Professor of Surgical Pathology
Virginia Commonwealth University
Health Sciences Division
Medical College of Virginia
Richmond, Virginia

THIN-NEEDLE
ASPIRATION
BIOPSY

Volume 14 in the Series
MAJOR PROBLEMS IN PATHOLOGY

JAMES L. BENNINGTON, M.D., *Consulting Editor*
Chairman, Department of Pathology
Children's Hospital of San Francisco
San Francisco, California

1983
W. B. Saunders Company
Philadelphia, London, Toronto, Mexico City, Rio de Janeiro, Sydney, Tokyo

W. B. Saunders Company: West Washington Square
Philadelphia, PA   19105

1 St. Anne's Road
Eastbourne, East Sussex BN21 3UN, England

1 Goldthorne Avenue
Toronto, Ontario M8Z 5T9, Canada

Apartado 26370—Cedro 512
Mexico 4, D.F., Mexico

Rua Coronel Cabrita, 8
Sao Cristovao Caixa Postal 21176
Rio de Janeiro, Brazil

9 Waltham Street
Artarmon, N.S.W. 2064, Australia

Ichibancho, Central Bldg., 22-1 Ichibancho
Chiyoda-Ku, Tokyo 102, Japan

Library of Congress Cataloging in Publication Data

Frable, William J.

Thin-needle aspiration biopsy.

(Major problems in pathology ; v. 14)

1. Biopsy, Needle.   I. Title.   II. Series. [DNLM:
   1. Biopsy, Needle. W1 MA 492X v. 14 / WB 379 F797t]

RD35.F7   616.07'58   81–48536

ISBN 0–7216–3835–X   AACR2

Thin Needle Aspiration Biopsy

ISBN   0-7216-3835-X

Last digit is the print number: 9   8   7   6   5   4   3   2   1

DEDICATED TO
Mary Ann, Deborrah, and Geraldine

FOREWORD

The thin-needle aspiration biopsy, employed primarily for the cytologic diagnosis of deep-seated neoplasms in various tissues and organs, has been used widely in Europe for many years. In spite of numerous publications documenting its advantages and diagnostic accuracy, pathologists and clinicians have been slow to accept the thin-needle aspiration biopsy in the United States.

After years of studious neglect in this country, the thin-needle aspiration biopsy has suddenly come into favor, as indicated by the great number of publications on this subject in the American literature and a proliferation of workshops and continuing education programs on its use and interpretation. During this same period, a dramatic increase has occurred in the number of medical centers offering the thin-needle aspiration biopsy as a routine diagnostic service.

As with almost any medical innovation, the early phase of transition from development to routine application is characterized by conflicting reports of clinical efficacy. With his vast experience in the performance and cytologic interpretation of the thin-needle aspiration biopsy, Dr. Frable is ideally suited to offer an objective evaluation of the strengths and limitations of this diagnostic technique. In this monograph, Dr. Frable provides a comprehensive review of the current status of our knowledge about the use and interpretation of this valuable procedure. *Thin-Needle Aspiration Biopsy* is an indispensable resource and guide for all clinicians, surgeons, radiologists, and pathologists who deal with this procedure.

JAMES L. BENNINGTON, M.D.

PREFACE

This monograph represents my experience with fine-needle aspiration biopsy during the past nine years. Its genesis probably occurred during 1964 and 1965, when I was first introduced to aspiration biopsy while serving a fellowship in surgical pathology at Memorial Center for Cancer and Allied Diseases in New York City. A few aspirations were still being performed at that institution, where it was introduced by Dr. Hayes Martin more than 30 years before. My responsibility as the fellow was to return each evening to stain the aspiration smears so that they would be ready to read the following morning. The pathology attending staff expressed no great enthusiasism for the procedure, vigorously cautioning against overdiagnosing the smears.

Although my interest in exfoliative cytology was greatly stimulated by the training I received at Memorial, it was not until 1972, when a chance opportunity arose to visit the Karolinska Institute in Stockholm, that I was re-exposed to aspiration biopsy. By this time, some of the papers from the cytology laboratory of Dr. Zajicek and his colleagues were beginning to appear in the American literature. He and Dr. Franzen were most generous in allowing me to visit with them over the course of a single day to observe the actual performance of several aspirations followed by interpretation of the smears. Seeing their success first hand stimulated me to attempt to introduce the method at the Medical College of Virginia.

Armed with little more than the equivalent experience of "see one, do one, teach one," I began to practice on surgical specimens while attempting to stimulate interest by attending meetings of the tumor board and discussing possible applications with our oncology staff. A few cases were referred, and, most fortunately, they were easy to diagnose. Word spread to the house staff that the procedure was fast and accurate. Despite the criticism of some skeptics, we began to make progress.

By 1973, there were enough cases and adequate interest to attempt a workshop. This was suggested by Dr. George Stevenson, Scientific Director of the American Society of Clinical Pathologists, and by members of the Council on Cytopathology. The first few tries were not overwhelmingly successful. This did not surprise me, since many pathologists remained unconvinced that an accurate diagnosis could be made from a cell spread of a tumor. It has been gratifying to watch negativism give way to great interest on the part of pathologists. Dr. Martin Rush, a practicing pathologist who had studied with Dr. Zajicek, joined forces with us for some of the first workshops. Dr. Joseph Linsk, a medical oncologist using aspiration biopsy in his own practice, provided encouragement. The workshop now requires a full day. Two faculty members have been added: Dr. David Kaminsky and Dr. Philip Feldman, who offer additional expertise and interesting cases. Other cytopathologists have introduced aspiration biopsy into their institutions, and several now provide excellent workshops. Radiologists, with their new imaging equipment, have joined the ranks of the aspirators, placing the burden of interpretation squarely on the pathologist. The American Society of Cytology has provided guidance in developing training programs and in making room for the large number of papers concerning aspiration biopsy that have suddenly appeared in the literature. The International Academy of Cytology has devoted an expanding proportion of its tutorials in clinical cytology to aspiration biopsy. With the expertise and guidance of Dr. Myron Melamed and Dr. Steven Hajdu, there has been a rebirth of aspiration biopsy at Memorial Sloan-Kettering Cancer Center.

We have all learned together. This monograph attempts to reflect that accumulated experience. Chapters arranged according to systems or organs, where appropriate, follow an introductory chapter devoted to history and a chapter on techniques. The latter is detailed to enable the readers to understand the necessary fine points of the performance of the actual aspiration and the preparation of the smears so that they can begin to practice on suitable specimens, building up a library of case material for future reference. Various staining methods are presented, since the chapters that follow are illustrated with smears from the same cases stained by both Romanovsky and Papanicolaou methods for comparison.

Europeans stress the use of the May-Grunwald-Giemsa stain while neglecting the Papanicoloau stain. The opposite is true in the United States. I believe that both stains are valuable and that when used together they provide a better opportunity for making a more accurate histopathologic diagnosis from the smear. A specific diagnostic approach is stressed throughout this book. It should be remembered that aspiration biopsy is a hybrid technique, not actually a method of either exfoliative cytology or tissue pathology but a logical bridge between the two. To this end, corresponding tissue sections are illustrated for comparison with the aspiration smears.

An attempt has been made to survey as much of the literature as possible, particularly to summarize results of large series and to make comparisons in an effort to document accuracy of the method. Finally, a review of the applications of aspiration biopsy in research and special methods useful in both research and diagnosis are presented.

I believe it is now time to predict that aspiration biopsy will become an important part of the pathologist's practice and skill. It is hoped that those whose particular interest is surgical pathology will look more favorably upon aspiration biopsy as a powerful clinical tool in the diagnosis and management of patients with tumors. If this book can bring that interest to focus and be of help to those already engaged in using fine-needle aspiration biopsy, its purpose will have been fulfilled. The practicing cytopathologist will find interesting and challenging cases in this presentation, while those unfamiliar with aspiration biopsy will be encouraged to learn it and try it.

ACKNOWLEDGMENTS

I gratefully acknowledge the faith and confidence of many physicians of Virginia Commonwealth University, Medical College of Virginia and of the Richmond metropolitan area as well as the house staff of the Medical College of Virginia for referring their patients for aspiration biopsies. Special thanks are due to Dr. Walter Lawrence, Jr., Professor of Surgery and Director of the Cancer Center, Dr. J. Shelton Horsley, Professor of Surgery and Associate Director of the Cancer Center, Dr. James W. Brooks, Professor of Surgery, Dr. Alton Sharpe, Professor of Medicine, Dr. William J. Brewer, Assistant Professor of Radiology, and Dr. James W. Walsh, Assistant Professor of Radiology, Virginia Commonwealth University, Medical College of Virginia.

There are many pathologists who have contributed cases for review and study and who have shared their experiences with me during workshops and informal discussions while we have all learned about aspiration biopsy. I wish to thank particularly Dr. David B. Kaminsky, Director of Laboratories, Eisenhower Medical Center, Palm Desert California, and Dr. Philip Feldman, Director of the Cytology Service, University of Virginia Medical Center, Charlottesville, Virginia, for their workshop collaboration and support. Present and former Fellows in Surgical and Cytopathology, Medical College of Virginia, Dr. John Spahr, Dr. Richard DeMay, Dr. Ernie Kawamoto, and Dr. Gerard O'Dowd, provided countless hours of coverage of the aspiration biopsy service as well as inspiration and advice while I completed this monograph. Dr. DeMay and Dr. Saul Kay were invaluable contributors to the ultrastructural studies.

Specific contributions of illustrated case material were provided by the following: Dr. J. Valacenti, Medical University of South Carolina, Charleston, South Carolina (Fig. 4–34); Dr. L. Mohanty, McGuire Veterans Administration Hospital, Richmond, Virginia (Figs. 5–15 and 5–27); Dr. R. Lawrence Smith, General Hospital of Virginia Beach, Virginia Beach, Virginia (Fig. 7–11); Dr. F. Gutierrez, Chippenham Hospital, Richmond, Virginia (Figs. 7–28 and 7–29); Dr. Rene Vauclair, Hospital Notre-Dame, Montreal, Quebec, Canada (Figs. 7–16 and 7–17); Dr. J. Chenard, Hospital St-Sacrement, Montreal, Quebec, Canada (Figs. 7–18 and 7–19); Dr. Y. Boivin, Hotel-Dieu de Montreal, Montreal, Quebec, Canada (Figs. 7–31, 7–32, and 7–33); and Dr. Alan Handy, Pagosa Springs, Colorado (Figs. 9–19 and 9–20).

I am most grateful for the permission of Georg Thieme Verlag, Stuttgart, to use and reproduce the title and first nineteen lines of the article by O. O. Leyden, which appeared in Medicinische Wochenschrift, Vol. 9, page 52, 1882. I would like to thank the J. B. Lippincott Co., Philadelphia, Pa., for permission to reproduce and use Figures 2 and 3 from the article "Thin-Needle Aspiration Biopsy. A Personal Experience with 469 Cases," which appeared in the American Journal of Clinical Pathology, Vol. 65, No. 2, pages 168–182, 1976. I am also grateful to Masson Publishing, USA, Inc., New York, New York for allowing me to reproduce and use Figures 11–12 and

11–13 from *Diagnostic Respiratory Cytopathology*, pages 302 and 303, 1979, by W. W. Johnston, and W. J. Frable.

Many hours of superb secretarial and editorial assistance were provided by Ms. Janice G. Brammer, Section of Surgical Pathology, Medical College of Virginia. Likewise, Mr. David Bennett, Department of Visual Education, Medical College of Virginia, provided his time and talent in taking the many photomicrographs. Unlimited technical assistance was provided by Ms. Grace Hasenfang CT(ASCP) and Ms. Carol Trew CT(ASCP), Chief Cytotechnologists, and their entire staff of the cytopathology laboratory, Mr. Jerry Coates, Chief Histotechnologist, and Mr. Virgil Mumaw, Director of the electron microscopy laboratory, Medical College of Virginia.

CONTENTS

COLOR PLATES

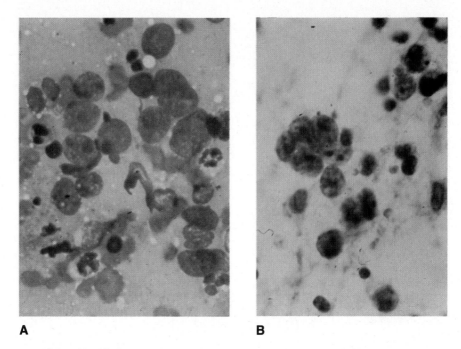

A

B

Plate 1 (*A* and *B*).   Lymphoepithelioma metastatic to cervical lymph node. Large round neoplastic cells are present in *A* and *B*. Note the metachromasia of the chromatin and the large nucleoli in the smear stained with Diff-Quik (*A*). The clumping of these undifferentiated epithelial cells is more obvious in the fixed smear (*B*). *A*, Diff-Quik × 400. *B*, Papanicolaou × 400.

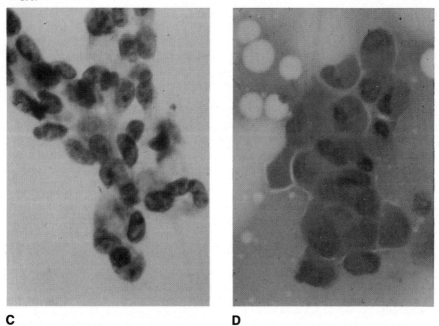

C

D

Plate 1 (*C* and *D*).   Signet cell carcinoma of the colon, metastatic to inguinal lymph node. Malignant features of the cells are easily appreciated in *C*, but vacuolization is not prominent. The nuclei are eccentric. Mucicarmine stain confirmed the presence of mucin (*D*). *C*, Papanicolaou × 400. *D*, Mucicarmine × 400.

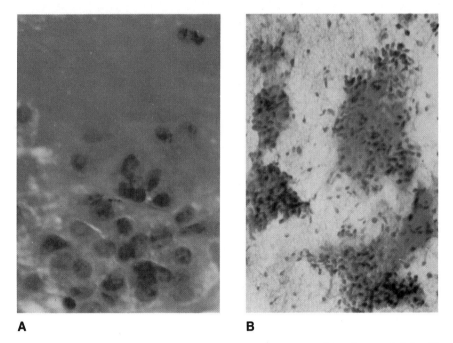

A **B**

Plate 2 (*A* and *B*).   Benign mixed tumor of parotid salivary gland. Uniform epithelial cells are visible within an intensely metachromatic stroma, revealed with the Diff-Quik stain (*A*). At lower-power magnification (*B*), the relationship between the epithelial and stromal components resembles that evident in a tissue section. *A*, Diff-Quik × 400. *B*, Papanicolaou × 175.

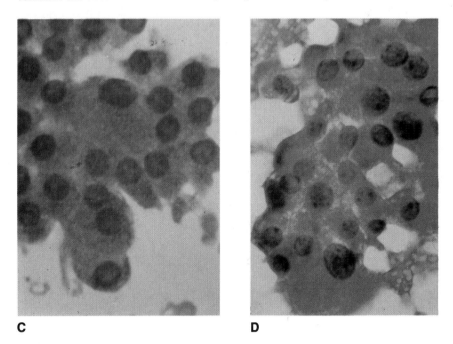

C **D**

Plate 2 (*C* and *D*).   Hürthle cell adenoma of thyroid. The granularity of the cell cytoplasm is evident in both *C* and *D*, but it is more vivid with the Papanicolaou stain (*D*). *C*, Diff-Quik × 400. *D*, Papanicolaou × 400.

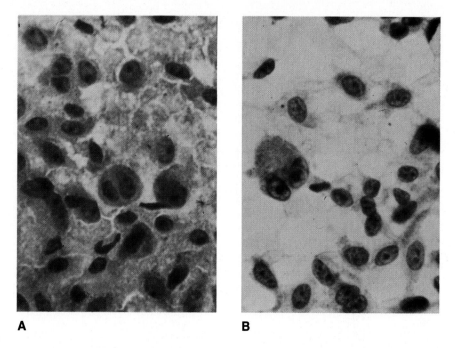

A   B

Plate 3 (*A* and *B*). Malignant melanoma metastatic to cervical lymph node. The double-nuclei cell pattern is evident in both *A* and *B*. More prominent nucleoli are visible in the fixed, Papanicolaou-stained preparation (*B*). *A*, Diff-Quik × 400. *B*, Papanicolaou × 400.

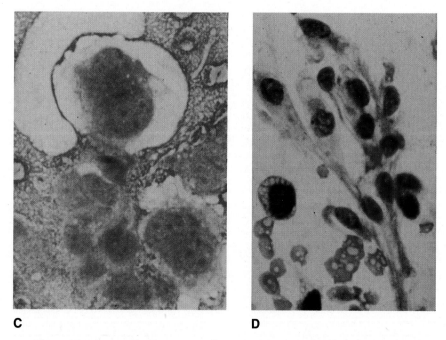

C   D

Plate 3 (*C* and *D*) Chondrosarcoma of the tibia. The metachromasia of the cartilaginous matrix surrounding some large and double-nuclei chondrocytes is better demonstrated with the Diff-Quik stain (*C*). Less differentiated and spindle-shaped malignant cartilaginous cells are evident in the fixed smear (*D*). *C*, Diff-Quik × 400. *D*, Papanicolaou × 400.

Chapter One

Introduction and History

Not unlike the healing process, the evolution of important scientific contributions in medicine requires both the elixir of time and the synthesis of a number of observations.[1] There are probably additional social, economic, and even political considerations that influence the ultimate acceptance of medical facts and the development of medical procedures.[2, 3]

The history of aspiration biopsy was influenced by such factors. Its development in many ways parallels that of cytology and cytologic diagnosis, and its progress toward general acceptance by the scientific community is similar to that of such concepts as carcinoma in situ and preneoplastic, or dysplastic, states.

DEVELOPMENT OF DIAGNOSTIC CYTOLOGY

Papanicolaou's now famous monograph of 1943, *The Diagnosis of Uterine Cancer by Exfoliative Cytology,* ushered in the modern era of cytologic diagnosis. It was not until six years after the publication of this monograph that Papanicolaou's method received general acceptance as a screening and diagnostic technique. His work was preceded by his own publication in 1926 and by that of Babes in 1927. Babes, writing in the proceedings of a conference of the Gynecologic Society of Bucharest, described the diagnosis of uterine cancer by exfoliative cytology.[1] Perhaps, except for fate, we might now well be calling the Pap smear the Babes test.

However, to understand the history of cytology we must look even farther back to the publication of Schleiden's cell theory in 1838, and examine this work along with two of the earliest studies on microscopic examination of exfoliative cells, published by Donne and Mueller. Donne described the examination of fresh smears prepared from human colostrum, and Mueller, in 1838, described in detail the appearance of cancer cells.[4]

Webb has thoroughly reviewed this early history of cytology, particularly with regard to needle aspiration biopsy, recognizing that microscopy led first to the examination of cells rather than to the study of tissue, since at that time efficient methods of preparing histologic sections were unknown.[5] It was the eventual invention of the microtome along with the development of cultural methods for studying bacterial organisms that resulted in the remarkable decline in the cytologic method beginning in the twentieth century. Cytology was not to be revived until the landmark work of Papanicolaou.[1]

DEVELOPMENT OF NEEDLE ASPIRATION TECHNIQUE

EARLY HISTORY

Needle aspiration biopsy has had a very similar history. We must look back to the 1847 publication of Kun as probably the first report of a needle biopsy.[6] It is not entirely clear as to whether this material was examined in a histologic sense, but, as there were no microtomes at this time, the examination was probably cellular. Webb has cited the description of the procedure as follows: "An exploring needle, having at its extremity a small depression with cutting edges. On plunging this into the tumor one can extract a minute portion of tissue—in this manner a microscopic examination can be practiced."[5]

In all probability, the next significant contribution to the development of aspiration biopsy was the 1904 publication of Greig and Gray, a study of the aspiration of nodes for the identification of trypanosomes. This work provided one of the early descriptions of needle aspiration biopsy.[7] It was preceded, however, by several publications that also delineated aspiration biopsy. Skey, in 1851, strongly favored breast aspiration for cysts only. He discouraged microscopy of the contents, however.[8] Sir James Paget and Erichsen, in 1853, both favored aspiration biopsy.[5, 9] Paget gave a series of lectures at the Royal Academy of Medicine in 1853 on the surgical pathology of tumors. He was an excellent microscopist, as evident in the following quotation: "Many of the cells of cancer, for example, may be somewhat like gland cells or like epithelial cells, yet a practiced eye can distinguish them even singly and much more plainly their grouping distinguishes them; they are heaped together disorderly and seldom have any lobular or laminar arrangements such as exists in the natural glands or epithelia."[5] This is truly a cytologic description and in fact is in no way dissimilar from accounts of what is seen in the modern preparation of aspiration biopsy smears.

In 1863, Pritchard used a groove needle for breast aspiration. He provided an excellent description of the cytology of fat necrosis.[5] As dangerous as it might have been perceived at the time, transthoracic aspiration biopsy was attempted in 1883. Leyden reports the use of this diagnostic technique for the identification of pneumonia. The title of that communication is reproduced from the original journal in Figure 1–1.[10]

Publications about the aspiration technique appeared sporadically during the early twentieth century. Proscher, in 1907, employed the aspiration method to identify spirochetes in lymph nodes. Horder, in 1909, used aspiration biopsy of the lung for diagnostic purposes. Ward, in 1914, used aspiration biopsy of lymph nodes for the diagnosis of lymphomas.[11] Likewise, Dudgeon and Patrick, in 1927, emphasized the cytologic method applied to tissue biopsies in a paper entitled "A New Method for the Rapid Microscopical Diagnosis of Tumors." This is the scrape, or touch-preparation, essentially a duplicate of the typical method used in preparing a smear from a needle aspiration biopsy. Rapid staining was accomplished by hematoxylin and eosin or by other available staining methods. The authors reported 200 cases so examined with a diagnostic accuracy of 98.6 per cent.[12] There were, however, those in the scientific community who could not accept a cytologic diagnosis. This opinion may be found in the quotation of Sir John Bland-Sutton: "In the appearance of a cell from cancer—there is nothing characteristic of a disease, nothing that would lead a pathologist to identify it as a malignant cell."[5] Unfortunately, this negative attitude still exists in the minds of some modern pathologists and clinicians.

Physicians from two institutions, the Memorial Center for Cancer and Allied Diseases in New York and the Karolinska Institute in Stockholm, Sweden, must be given the credit for providing the major impetus in the development of needle

VII. Verhandlungen des Vereins für innere Medicin.

Sitzung am Montag den 20. November 1882.

Vorsitzender: Herr Frerichs.

Schriftführer: Herr Ewald.

Nach einem durch Herrn Wernich erstatteten Berichte über die Bibliothek spricht:

Herr Leyden: Ueber infectiöse Pneumonie.

M. H. Meine heutige Demonstration betrifft Präparate von parasitären Kokken, die von einem Falle von Pneumonie herstammen und liefern einen neuen Beweis dafür, dass auch die Pneumonie zu den infectiösen Krankheiten gehört. Diese Thatsache ist keineswegs etwas Neues, und doch habe ich es für angebracht gehalten, eine solche Demonstration hier anzukündigen, einmal weil die Thatsache in dieser Gesellschaft, welche ich für das eigentliche Forum halte, vor das sie gehört, noch nicht besprochen worden ist, und zweitens weil es mir gelungen ist, das bisher Gefundene um einen kleinen Beitrag zu fördern, die vorliegenden Mikroben sind nämlich dem Lebenden entnommen. Ich habe einem Pneumoniker mit der Pravaz'schen Spritze eine kleine Menge Blut und Exsudat aus der hepatisirten Lunge entnommen und konnte darin die Parasiten in ziemlich reichlicher Zahl nachweisen.

Figure 1–1 Title of first reported transthoracic aspiration biopsy. (From Leyden, O. O.: Ueber infectiöse Pneumonie. Dtsch. Med. Wochenschr. 9:52–54, 1883. Reprinted with permission of the publisher, Georg Thieme Verlag, Stuttgart.)

aspiration biopsy. It is interesting to note that the Memorial clinicians' efforts preceded the cytology publications of Papanicolaou by some 15 years. Their diagnostic methods combined both cytologic and histologic features from cell-block preparations.[13-15] The contributions of the Karolinska clinicians followed those of Papanicolaou by several years, and their emphasis is much more cytologic. This group's background of training in hematology is reflected in its approach, which emphasizes Romanovsky's staining method.[16, 17] Their work can be regarded as a revival of the theories discussed in two preceding monographs, one published by Lopes Cordozo in Holland in 1954, and another by Soderstrom in 1966. Both authors firmly established the technique in Scandinavia.[18, 19]

In the late 1920's, through the efforts of Martin, a clinician, and Stewart and Ewing, pathologists, the practice of needle aspiration of palpable lumps and tumors situated in deeper structures was begun at Memorial Hospital in New York. In each case, an attempt was made to procure amounts of material adequate not only for cytologic smears but also for the preparation of a clot for cell-block and histologic section. A standard 18-gauge needle was used, and local anesthesia was administered, at least in the early aspirations. The original publication tabulates some 65 cases that involve a variety of tumors and sites with an 80 per cent accuracy rate and no false-positive results.[13] Convenience and rapid diagnosis were stressed then as they are today, and the method must have been successful, for in 1934 the same authors published a total series of 1400 cases. The technique of aspiration used by Martin is quite similar to that practiced today, with the interesting difference that he removed the syringe from the needle prior to withdrawal of the needle and subsequent preparation of the smears.[15] The reasons for this procedure are fairly obvious in the modern description of the application of aspiration biopsy (see Chapter 2).

The original cytopathology article dealing with aspiration was published by Stewart in 1933, an accumulative series of 2500 cases studied over a period of three years. He stressed breast and lymph node aspiration and discussed the scope and limitations of this method in detail.[14] These efforts were followed by increased use of aspiration biopsy primarily in Memorial Hospital. A series of publications followed over the years, principally by clinicians trained at Memorial Hospital in the aspiration technique; yet, until recently, this biopsy method remained largely restricted to that institution.[20-22] The one exception is Godwin, whose excellent descriptions and illustrations thoroughly demonstrate many of the morphologic features of a variety of tumors and sites. His studies are just as appropriate and diagnostically useful today as they were at the time of their original publication.[11, 23] Seemingly, no organ was left untouched by the Memorial group in the use of aspiration biopsy. This is documented in the publications of Ferguson, 1930; Coley, Sharp, and Ellis, 1931; and Sharp, 1931.[20-22]

Historically, the lack of success in disseminating this biopsy method beyond what was at the time the major cancer hospital in the United States has been questioned often. Christopherson, in his discussion of a paper presented by Godwin as part of a symposium on diagnostic accuracy of cytologic techniques, provided what this author believes is a suitable answer:

> Looking back it seems rather strange that the cytologic diagnosis of aspiration material has not grown commensurately with its value as a diagnostic procedure. In analysing the reasons for this in our own institution it would seem that the ever-changing surgical resident has often not been familiar with the technique, and its extreme value in tumor diagnosis. Perhaps we have been too busy expounding the virtues of exfoliative cytology and have failed to effectively communicate on needle aspiration with our surgical colleagues. It is indigenous to surgical training that there is a preference for cutting over sticking, this in spite of the tremendous advantage the needle has in carefully selected instances.[23]

FACTORS ESSENTIAL TO ACCURACY AND SUCCESS

It is evident, however, that others were becoming enthusiastic about the procedure. Smith, for example, reports a 20-year experience at the Ontario Cancer Foundation, at the University of Western Ontario, where aspiration material was originally prepared by cut sections. However, smear preparation was eventually introduced and used in conjunction with the former method, and its value became established. Many instances of smear preparation's surprising superiority to the original technique were soon noted. As Smith points out, however, the following factors are essential to establishing accurate of evaluation of aspiration biopsy material: the experience of the pathologist and the clinician; their attitude towards achieving perfection; their acceptance of the challenge of pushing the cytologic diagnosis to its limit; and the clinician's ability and willingness to accept the responsibility for positive, negative, and equivocal reports, particularly for the latter two.[24]

In light of Christopherson's comments, it seems that the unique combination of clinician, hematologist, and pathologist at the Karolinska Institute led to the success of needle aspiration biopsy in that institution and to its subsequent resurgence not only in the Scandinavian countries but also, more recently, in the United States and in other parts of the world. The original publications of Franzen, Zajicek, Eneroth, and several others describe the scope of the thin-needle aspiration diagnostic technique, and an astonishing number of cases were reported during the period extending from 1950 to the present.[17, 25] It cannot be overemphasized that these individuals are primarily clinicians with hematologic and cytopathologic training, who not only interpret the material but also examine the patient and perform the biopsy. It is this thorough familiarity with the patient and his or her clinical problem that this author and many others now believe has contributed significantly to restoring the utility, accuracy, and overall success of this procedure.[2, 3, 26] There are many others, such as Lopes Cardozo, Soderstrom, Lowhagen, Nordenstrom, and Dahlgren, who have contributed in a similar fashion and who have the orientation of both clinician and cytopathologist. Important monographs have been published by the aforementioned authors and by Zajicek.[17-19, 25, 27] Those of Lopes Cardozo and Soderstrom are particularly thoughtful accounts of the utility of needle aspiration biopsy and the elements that make up the diagnostic evaluation accomplished with this method. The general principles that are very succinctly and beautifully presented in these monographs are equally applicable to the interpretation of aspiration smears and to the general problem of a pathologic interpretation of any small or limited biopsy material. These monographs are thought-provoking analyses of how any well-trained pathologist or cytopathologist organizes the mental process that constitutes a diagnostic interpretation.[18, 19]

CRITICISM AND OPPOSITION

Despite the recent successful application of needle aspiration biopsy, there have been obstacles to its development and general acceptance. Those who are critical of the technique base their arguments on (1) their belief that the procedure is inherently inaccurate because of the limited amount of material obtained and the difficulty of interpreting cytologic findings, and (2) the danger of seeding and spreading tumor by piercing it with needles. Thus, Ochsner and DeBakey, who initially favored the transthoracic aspiration biopsy in 1939, opposed it vigorously in 1942 on the basis of two cases in which implanted tumor apparently occurred in the needle tract site.[28] This latter article will probably best be remembered for its sweeping negative conclusions about aspiration biopsy and its lack of substantial scientific fact.[29] In later chapters of this monograph, this author will discuss in detail the theoretical and practical considerations of tumor spread in needle-tract seeding with the use of the aspiration biopsy.

CURRENT CONSIDERATIONS

The answer to the allegation that needle aspiration biopsy is inaccurate certainly has a historical parallel with exfoliative cytology of all types, particularly that most commonly practiced, cervical-vaginal cytologic diagnosis. Modern clinicians and pathologists must have interest in, dedication to, and a willingness to learn the interpretive methods of cytology, specifically, those used in the interpretation of biopsies. As noted by Ng, we are today faced with a major deficit of pathologists who are trained and interested in cytopathology.[30-32] Perhaps needle aspiration biopsy will provide the stimulus and interest necessary to make cytopathology a major diagnostic technique. Recent reviews of the literature suggest that this is the case, as there has been a dramatic increase in the number of aspiration biopsies performed during the last ten years in the United States as well as in the number of research papers reporting this method's utility and accuracy and, more recently, its substantial contribution to quantitative and other sophisticated research cytologic methodology.[25] This author believes that Stewart's statement regarding aspiration biopsy is as appropriate today as it was in 1933: "Diagnosis by aspiration is as reliable as the combined intelligence of the clinician and pathologist makes it."[14]

REFERENCES

1. Johnston, W. W., and Frable, W. J.: The cytopathology of the respiratory tract: A review. Am. J. Pathol. 84:372–406, 1976.
2. Fox, C. H.: Innovation in medical diagnosis: The Scandinavian curiosity. Lancet 1:1387–1388, 1979.
3. Koss, L. G.: Editorial. Thin needle aspiration biopsy. Acta Cytol. 24:1–3, 1980.

4. Grunze, H., and Spriggs, A. I.: *History of Clinical Cytology. A Selection of Documents.* Viernheim, G-I-T Verlag Ernst Giebeler, 1980, pp. 25, 33.

5. Webb, A. J.: Through a glass darkly. (The development of needle aspiration biopsy.) Bristol Med. Chir. J. *89*:59–68, 1974.

6. Kun, M.: A new instrument for the diagnosis of tumours. Monthly J. Med. Sci. 7:853, 1847 (cited by Webb).

7. Grieg, E. D. W., and Gray, A. C. H.: Note on the lymphatic glands in sleeping sickness. Br. Med. J. *1*:1252, 1904.

8. Skey, F. C.: *Operative Surgery.* Edinburgh, J. & A. Churchill, 1851, p. 392.

9. Erichsen, J. E.: *The Science and Art of Surgery.* London, Walton and Maberly, 1853 (cited by Webb).

10. Leyden, O. O.: Ueber infectiöse Pneumonie. Dtsch. Med. Wochenschr. 9:52–54, 1883.

11. Godwin, J. T.: Aspiration biopsy. Technique and application. Ann. N.Y. Acad. Sci. 63:1348–1373, 1956.

12. Dudgeon, L. S., and Patrick, C. V.: A new method for the rapid microscopical diagnosis of tumours. Br. J. Surg. *15*:250–261, 1927.

13. Martin, H. E., and Ellis, E. B.: Biopsy by needle puncture and aspiration. Ann. Surg. 92:169–181, 1930.

14. Stewart, F. W.: The diagnosis of tumors by aspiration biopsy. Am. J. Pathol. 9:801–812, 1933.

15. Martin, H. E., and Ellis, E. B.: Aspiration biopsy. Surg. Gynecol. Obstet. 59:578–589, 1934.

16. Franzen, S., Giertz, G., and Zajicek, J.: Cytological diagnosis of prostatic tumours by transrectal aspiration biopsy. Br. J. Urol. 32:193–196, 1960.

17. Zajicek, J.: *Aspiration Biopsy Cytology. Part I: Cytology of Supra-diaphragmatic Organs.* New York, S. Karger Publishers Inc., 1974.

18. Lopes Cardozo, P.: *Clinical Cytology.* Leiden, Stafleu, 1954.

19. Soderstrom, N.: *Fine Needle Aspiration Biopsy.* Stockholm, Almqvist & Wiksell, 1966.

20. Ferguson, R. S.: Prostatic neoplasms: Their diagnosis by needle puncture and aspiration. Am. J. Surg. 9:126–127, 1930.

21. Coley, B. L., Sharp, G. S., and Ellis, E. B.: Diagnosis of bone tumors by aspiration. Am. J. Surg. *13*:215–224, 1931.

22. Sharp, G. S.: The diagnosis of primary carcinoma of the lung by aspiration. Am. J. Cancer *15*:863–870, 1931.

23. Godwin, J. T.: Cytologic diagnosis of aspiration biopsies of solid or cystic tumors. Acta Cytol. 8:206–215, 1964.

24. Smith, I. H., Fisher, J. H., Lott, J. S., and Thomson, D. H.: The cytological diagnosis of solid tumors by small needle aspiration and its influence on cancer clinic practice. Can. Med. Assoc. J. 80:855–860, 1959.

25. Zajicek, J.: *Aspiration Biopsy Cytology, Part II: Cytology of Infra-diaphragmatic Organs.* New York, S. Karger, 1979, pp. 152–159, 195–211, 213, 214.

26. Editorial: Utility of needle aspiration biopsy of tumours. Br. Med. J. *1*:1507–1508, June, 1978.

27. Dahlgren, S. E., and Nordenstrom, B.: *Transthoracic Needle Biopsy.* Stockholm, Almqvist & Wiksell, 1966.

28. Gledhill, E. Y., Spriggs, J. B., and Binford, C. H.: Needle aspiration in the diagnosis of lung carcinoma. Report of experience with 75 aspirations. Am. J. Clin. Pathol. *19*:235–242, 1949.

29. Ochsner, A., and DeBakey, M.: Significance of metastases in primary carcinoma of the lung. J. Thorac. Surg. *11*:357–387, 1942.

30. Ng, A. B. P.: Presidential Address, Annual Meeting, American Society of Cytology. Acta Cytol. 22:121–123, 1978.

31. Ng, A. B. P.: Current status of practice and training in cytology. I: A survey of the practice of cytology in anatomic pathology laboratories. Am. J. Clin. Pathol. 73:202–216, 1980.

32. Ng, A. B. P.: Current status of practice and training in cytology. II: A survey of cytology training in pathology training programs. Am. J. Clin. Pathol. 73:217–231, 1980.

Chapter Two

Techniques of Thin-Needle Aspiration Biopsy

Techniques to be described in this chapter include actual performance of the thin-needle aspiration procedure, preparation of smears, and routine staining methods. Special procedures that can be useful in diagnosis but that have more application to research will be reviewed and described in Chapter 11.

THE THIN-NEEDLE METHOD

The method of aspiration biopsy employed by the author involves the use of the thin needle as described by Franzen, Zajicek, and their colleagues.[1,2] Needles of external diameter of 0.6 to 1.0 mm (essentially 22-gauge) are used in this method. There have been variations in the size of the needle employed; for example, the standard needle used by the Memoral Sloan Kettering Cancer clinicians is an 18-gauge.[3] A thorough review of the subject of needle biopsy is provided in a monograph by Deeley, in which he discusses not only a range of needle sizes up to 12-gauge but also remarkable variations in configurations of cutting edges, with an emphasis on those used for obtaining tissue fragments.[4] Although this latter subject is well beyond the scope of this monograph, it can be said unequivocally that the larger the external diameter of the needle, the greater the likelihood of complications. The thin-needle technique that is to be described presents virtually no problems, except for transthoracic and, rarely, transabdominal aspiration.[1,4]

PRELIMINARY TRAINING AND PLANNING

Even before the practice of thin-needle aspiration biopsy is begun, it should be obvious that a thorough knowledge of anatomy is necessary. For the interested cytopathologist without such knowledge, this requirement may constitute a major obstacle that can, however, be overcome by both study and clinical practice.[5] Although most "lumps and bumps" are superficially located, or at least in such a position that they are not directly in relation to potentially hazardous sites for biopsy, the aspiration should be planned in such a way that subsequent treatment is not compromised. Thus, when primary malignant tumors are aspirated, it is best for the needle tract to be placed in a location that will probably be included in a subsequent excision, despite the fact that documentation of needle-tract implants following thin-needle aspiration biopsy is quite rare.[1, 4, 5]

It should also be evident that knowledge of the clinical problem of any patient undergoing needle aspiration biopsy is important. This author believes that the surgical pathologist-cytopathologist is uniquely trained to perform needle aspiration biopsy because of his or her general interest in biopsy interpretation, much of which, in any large general hospital, likely involves the study of malignant tumors. Aspiration biopsy is also very valuable for diagnosing malignant tumors. The surgical pathologist-cytopathologist with a special interest in oncology should therefore find the technique a useful and rewarding contribution to the management of patients with such tumors. However, because surgeons are trained primarily to cut and surgical pathologists have been reluctant to see patients, aspiration biopsy did not become popular in the United States until recently. Indications and contraindications for aspiration biopsy will be described in subsequent chapters in conjunction with a review of results, from both the literature and this author's own series.

BASIC EQUIPMENT

The following equipment (Fig. 2–1) is required for rapid and efficient performance of thin-needle aspiration biopsy:

1. Cameco Syringe Pistol or Aspir-Gun.
2. 20.0 ml disposable plastic syringe with Luer Lok Tip.
3. 22-gauge 0.6 to 1.0 mm external diameter disposable needles, 3.8 cm and 8.8 cm (1-1/2 in and 3-1/2 in) long, with or without mandrin.
4. Alcohol prep sponges.
5. Sterile gauze pads.
6. Microscopic glass slides with frosted ends.
7. Suitable spray fixatives or a bottle with 95 per cent methyl, ethyl, or isopropyl alcohol, to hold glass slides for immediate fixation of wet smears.

The necessary equipment for aspiration biopsy of "lumps and bumps" can be carried in a coat pocket. A small plastic tray easily holds all the equipment as well as longer biopsy needles measuring 15 cm and 20 cm (6 in and 7 in), employed for

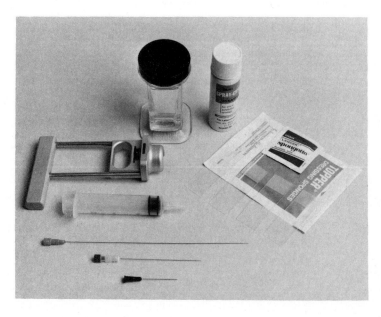

Figure 2–1 Basic equipment required for aspiration biopsy. Needles of various lengths, all 22 gauge; syringe holder (Cameco Syringe Pistol. Precision Dynamics Corp., Burbank, California.); 20 ml disposable syringe; alcohol skin prep pad; sterile gauze pad for hemostasis; Coplin jar of 95 per cent ethyl alcohol or aerosol spray fixative for fixation. Spray fixation is preferred by the author for slides to be stained by the Papanicolaou technique.

transthoracic and transabdominal aspiration. Local anesthesia, 1 per cent or 2 per cent xylocaine or lidocaine, may be required for needle aspiration of transthoracic or transabdominal masses but is rarely necessary for other clinically palpable lumps. This author usually has available a small vial of buffered glutaraldehyde for fixing part of the aspirate for electron microscopy and a tube of tissue culture transport media for obtaining cells for tissue culture studies.[6, 7] Since the aspiration biopsy is virtually nontraumatic, it may be repeated frequently enough to procure amounts of material adequate not only for diagnostic purposes but also for a variety of research applications.[6-9]

ASPIRATION TECHNIQUE

The consultative nature of the aspiration biopsy necessitates reviewing the history of the patient, determining the clinical problem in relation to the lesion to be biopsied, and, finally, deciding whether the biopsy is justified. During palpation of any mass to be biopsied, attempt to determine its location in relation to surrounding structures, estimate its depth, and assess the optimal direction for approach to accomplish the aspiration biopsy. Deeply seated lesions are usually best approached directly and perpendicularly to the skin surface. Superficially lying and small tumors, however, may best be approached by penetrating the skin at a nearly horizontal plane and subsequently feeling for the mass with the tip of the needle. This is particularly true of metastatic nodules in the skin and subcutaneous tissue. Breast "lumps," in contrast, may feel deceptively more superficial.

Preparing the Patient for Aspiration

Positioning. When positioning the patient for the aspiration biopsy, he or she should be comfortable, but the mass must be readily palpable and easily grasped during the biopsy. This is of utmost importance in head and neck lesions, where the prominence of an enlarged lymph node, or lump, may depend on whether the patient is lying down or sitting up. In the head and neck area, the prominence of the sternocleidomastoid muscle and its relationship to the cervical lymph nodes mandate positioning the patient so that a minimum of soft tissue is traversed before reaching the target. Penetrating the sternocleidomastoid muscle is to be avoided. Biopsies taken through this muscle may occasionally cause plugging of the needle and are painful. When aspirating thyroid lesions, place a small pillow under the patient's upper back and extend the neck and tilt the head back, so the nodule will be more prominent and easier to penetrate. This position will also provide fairly easy access to a low-lying thyroid mass, which may be brought up into range by having the patient swallow.

Obtaining Informed Consent. The examiner should avoid rushing the aspiration biopsy, taking time to examine the patient thoroughly while describing the technique and what is to be accomplished with it. This allows the patient to gain some measure of confidence in the physician, who is perhaps seeing him or her for the first time as a consultant but who is going to perform a procedure that the patient may well view as surgical in nature. Although the aspiration is considered a type of biopsy, this author has not obtained written legal consent from patients prior to performing this procedure, except for thyroid biopsies. However, obtaining permission for thyroid aspiration has likewise recently been deemed essentially unnecessary and has been discontinued. Written permission is still obtained for transthoracic and transabdominal aspiration as well as for all biopsies in children. Fine-needle aspiration biopsy is no more traumatic than a venipuncture; in fact, it is usually atraumatic. The needle used for aspiration biopsy is substantially smaller than the 16-gauge needle traditionally employed for procurement of blood samples. The matter of obtaining biopsy permission, however, is a matter of personal choice depending upon exposure to medical liability.

Performing the Aspiration

Palpating and Puncturing the Mass.   With the patient in a position that is comfortable as well as suitable for successful aspiration, the lesion is grasped with one hand, usually with two fingers, or pushed into a position where it seems fixed and stable. With the other hand, the skin is prepared with an alcohol sponge as for a venipuncture. The syringe pistol with attached needle is laid against the skin at the determined puncture site (Fig. 2–2). A quick motion should then be used to insert the needle through the skin. This is followed by advancing the needle into the mass. Actual puncture of the target may be tested by a slight lateral motion of the syringe pistol. The mass will move under the palpating fingers of the other hand if it has been penetrated by the needle. After the mass has been punctured, full suction is continuously applied to the aspirating syringe while the needle is moved back and forth in the tumors with short, quick strokes and in *slightly* different directions. For illustrative purposes, the variation in direction of the needle has been greatly exaggerated (Fig. 2–3C). This alteration in direction should be fairly minimal in actual practice, and, coupled with the forward and backward motion, it is carried out only within the mass.

Critical Considerations During Aspiration.   While performing the actual aspiration, the practitioner observes the junction of the needle and the hub of the syringe for the appearance of any specimen. This is a critical step, as it is absolutely essential to the procurement of high quality aspirates to keep the material within the needle and not aspirate excessive blood or fluid, which dilutes the cellular composition of the specimen. At the first appearance of any sample at the junction of the syringe and the needle, the aspiration is stopped by releasing the trigger of the syringe pistol and letting the vacuum in the syringe equate to normal. It is possible that no specimen will appear in the hub of the syringe during 10 or 12 passes within the lesion, but this does not indicate an unsuccessful aspiration. After this number of passes, if no sample is seen, the aspiration is stopped by allowing the air pressure in the syringe to return to normal. The absolutely important principle is to avoid diluting the aspirate with blood or fluid. It cannot be overemphasized that this is the point at which those who

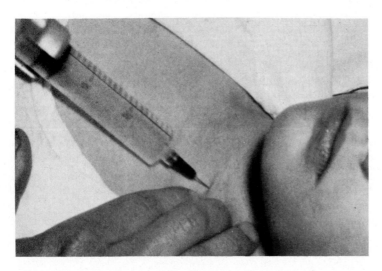

Figure 2–2 Actual aspiration biopsy of thyroid mass.

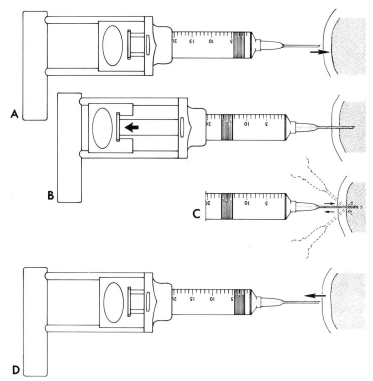

Figure 2–3 Steps in aspiration biopsy of palpable mass. *A*, Introduction of the needle into the mass after preparation of the skin with alcohol. *B*, Application of full vacuum to the syringe with needle in the mass. *C*, Back and forth motion of needle within the mass while full vacuum of the syringe is maintained and position of the needle is varied. For purposes of illustration, the variation in needle position during aspiration has been greatly exaggerated. *D*, Withdrawal of needle from the mass *after* vacuum has been released. See text of Chapter 2 for additional details of the procedure.(From Frable, W. J.: Thin-needle aspiration biopsy. A personal experience with 469 cases. Am. J. Clin. Pathol. 65:2, 1976.)

are unfamiliar with the procedure or who are just learning the aspiration biopsy technique go wrong.

When the air pressure in the syringe is equalized, the needle is withdrawn from the mass, and pressure is applied to the puncture site with a sterile gauze pad. *Never* withdraw the needle from the mass with any vacuum in the syringe pistol. The important consideration in this caution is not that tumor cells will be pulled into the needle tract, as that is both a theoretical and an unsubstantiated claim. What does happen of vital importance, however, is that the small aspirate biopsy will be pulled into the syringe and diluted with air, which immediately causes drying artefacts. The specimen, in all probability, will be irretrievably lost. If a cyst is detected, as may frequently be the case with breast aspirations, it should be evacuated as completely as possible. The fluid obtained from cysts may be processed in the same way that any fluid specimen is prepared for cytologic examination. In the case of breast cysts, it may even be discarded.[1, 10] Discarding breast-cyst fluid, however, should be limited to those specimens that are clear yellow and otherwise devoid of any obvious particulate matter. Cyst fluids that are turbid or that in any way reflect bleeding, recent or remote, should be processed for cytologic examination.[1] After aspiration of any cyst, it is essential that the area be reexamined for any residual mass. If such a mass is found, it should be aspirated a second time with a new needle and a new syringe, and appropriate smears should be prepared from any specimen obtained. This procedure is vitally important in the performance of needle aspiration biopsies of breast masses

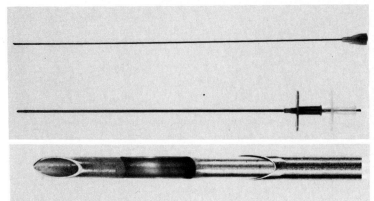

Figure 2–4 Lee Biopsy Needle (Becton Dickinson & Co., Rutherford, New Jersey). Inner stylus has been removed. Details of slotted end of the needle are visible (inset).

but is equally applicable to aspirations of all other sites in which cysts may be encountered.[5]

Technical Variations. Variations in this basic aspiration procedure occur in selected cases such as transabdominal and transthoracic aspirations, where one is dealing mostly with nonpalpable lesions or is using special biopsy guidance techniques such as fluoroscopy, ultrasound, or CAT scanning.[11] These methods will be described in subsequent chapters dealing with the diagnostic aspects of particular organ sites.

The utility of needle aspiration biopsy for the diagnosis of lung tumors has also led to variations in needle design. One that is gaining some acceptance is the slotted design of the Lee needle (Fig. 2–4), which allows procurement of both tissue fragments and material for aspiration.[12] Although the author has no experience with this needle, he finds it difficult to believe that its size (16-gauge) and stiffness do not cause significant complications, despite reports to the contrary.[12]

Various authors also advocate using a rotating motion of the needle once it is in place within the tumor rather than a back-and-forth motion. This preference probably reflects their orientation to performing needle biopsies in which rotation is a standard part of the technique.[4, 13] This author has tried both methods and finds the to-and-fro motion, perhaps best described as the "jackhammer method," preferable.

Practice. The primary factor for becoming adept at needle aspiration biopsy is practice. This is possible using both cadavers and surgical specimens, from which a collection of biopsies from normal tissues as well as tumors may be procured. Practice enables one not only to acquire skills in the technical aspects of aspiration biopsy and in preparation of smears but also to accumulate a valuable library of reference slides for comparison with actual cases.[5]

SMEAR PREPARATION

Smears are prepared from a small drop of semi-solid aspirate placed on a glass slide. This is best accomplished by detaching the needle from the syringe and filling the syringe with air. The needle is then reattached. Advancing the plunger of the syringe will express a small drop of the aspirated material in the center of a glass slide. Care must be taken to place the bevel of the needle against the slide while expressing this drop so that there is no intervening air gap allowing the material either to be splattered onto the slide or to cross any intervening air space. Failure to observe this caution results in significant drying artefacts in alcohol- or spray-fixed smears. With sufficient skill and practice it is possible to place all the aspirated material—normally

4 or 5 drops in a 3.8 cm (1-1/2 in) needle—on a sequence of slides and then begin actual smear preparation without encountering significant drying artefacts in those smears that are eventually alcohol- or spray-fixed.

To make the smear, place a coverglass or another slide over the drop and quickly pull the top and bottom glass plates apart as the drop spreads from the weight of the top slide or coverglass (Fig. 2–5, A and B). The principle is identical with that used in making bone marrow smears. Clinicians and pathologists trained in hematology will readily recognize it. For those without this expertise, practice is again required. As will be subsequently seen, the critical importance of this step cannot be overemphasized because it directly affects how easy or difficult it may be to interpret individual smears cytologically. The final important point is that the smear should occupy only a small area of the slide. This provides a simulated tissue pattern and also materially reduces the area of the smear that must be screened for diagnostic features. Examples of both well- and poorly-prepared smears are illustrated in Figure 2–6.

Diluted Biopsies

Aspiration biopsies that are diluted by fluid or blood do not provide good smears and of necessity occupy large areas of the slide. Diagnostic cells are usually found at the edges of such smears and consist principally of single cells or cells in groups of twos or threes. These patterns may materially affect one's ability to make an accurate cytologic-histopathologic diagnosis. Since aspirates are occasionally diluted by blood or fluid, the principle for differential blood smears may be employed in preparing this type of material (Fig. 2–5, C to F). With the edge of a coverglass or slide pushed

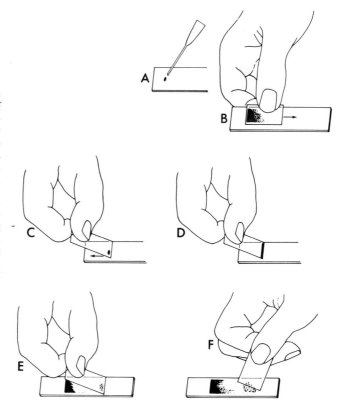

Figure 2–5 Preparation of smears from aspiration biopsies. *A* and *B*, Drop of semi-solid aspiration from neoplasm is expressed on a slide. A thick coverglass or another slide is used to compress the drop of aspirate and spread it over a small area of the slide. The technique is identical with that used in the preparation of smears from bone marrow aspirations. *C, D, E,* and *F,* Drop of aspirate from vascular neoplasms or organs such as the thyroid prepared by method similar to that used in making smears of peripheral blood for differential counting. Diagnostic cells will collect along the edges of the smear or in aggregates at the ends of the last smear after the blood or fluid has been left behind. (From Frable, W. J.; Thin-needle aspiration biopsy. A personal experience with 469 cases. Am. J. Clin. Pathol. 65:2, 1976.)

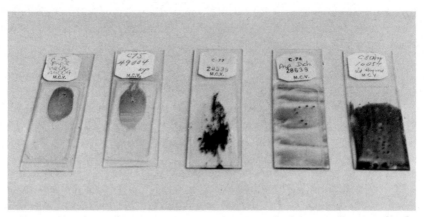

Figure 2–6 Examples of good and bad smears. The two on the left are well prepared and occupy a small area of the slide. The middle smear results from plugging of the needle and splattering of aspirate, usually unavoidable in making the smear. The two smears on the right result from aspirates diluted with blood and from uneven smear techniques. Screening is required of these last two smears to detect any diagnostic cells.

against the drop of fluid aspirate, the specimen will immediately spread along the edge of this slide. Gradually pulling this slide or coverglass over the surface of the horizontal slide will tend to leave the blood or fluid behind and concentrate the cells. This usually results in a large number of smears with very few cells, but the final few smears or the remnants of some of the final smears will contain most of the cells of interest.

Obviously, it is necessary to screen all the slides, or diagnostically significant cells may be missed. For specimens that are largely fluid, this author has relied more heavily on standard cytologic technique, using, for example, filter preparations (Millipore or Nucleopore) or smears prepared from the cell sediment that remains after centrifugation. Both techniques are extremely useful for examining cyst fluid encountered in aspiration, particularly that obtained from breast and thyroid. For excessively bloody specimens, after an adequate number of smears are prepared, the remaining specimen may be allowed to clot. It can then be fixed with standard tissue fixatives, such as Zenker's or formalin, and prepared as a cell block. The author prefers the Harris method of using bacterial agar as a temporary coagulating and mounting media for the preparation of cell blocks. The details of this procedure are included in the appendix to this chapter.[14]

Fixatives

Smears should be air-dried for Romanovsky staining. For Papanicolaou staining or other special staining techniques, smears can be fixed wet in 95 per cent ethyl, methyl, or isopropyl alcohol or spray-fixed. Initially, wet fixation in 95 per cent ethyl alcohol was used for all Papanicolaou-stained smears. Considerable cell loss occurred with aspirates from thyroid and, occasionally, from breast. The recent use of spray fixatives has resulted in improved retention of cells on the slide. Either inexpensive commercial hair spray or spray fixative prepared by scientific supply companies is suitable.[15] Spray-fixed aspiration biopsy smears should dry at least one hour prior to staining. It is very important when using aerosol-spray fixatives to avoid holding the can closer than one foot from the slide to prevent freezing artefacts.[16]

The author has tended to use air-dried smears for special staining techniques, and these have so far proved satisfactory. No standard histologic special stain has yet been encountered that cannot be applied, with some slight variation in staining times, to aspiration biopsy smears. Tissue controls for special stains should be used.

Stains

Both history and the personal preference of various authors seem to dictate, for the most part, what standard stains are used on aspiration biopsy smears. The Memorial group has traditionally used hematoxylin and eosin, probably because of their experience with surgical biopsy interpretation. Those individuals in the Stockholm group, influenced by their hematologic background, have preferred May-Grünwald-Giemsa. Cytopathologists whose experience is based on exfoliative cytology will find the Papanicolaou stain extremely helpful. This stain seems to be used in conjunction with the hematologic stains or hematoxylin-eosin or both at most laboratories in which needle aspiration biopsy is currently practiced. This author has also used a quick stain employed in frozen section diagnosis, metachrome B, which is very rapid and which, like the Giemsa stain, can lead to an immediate diagnosis after the aspiration biopsy. The clinical utility of this is obvious. For outpatients, if there is a question about the quality of aspirated material, the biopsy can be repeated.

Metachrome B has the same limitations in aspiration biopsy as it does in frozen sections. Therefore, this author now prefers the Diff-Quik stain, a recently available commercial product that is very analogous to May-Grünwald-Giemsa. The Diff-Quik stain is a three-step procedure that takes less than 20 seconds to perform and is very useful not only for interpreting aspiration biopsy smears but also for general performance of hematologic work, including examination of both peripheral blood smears and bone marrow aspirations.

A list of equipment, where to procure it, and directions for preparation and actual staining techniques for those stains used in standard practice in this author's laboratory is included in the appendix to this chapter.

REFERENCES

1. Zajicek, J.: *Aspiration Biopsy Cytology. Part I. Cytology of Supradiaphragmatic Organs.* Monographs in Clinical Cytology. Vol. 4. New York, S. Karger, 1974, pp. 1–15, 20–26.
2. Soderstrom, N.: *Fine Needle Aspiration Biopsy.* Almqvist & Wiksell, Stockholm, 1966, pp. 13–18.
3. Martin, H. E., and Stewart, F. W.: Advantages and limitations of aspiration biopsy. Am. J. Roentgenol. 35:245–247, 1936.
4. Deeley, T. J.: *Needle Biopsy.* London, Butterworth & Co. (Publishers), Ltd., 1974.
5. Frable, W. J.: Thin-needle aspiration biopsy. A personal experience with 469 cases. Am. J. Clin. Pathol. 65:168–181, 1976.
6. Kaneshima, S., Kiyasu, Y., Kudo, H., et al.: An application of scanning electron microscopy to cytodiagnosis of pleural and peritoneal fluids. Comparative observation of the same cells by light microscopy and scanning electron microscopy. Acta Cytol. 22:490–499, 1978.
7. Plesnicar, S., Rubio, C., Sigurdson, A., et al.: Studies on the effect of aspiration biopsy on aspirated cells. Determination of cell viability by dye permeability and trypsin digestion tests on aspirates from lymph nodes, spleen and bone marrow and by lymph node cell cultures with phytohemagglutinin. Acta Cytol. 12:454–461, 1968.
8. Pollock, P. G., Valicenti, J. F. Jr., Meyers, D. S., et al.: The use of fluorescent and special staining techniques in aspiration of nocardiosis and actinomycosis. Acta Cytol. 22:575–580, 1978.
9. Zajicek, J.: Aspiration biopsy cytology. Lymphology 10:940–1001, 1977.
10. Haagensen, C. D.: *Diseases of the Breast.* Philadelphia, W. B. Saunders Co., 1971, pp. 172–175.
11. Bartrum, R. J. Jr., and Crow, H. C.: Gray-Scale Ultrasound. A Manual for Physicians and Technical Personnel. Philadelphia, W. B. Saunders Co., 1977, pp. 191–202.
12. Lee, L. H.: A new biopsy needle and its clinical use. Am. J. Roentgenol. Radium Ther. Nucl. Med. 121:854–859, 1974.

13. Dahlgren, S. E., and Nordenstrom, B.: *Transthoracic Needle Biopsy.* Stockholm, Almqvist & Wiksell, 1966.
14. Harris, M. J.: Cell block preparation. Three-percent bacterial agar and plasma-thrombin clot methods. Cytotech. Bull. *11:*6–7, 1974.
15. Freeman, J. A.: Hair spray: An inexpensive aerosol fixative for cytodiagnosis. Acta Cytol. *13:*416–419, 1969.
16. Holmquist, M. D.: The effect of distance in aerosol fixation of cytologic specimens. Cytotech. Bull. *15:*25–27, 1979.
17. Geschickter, C. F.: Fresh tissue diagnosis in the operating room. Stain Technol. 5:81–86, 1930.
18. Hajdu, S. I., and Melamed, M. R.: The diagnostic value of aspiration smears. Am. J. Clin. Pathol. *59:*350–356, 1973.

APPENDIX

EQUIPMENT

1. Cameco Syringe Pistol. Available from Precision Dynamics Corporation, 3031 Thornton Avenue, Burbank, California 91504.
2. Aspir-Gun. Available from Everst Company, 5 Sherman Street, Linden, New Jersey 07036.
3. 20.0 ml disposable plastic syringe with Luer Lok Tip. Available from Becton Dickinson Division of Becton Dickinson & Company, Rutherford, New Jersey 07070.
4. 22-gauge 0.6 to 1.0 mm external diameter disposable needles 3.8 cm and 8.8 cm long, with or without mandrin. (Used for most aspirations of palpable lumps.) Available from Becton Dickinson, Division of Becton Dickinson & Company, Rutherford, New Jersey 07070.
5. Aspiration biopsy needles 15 cm and 20 cm (6 in and 7 in) long, 22-gauge, with or without mandrin. (For biopsy of lung, transabdominal and pelvic masses, and prostate.) Available from Becton Dickinson, Division of Becton Dickinson & Company, Rutherford, New Jersey 07070. Catalogue numbers for 6-in and 7-in needles are SH-2686 6″ and 7″. Also available with mandrin from C. I. Cook, Inc., P. O. Box 489, Bloomington, Indiana 47401 as CHIBA Biopsy CHN 22 15.0 cm and 20.0 cm with mandrin.

STAINING TECHNIQUES

1. *Papanicolaou Stain.* Any of the modifications available in most laboratories are satisfactory.
2. *Metachrome B Stain.*[17] Available as Azure A, French, or MacNeal formula. To four parts of previously filtered, 1 per cent aqueous solution azure A (Azure 1)* very rapidly add one part of filtered 0.5 per cent aqueous Erie Garnet B.† The mixture is immediately filtered to prevent precipitation. Occasional refiltering is necessary if the mixture has been standing a month or more.

   Staining Procedure. The air-dried aspiration smears are placed in the stock stain, which is diluted with an equal volume of distilled water in a Coplin jar for 8 to 10 seconds. Wash gently for a few seconds in running tap water. The smears may be examined wet or mounted with a coverslip using a few drops of 40 per cent glucose solution (Brun's media). The smears may be made permanent by soaking off the coverslip in water and allowing them to dry completely. When dry, dip in xylol for several seconds and coverslip with Permount or another similar mounting media.
3. *Diff-Quik Stain Set 64851.*‡ This commerical stain kit, a modified Wright stain, is a three-solution, three-step method that is both fast and practical. It has also provided this author with good cell detail. This stain is comparable to the May-Grünwald-Giemsa and the Wright-Giemsa, but it is much quicker.

---

*Azure A available from MCB Manufacturing Chemists, 2902 Highland Avenue, Norwood, Ohio 45202. Catalogue number AX 1875.

†Erie Garnet B available from City Chemical Co., 132 W. 22nd St., New York, New York 10011. Congo Corinth color index 22145 is a suitable substitute for Erie Garnet B, which has been in short supply. It can be obtained from Roboz Surgical Instrument Co., 810 18th St. N.W., Washington, D.C. 20006.

‡Available from Harleco, Division of American Hospital Supply Corp., 480 Democrat Rd., Gibbstown, New Jersey 08027. For deeper staining, increase the number of dips in solutions I and II. For paler staining, decrease the number of dips to not less than three full one-second dips. To increase eosinophilia, increase the number of dips in solution I. To increase basophilia, increase the number of dips in solution II. Stain solutions should be tightly covered when not in use.

Staining Procedure.   The air-dried smears are dipped for five seconds (five dips) in solutions I, II, and III, respectively, and the excess stain is drained from the slides between solutions. After the smear is immersed in the third solution, the slide is rinsed with water and either allowed to dry or examined wet. After the smear completely dries, it may be made permanent by immersing it in xylol for several seconds and mounting it with Permount and a coverslip.

4. *Modified May-Grünwald-Giemsa Stain*

May-Grünwald stock stain*	1.0 gm. eosin-methyl blue. 1000 ml methyl alcohol.
Giemsa stock stain†	Add 1.0 gm Giemsa powder to 66.0 ml glycerin. Incubate at 37° for 3 hours, mixing occasionally. Add 66.0 ml methyl alcohol to the incubated stain. Store in the refrigerator.
May-Grünwald working stain	To 40.0 ml of stock stain add 20.0 ml methyl alcohol in a Coplin jar.
Giemsa working stain	Add 45.0 ml of Giemsa stock stain to 45.0 ml of distilled water in a Coplin jar.

Staining Procedure.   Immerse the air-dried aspiration smears in May-Grünwald working stain for 15 minutes. Rinse gently in tap water. Immerse the smears in Giemsa working stain for 15 minutes. Rinse gently with tap water. Allow to air-dry. Dip in xylol for 10 seconds and mount in Permount.

Prepare May-Grünwald working stain fresh once per week. Prepare Giemsa stain fresh daily. The stock Giemsa stain is good for six months if refrigerated. The stock May-Grünwald stain is good indefinitely and does not require refrigeration.

5. *Modified Wright-Giemsa Stain*

Wright Stain‡	Any formula in standard laboratory use is satisfactory.
Giemsa stain	Formula previously outlined is satisfactory.
Buffer solution pH 6.4 and pH 6.8§	
Giemsa working stain	Dilute 1 part Giemsa stock stain with 9 parts of buffer pH 6.8. Prepare fresh daily.

Staining Procedure.   Flood the air-dried aspiration smears with methyl alcohol and allow the alcohol to evaporate completely. Then flood the smears with Wright's stain for 3 minutes. Add buffer solution pH 6.4 drop by drop to the Wright's stain, blowing on the slide to mix stain and buffer. The stain should develop a green sheen when sufficient buffer has been added. Allow to stand for 4 minutes. Wash in tap water and dry completely. Stain with working Giemsa solution for 3 minutes.

---

*Available as Jenner stain from Paragon C&C Co., Inc., 190 Willow Ave., Bronx, New York, 10454.

†Giemsa stain available as the tissue stain Wolbach modification or as the blood stain from Harleco. Either is satisfactory.

‡Wright's stain available from Harleco (in dry pack). A division of American Hospital Supply Corp., 480 Democrat Rd., Gibbstown, N.J. 08027.

§Giemsa stain available as the tissue stain Wolbach modification or as the blood stain from Harleco. Either is satisfactory. Buffer solution also available from Harleco as the salt in stable dry pack.

Wash with tap water and dry completely. Dip in xylol for 10 seconds and mount in Permount and coverslip.

6. *Hematoxylin-eosin stain*[18]

Eosin Y solution*
Harris Hematoxylin†
Dilute ammonium hydroxide

Add one drop of concentrated ammonium hydroxide to 100.0 ml of distilled water.

Staining Procedure.   Use on air-dried aspiration smears.

1.	Absolute ethyl alcohol	1 minute
2.	95 per cent ethyl alcohol	1 minute
3.	Tape water	several dips
4.	Harris Hematoxylin	2 minutes
5.	Tap water	several dips
6.	Dilute ammonium hydroxide	1 to 2 dips
7.	Eosin Y	30 seconds
8.	Tap water	several dips
9.	Tap water	several dips
10.	95 per cent ethyl alcohol	several dips
11.	95 per cent ethyl alcohol	several dips
12.	Absolute ethyl alcohol	several dips
13.	Acetone	several dips
14.	Xylol	1 minute
15.	Mount with Permount and coverslip.	

---

*Eosin Y aqueous 5 per cent pure dye solution, available from Harleco, Division of American Hospital Supply Corp., 480 Democrat Rd., Gibbstown, N.J. 08027.

†Harris Hematoxylin also available from Harleco.

Chapter Three

Breast

NON-NEOPLASTIC LESIONS

One of the oldest and most frequently attempted needle aspiration biopsies is that which is performed on tumors of the breast.[1, 2] In this author's personal series, aspiration biopsies of breast masses and enlarged lymph nodes (see Chapter 4) have been performed in approximately equal numbers. Combined, aspiration biopsies of these two sites constitute nearly two thirds of the total aspirations performed. Despite the utility of the procedure, aspiration biopsy for diagnosis of a breast lump has not been without controversy.[3-6] In this author's opinion, many critiques of the procedure either are anecdotal and based on individual biases and orientations[6] or show significant variation in aspiration technique. These technical modifications plus the failure to correlate clinical findings with the results of the needle aspiration biopsy virtually ensure the failure that critics anticipate.[3-7] Proponents, however, have scrupulously adhered to the correct thin-needle aspiration biopsy method and have succeeded in closely correlating cytologic and clinical findings. In these series, 10 per cent or less of test results for aspirations from breast cancer are false-negative, and false diagnoses of carcinoma are also very rare.[8-25] To emphasize the correlation of various methods for the diagnosis of breast tumors, several authors have combined aspiration biopsy with mammography and thorough clinical examination. Further reduction in false-negative reports for aspirates from malignant tumors and in false-positive reports for aspirates from benign breast disease has thus occurred; data obtained from these series are nearly as accurate as those provided by frozen section diagnosis.[26-30]

Normal cellular elements from aspiration biopsy of the breast may be described as similar to those from non-neoplastic lesions, particularly cysts. In this author's opinion, there is no clinical indication to aspirate a breast without a clearly defined mass. Most of these masses will be either gross cysts or lesions collectively known as mammary dysplasia (fibrocystic disease, sclerosing adenosis, and various degrees of lobular and intraductal hyperplasia). The epithelial cells, derived from ducts and lobules in these conditions, are uniform and round to oval, containing relatively little cytoplasm and densely hyperchromatic nuclei with smooth uniform borders. The cells occur in sheets scattered randomly over the smear and are relatively scarce (Fig. 3–1). Nucleoli may be observed in both Romanovsky and Papanicolaou-stained smears. They are easier to see in the latter and are uniformly small and round. The cells in sheets fit together in an extremely regular and cohesive pattern with well-defined cell boundaries.

Small amounts of fibrous tissue and fat, including individual cells, may be seen in breast aspirates. Such aspirates constitute microbiopsies, readily identified by their

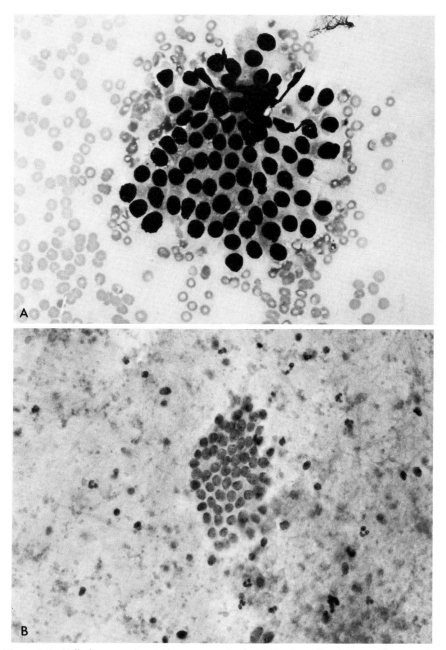

Figure 3–1   Cells from a patient with mammary dysplasia, histologically sclerosing adenosis. The cells are present in flat sheets. Nuclei are uniform and small with a smooth nuclear border. Very small nucleoli are visible in *B*. A few red blood cells and inflammatory cells make up the background. *A*, Diff-Quik × 375. *B*, Papanicolaou × 375. (All Diff-Quik smears are air-dried. All Papanicolaou-stained smears are alcohol-wet or spray-fixed.)

normal histologic appearance with either the Papanicolaou stain or hematoxylin and eosin.

   Bipolar Nuclei.   A few naked bipolar nuclei may also be seen in smears from non-neoplastic lesions of the breast. Such nuclei are very common in fibroadenomas (to be described) and have a uniform hyperchromatic pattern, a condensed chromatin structure, or both. Nucleoli are not usually visible. According to some authors, these nuclei possibly derive from myoepithelial cells.[31,32]

Foam cells and apocrine cells are very frequently seen in breast aspirates, most commonly from gross cystic disease. The former have a typical histiocytic appearance with small, eccentric nuclei and finely vacuolated cytoplasm (Fig. 3–2). While foam cells may represent true histiocytes, their most frequent origin seems to be degenerated duct epithelial cells, reflecting some degree of proliferative activity of the ductal epithelium with subsequent degeneration. The apocrine cells have abundant, finely granular cytoplasm that stains slightly metachromatic with the Romanovsky dyes and

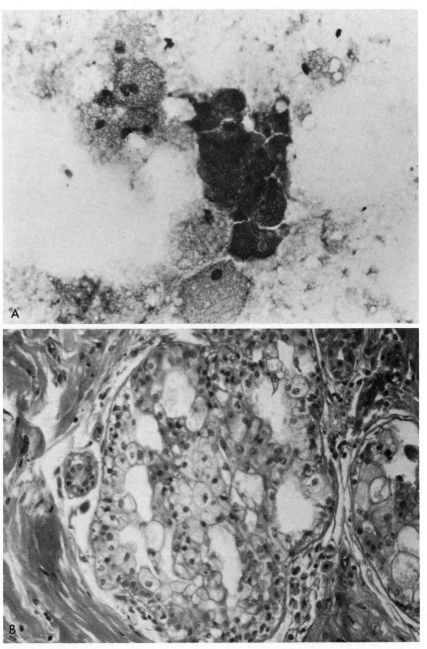

Figure 3–2 Cells and corresponding tissue from a patient with mammary dysplasia, histologically fibrocystic disease, with some duct proliferation and histiocytic metaplasia. Histiocytic cells are evident in the smear and correlate with the tissue findings. *A*, Metachrome B × 375. *B*, Hematoxylin and eosin × 240.

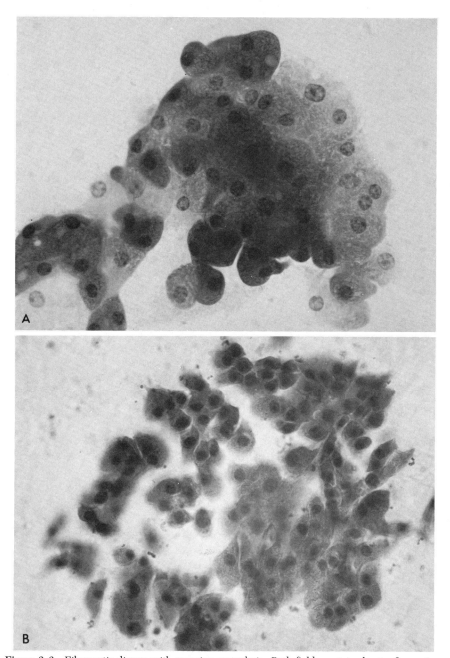

Figure 3–3 Fibrocystic disease with apocrine metaplasia. Both fields contain sheets of apocrine cells with evident granular cytoplasm and uniform small nuclei with prominent but round nucleoli. Cytoplasmic granularity is more evident with the Diff-Quik stain *(A)* than with the Papinicolaou stain *(B)*. The latter stain usually shows intense eosinophilia of the cytoplasm. A, Diff-Quik × 375. B, Papanicolaou × 375.

uniformly eosinophilic with the Papanicolaou stain. The nuclei have a relatively dense chromatin structure with readily visible, uniform, round nucleoli that stain dark purple (Fig. 3–3). These nucleoli may appear more distinct in Papanicolaou-stained aspirates. The cytoplasm of these cells may also occasionally stain either cyanophilic or frankly basophilic. In the latter situations, the relatively abundant cytoplasm and its granular texture are the major diagnostic features that identify these cells of apocrine-metaplastic type.

Large multinucleated cells have been detected in a variety of breast diseases.[31] These cells are probably multinucleated histiocytes or duct cells similar to those seen in aspirates from fibrocystic disease. This author has seen them only rarely. Vassilakos illustrates numerous multinucleated giant cells, some of the Langhans type, from a case of tuberculosis of the breast that radiographically mimicked a carcinoma. Although all the elements in the aspirate suggested a granuloma, possibly of tuberculous type, the diagnosis was not made. Excisional biopsy and frozen section were recommended.[33]

ASPIRATION OF BREAST CYSTS

Surgeons, in general, now seem to agree that aspiration of gross breast cysts is an excellent procedure for both diagnosis and treatment, since in the majority of cases the cyst will disappear after aspiration. Haagensen emphasizes the importance of aspiration of cysts, although he objects to aspirating solid lumps for diagnosis, basing his opposition on what this author believes is speculation concerning the spread of cancer cells.[34,35] Whether performed only on cysts or as part of an evaluation of all breast masses, aspiration is simple, inexpensive, convenient for the patient, and highly accurate in experienced hands.[36,37]

EXAMINATION OF CYST FLUID

It has been the policy of most authors to examine cyst fluid cytologically; however, two reports indicate that if the fluid is clear and yellow there is nothing to be gained by a cytologic study.[35,38] This author concurs in that opinion. Although he examines cyst fluid, he has not seen a case demonstrating malignant cells. Most fluid that is clear and light yellow from breast cysts is essentially acellular or contains a few duct cells, foam cells, or apocrine cells. As pointed out by Haagensen, however, gross cystic disease does predispose one to the subsequent development of breast cancer. This is no way implies that the cancer will be either in or near the cyst, and, in fact, in Haagensen's own series, it occurred more frequently in the opposite breast.[34]

While intracystic carcinoma can occur, it is extremely rare.[38,39] When aspirating cysts, if the fluid is anything other than clear and yellow in color, that is, if it contains blood or evidence of exudate, it should be examined cytologically. Of equal importance is careful reexamination of the patient for any residual breast mass. If such a mass is found, a second aspiration should be performed.[18,40] Careful follow-up by mammography and clinical examination will also essentially prevent overlooking any cases of intracystic carcinoma or carcinoma adjacent to an aspirated breast cyst. Review of one report that does not include findings of variation in cyst fluid color or the presence of a residual mass in three cases of carcinoma associated with breast cysts reveals that significant abnormalities were present, indicating need for immediate follow-up in all three cases.[38]

Mastitis.   Various forms of mastitis, including fat necrosis, may present as firm breast lumps or diffuse swelling of the mammary gland. Cysts can likewise exhibit variable degrees of inflammation, including abscess formation, that may present clinically with many of the signs of advanced breast cancer. Aspiration biopsy can provide significant information about the nature of these clinical problems and may also reveal some degrees of cellular atypia of the duct epithelium that may suggest a carcinoma. As a general feature, however, the presence of large numbers of inflammatory cells does not support an aspiration diagnosis of carcinoma. This also applies to cases of inflammatory breast cancer.

Fat Necrosis.   Fat necrosis will demonstrate areas of amorphous material, including fat and inflammatory cells, some histiocytes, and, occasionally, foreign-body-type giant cells of various sizes. Fat from the normal breast occurs in distinct microbiopsies but is disassociated in cases of fat necrosis (Fig. 3–4).

Acute Mastitis.   Cases of acute mastitis have usually been observed by this author in the post-partum patient. They are of some concern not only because of the obvious clinical signs of inflammation but also because the engorged breast may be hiding a neoplasm. Aspiration yields either large numbers of inflammatory cells or, in the case of abscess formation, frank pus. This may be associated with isolated clusters

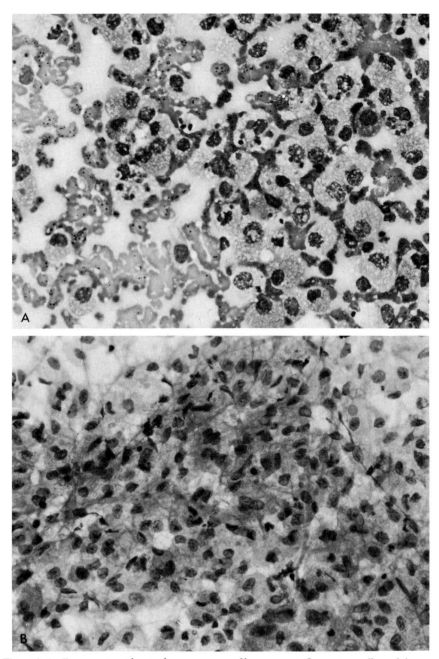

Figure 3–4   Fat necrosis with mixed smear pattern of histiocytes, inflammatory cells, and degenerating fat. An almost granulomatous sheet of cells with some multinucleated cells and fibroblasts is seen in panel *B. A,* Diff-Quik × 375. *B,* Papanicolaou × 375.

or sheets of atypical ductal epithelial cells showing vacuolization, some hyperchromasia, and prominence of nucleoli (Fig. 3–5).

CELL ATYPIA. The extremes of epithelial atypia are visible in Figure 3–6, which depicts the aspirate from a relatively discrete breast mass in a 45-year-old female with reddening of the overlying skin. The patient was afebrile, and the mass appeared to be partially fixed to the chest wall, reinforcing the clinical impression of carcinoma. Note the very active nuclei and the prominent nucleoli. The nuclear-cytoplasmic ratio

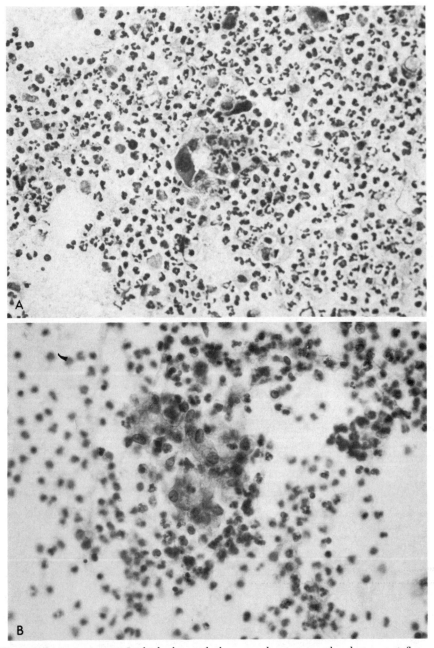

Figure 3–5 Acute mastitis. In the background, the smear demonstrates abundant acute inflammatory exudate containing a few degenerated atypical cells, probably of duct origin. Nuclear detail is lacking. The cells appear much more quiescent and more obviously histiocytic with the Papanicolaou-stained preparation. A, Diff-Quik × 375. B, Papanicolaou × 375.

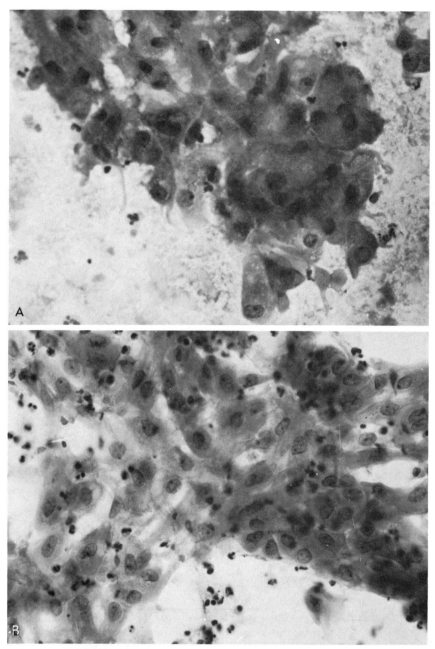

Figure 3–6   Acute mastitis with breast abscess. After partial removal of purulent material from a cystic mass, a second aspirate of a residual thickening revealed a few sheets of atypical cells with irregular nuclei and prominent nucleoli. Even for active cells, the nuclear cytoplasmic ratio is about normal. The much more orderly arrangement of the cells in the Papanicolaou-stained preparation (B) compared with that in the Diff-Quik–stained, air-dried smear A) suggests that carcinoma is unlikely. There are also too few atypical cells on this smear and too much acute inflammatory exudate to support a diagnosis of carcinoma. A, Diff-Quik × 375. B, Papanicolaou × 375.

of these cells is essentially normal for active epithelium. In addition, there is abundant acute inflammatory exudate in the background, with inflammatory cells actually within the dense cytoplasm of these cells. Cytopathologists familiar with the atypias of regeneration repair will readily recognize these features. The cellular atypia is much more impressive on the Romanovsky-stained smears than on the Papanicolaou-prepared material, the latter cells demonstrating sharply defined borders and much more quiescent nuclei. This contrasting pattern between the air-dried smears and the alcohol-fixed smears also supports a benign diagnosis.

In this particular case, after aspiration of both fluid and thick, green, purulent-looking material, there was still a residual mass. A second aspiration also yielded inflammatory cells and some atypical duct epithelium. One might proceed with antibiotic therapy in this patient, but the more realistic approach is to explore and biopsy the tumor, even though in all probability it is benign. This approach helps prevent the few but persistent false-negative diagnoses of breast cancer.

Comedomastitis.   Comedomastitis yields a greater amount of duct epithelium, also with a variable degree of atypia (Figs. 3–7 and 3–8). The same discrepancy in degree of atypia is noted when one compares the Romanovsky-stained, air-dried smears with the Papanicolaou-stained, alcohol-fixed smears. There is significant cellular degeneration, which leads to much of the variation of the cell pattern. When compared with carcinomas of the breast, this condition reveals a similar degree of marked cellularity, with small sheets, clusters, and single cells. Combined with these duct elements are histiocytes and scattered acute inflammatory cells, a pattern similar to that of duct carcinomas with a large number of comedo features. (Compare with Fig. 3–25.)

Plasma Cell Mastitis.   This author has not personally seen a case of plasma cell mastitis on aspiration biopsy. In such a case, there would presumably be a large component of plasma cells, with or without duct epithelium. Histologically, the duct epithelium can also be proliferative and somewhat atypical. It would not be unexpected that the aspiration would yield similar findings. The general principle in all cases of proliferative inflammatory lesions of the breast observed during aspiration biopsy is that the epithelial cells show degenerative changes as the cause of their atypia. The nuclear chromatin is not distinct but is clumped and fragmented. The nuclear outlines are still relatively smooth, and the nuclear cytoplasmic ratios of the duct cells are essentially normal. Large cell sheets, numerous pleomorphic cells, and cells with distinctly abnormal chromatin patterns as seen in carcinoma are lacking.

BENIGN NEOPLASMS

Fibroadenoma.   Fibroadenoma, subareolar adenoma (or duct papillomatosis), and intraductal papillomas are benign neoplasms that may present for needle aspiration. Fibroadenoma is by far the most common. It exhibits a smear pattern composed of large sheets and clusters of epithelial cells with some degree of nuclear atypia. The key to the diagnosis of fibroadenoma is the detachment of oval naked nuclei from the cell clusters and sheets (Figs. 3–9 and 3–10). Note that despite the relatively high cellularity of these smears and the prominent degree of cell activity, the cells are very uniform in size and shape and in consistency of chromatin and nucleolar detail. The *large number* of oval naked nuclei occurring with the active ductal epithelial cells is also very characteristic. Although oval naked nuclei may be seen in aspirates from mammary dysplasia, there are far fewer of them in those cases.[41] Uniformity of the smear pattern is evident on both the air-dried and the fixed smears, with the latter

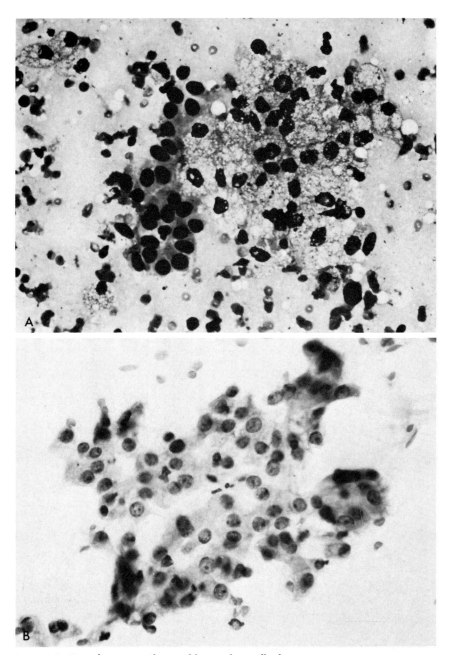

Figure 3–7 Comedomastitis. Sheets of breast duct cells demonstrating some variation in size and shape. This picture simulates carcinoma, but in this condition the cells are usually smaller than those of typical comedocarcinoma. There is a contrast between the more atypical appearance of the cells in the air-dried preparation (A) and that of the cells in the Papanicolaou-stained smear (B). These cases are difficult to interpret and require a conservative cytologic diagnosis and an excision of the mass. A, Diff-Quik × 375. B, Papanicolaou × 375.

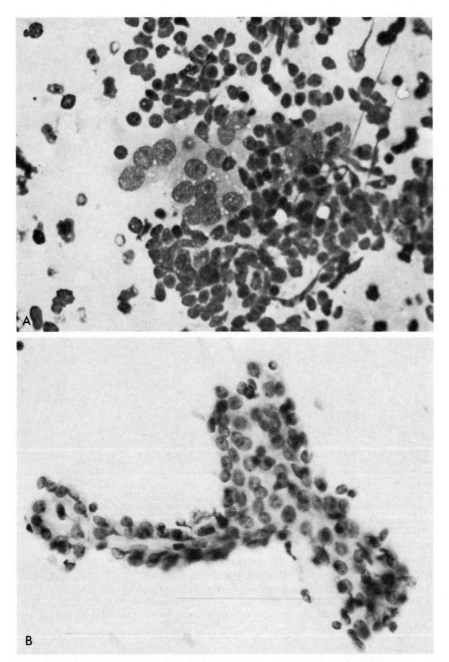

Figure 3–8   Comedomastitis. Another example of this smear pattern with marked contrast in atypia between the air-dried, Diff-Quik–stained smear and the Papanicolaou preparation. Exudate is evident in *A*, with a few cells having prominent nucleoli. In *B*, the large cohesive fragment of duct epithelium has a much more uniform appearance. *A*, Diff-Quik × 475. *B*, Papanicolaou × 375.

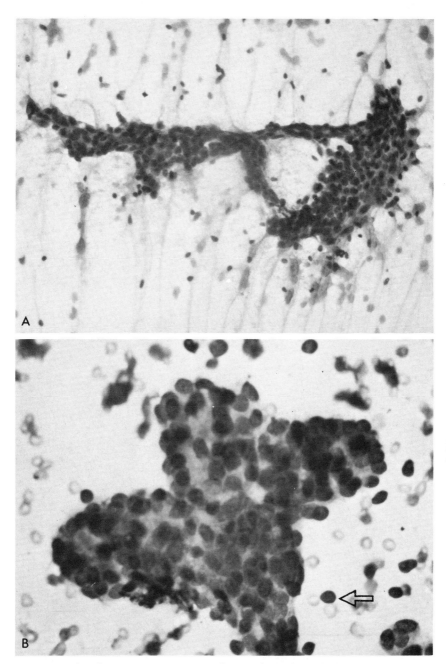

Figure 3–9   Fibroadenoma. Low-power magnification shows sheet of cohesive cells that mimics the configuration of duct epithelium seen with fibroadenoma. Note the scattered oval naked nuclei falling away from the epithelial cells. The air-dried preparation (B) also shows uniform cells with smudged chromatin. Note oval naked nuclei (arrow). A, Papanicolaou × 304. B, Diff-Quik × 475.

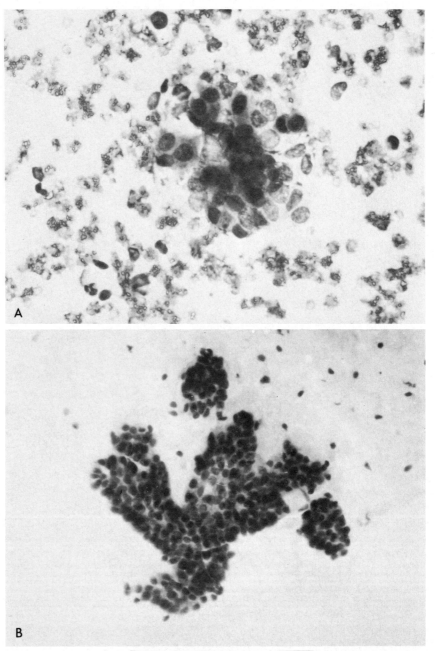

Figure 3–10   Fibroadenoma. Some variation in size and shape of the cells is evident in the air-dried smear (A). These atypical cells can be confused with carcinoma cells. In B, a much more uniform cell pattern is evident, with branching of the epithelial cells that is similar to the configuration of the duct structures of a fibroadenoma. Oval naked nuclei are also readily identified. A, Diff-Quik × 475. B, Papanicolaou × 304.

providing a greater degree of cell detail, a more obviously quiescent chromatin pattern, and a nuclear-cytoplasmic ratio that is essentially normal.

Fibroadenoma has been considered a significant cause of false-positive diagnoses.[42] The overall activity of the epithelial cells in this tumor is probably the reason. For the experienced observer, recognition of the consistent smear pattern and detection of oval naked nuclei readily lead to the correct diagnosis. For diagnosing a discrete mass in a young patient, knowledge of the clinical considerations of the case is also a definite aid. The stroma of fibroadenoma is infrequently seen in aspiration biopsy smears, and never abundantly. Its identifying feature is its metachromasia with the Romanovsky stains. Its presence is not necessary for the diagnosis. A similar stroma may also be seen in a small number of aspirates from mammary dysplasia.[41]

Adenoma. Because true adenoma of the breast is rather rare, there has been little experience with its pattern on aspiration biopsy. A case reported by Zajicek and two cases studied by this author reveal a pattern identical with that of fibroadenoma with no stromal elements[40] (Fig. 3–11).

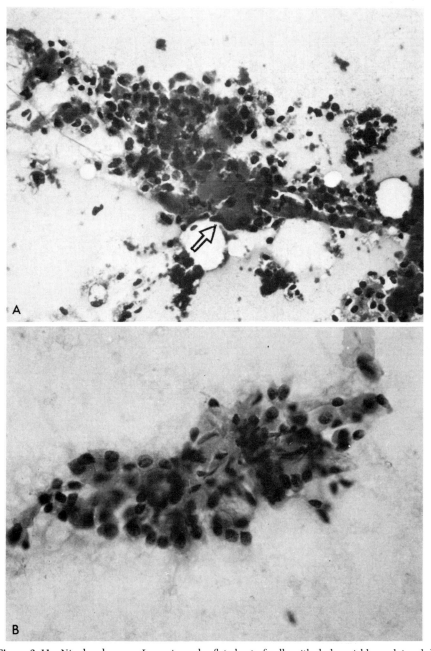

Figure 3–11 Nipple adenoma. Large irregular flat sheet of cells with dark variable nuclei and dense intervening metachromatic stroma (*A*, arrow). Similar findings are apparent in the Papanicolaou-stained aspirate with uniform nuclei and a true papillary configuration (*B*). The lesion was directly beneath the nipple. The aspiration pattern is similar to that of fibroadenoma; the most likely diagnosis is therefore adenoma of the nipple. *A*, Diff-Quik × 475. *B*, Papanicolaou × 475.

Intraductal Papillomas.   Intraductal papillomas, usually arising in the main secretory ducts, present most frequently with nipple discharge that may be bloody. This author has aspirated only one case, which provided large branching clusters of epithelial cells. Two fragments of the tumor (Fig. 3–12) were essentially microbiopsies that suggested the correct diagnosis.

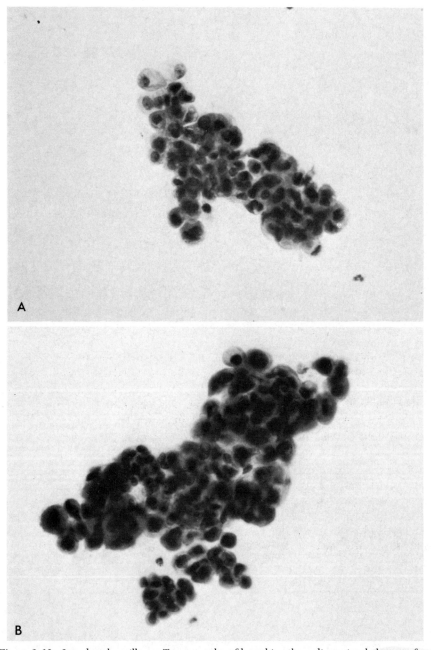

Figure 3–12   Intraductal papilloma. Two examples of branching three-dimensional clusters of uniform but hyperchromatic cells with a clean smear background. Where it is visible, the nuclear chromatin is somewhat granular. Bleeding from the nipple coupled with the aspiration pattern suggests an intraductal papilloma. Differential diagnosis from low-grade papillary carcinoma is not possible cytologically. *A* and *B*, Papanicolaou × 375.

There was also some cellular atypia. A fair amount of blood was present on the aspirate. This finding more often suggests carcinoma. The clinical picture of a patient with bloody nipple discharge and a subareolar mass combined with the aspiration smear findings reinforced the correct diagnosis.

Intraductal papillomas have been described with a variety of cell types, most of them benign in appearance. Some of the cells have large vacuoles and may have apocrine features. In the large series of aspiration biopsies reported by Franzen and Zajicek, there were eleven cases of intraductal papilloma. Three of these eleven aspirations provided only fat and blood or no cellular elements, six aspirations yielded benign duct epithelium, and two aspirations provided only cystic fluid with essentially no definite diagnostic cellular elements. There were no false-positive diagnoses in this small number of cases.[8]

SUMMARY

Benign lesions of the breast will yield scanty cellular material, except in cases of mastitis, fibroadenoma, and pure adenomas. In mastitis, the majority of the cells are inflammatory, with scant but sometimes atypical duct epithelial cells. In all other lesions, the breast duct cells are very quiescent, with an occasional fibroadenoma providing some usually uniform degree of active epithelium.

MALIGNANT EPITHELIAL NEOPLASMS (CARCINOMAS)

Unless convinced that only breast cysts should be aspirated, one will agree that the most important diagnosis to be made from fine-needle biopsies of solid breast tumors is carcinoma. Most reported series emphasize the diagnosis of carcinoma.[2,31,32,42-48]

Infiltrating Duct Carcinoma. Infiltrating duct carcinoma is the most common neoplastic lesion and therefore provides the best and most typical aspirates. The smears are highly cellular and composed of clusters and sheets with single cells dispersed over much of the smear. There is a background of degeneration and necrosis mixed with blood in some instances, although the background may be relatively clean. The individual cells are usually variable in size and shape, having a very granular, lightly metachromatic red-purple chromatin pattern with Romanovsky stains and a distinct, irregular chromatin pattern throughout the nucleus after alcohol fixation and Papanicolaou staining. A similar morphologic appearance, although lacking detail, may be seen on smears that are air-dried and stained by hematoxylin and eosin.

This author and others have observed several variations in the smear pattern from nonspecific infiltrating duct cancer that relate to both the cell size and the degree of stromal fibrosis.[40,49] The medium and small duct cell carcinomas with a nonspecific infiltrating pattern have more uniform cells. The same loss of cohesiveness between the cell sheets and clusters occurs throughout the smear. The chromatin pattern is similar to that of the large-cell infiltrating duct carcinoma, with an extremely high nuclear cytoplasmic ratio.

Other variations in cell type among the duct carcinomas have also been detected, including apocrine carcinomas in a cribriform pattern (Figs. 3–13 and 3–14) and squamous cell carcinoma (Figs. 3–15 and 3–16). This latter tumor, which most often occurs as metaplasia within a duct carcinoma, is quite rare. Six cases have recently been reported by Leiman.[56] While these variations have little or no clinical significance, they do demonstrate the excellent cytologic and histologic correlation that can be obtained with a needle aspiration biopsy that is well prepared and carefully evaluated.

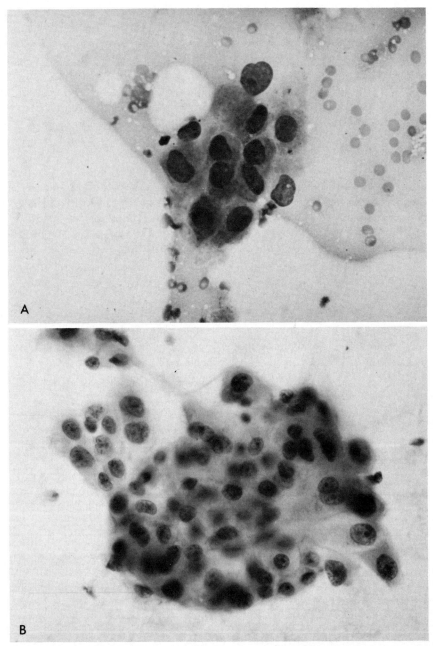

Figure 3–13   Infiltrating duct carcinoma with apocrine cells. These smear patterns also resemble those of the large cell type of infiltrating duct carcinoma, but there is a pronounced granularity to the tumor cell cytoplasm and unusually prominent nucleoli, as in apocrine cells in fibrocystic disease. With the Papanicolaou stain, the cytoplasm also appears granular but may stain either eosinophilic or basophilic. *A*, Diff-Quik × 375. *B*, Papanicolaou × 375.

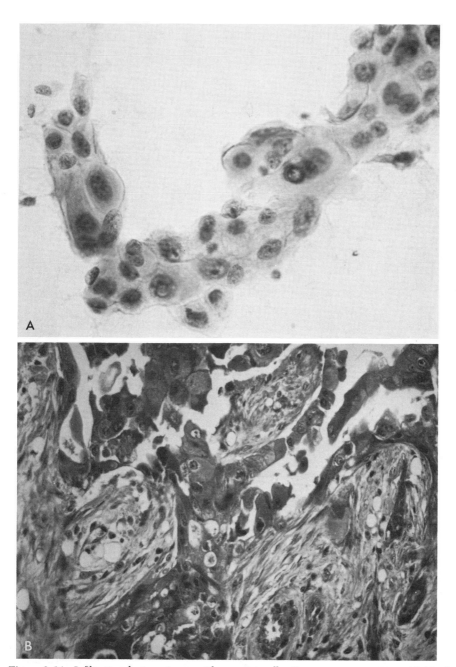

Figure 3–14 Infiltrating duct carcinoma with apocrine cells. Compare smear pattern with histologic section. *A*, Papanicolaou × 375. *B*, Hematoxylin and eosin × 240.

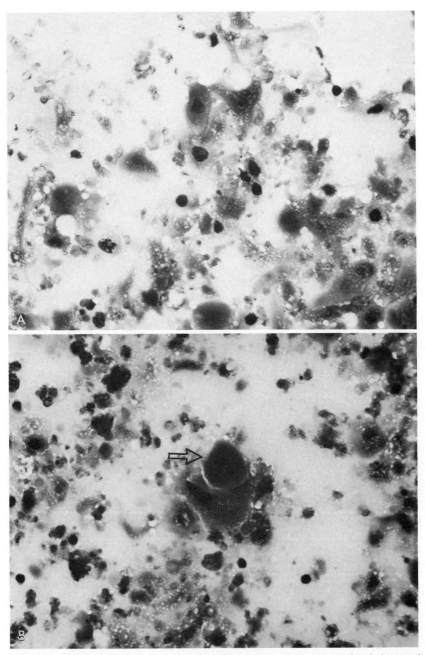

Figure 3–15   Squamous cell carcinoma, metaplastic type. Scattered degenerated and pleomorphic cells are seen in this smear within a necrotic background. Cytoplasm is very dense and will stain deep blue with Romanovsky stains, a characteristic of squamous cells that are keratinized. Even squamous ghost cells are visible (*B*, arrow). *A* and *B*, Diff-Quik × 375.

The small infiltrating duct carcinomas are usually seen as very scirrhous tumors and yield aspiration smears with a relatively low overall cellularity. These tumor cells appear to be more cohesive, but they are still irregular in size, shape, and nuclear margin. There is a linear arrangement with distinct nuclear molding, the so-called "Indian-file" arrangement, that cannot be distinguished from the pattern of infiltrating lobular carcinoma, a neoplasm with cells of similar size. This is not surprising, since ultrastructural studies suggest that the infiltrating lobular carcinoma originates from terminal duct epithelium.[50,51]

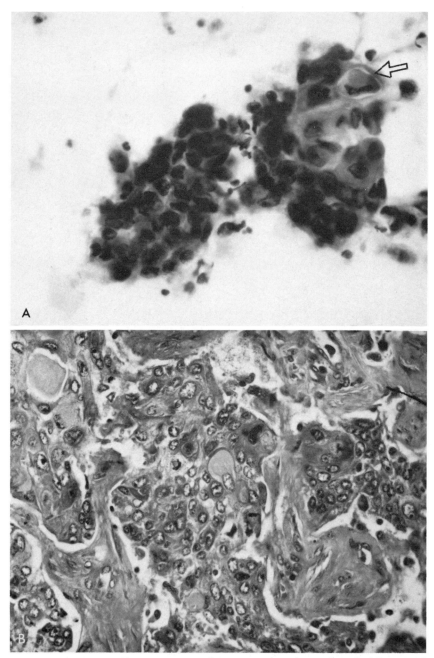

Figure 3–16   Squamous cell carcinoma, metaplastic type. Large cluster of poorly differentiated tumor cells, with some showing well-defined cell boundaries and masses of keratin (A, arrow) that stain intensely eosinophilic. Tissue from this case (B), with evidence of keratinized tumor cells. In other sections, this neoplasm was an undifferentiated large cell type of infiltrating duct carcinoma. A, Papanicolaou × 375. B, hematoxylin and eosin × 300.

Several examples of infiltrating duct carcinoma with variation in cell size and pattern are visible in Figures 3–17 through 3–24. One should compare these aspirates with those obtained from benign conditions and observe carefully the cellular patterns and arrangements, noting the lack of cohesiveness among the dissociated single cells, which, unlike the bipolar oval naked nuclei seen in fibroadenomas, retain their cytoplasmic outline. Note also the background presence of necrotic debris and, in some cases, disintegrating blood (Fig. 3–19).

Text continued on page 46

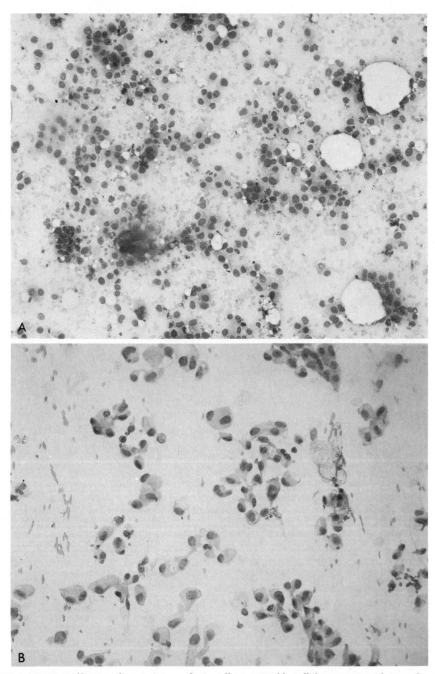

Figure 3–17   Infiltrating duct carcinoma, large-cell type. Highly cellular aspirate with irregular sheets and single cells is visible in *A*. Irregular patterns of the cells are apparent in *B*. Cellularity and nuclear abnormalities are consistent throughout the entire smear in typical cases of invasive duct carcinoma of the breast. *A*, Diff-Quik × 100. *B*, Papanicolaou × 200.

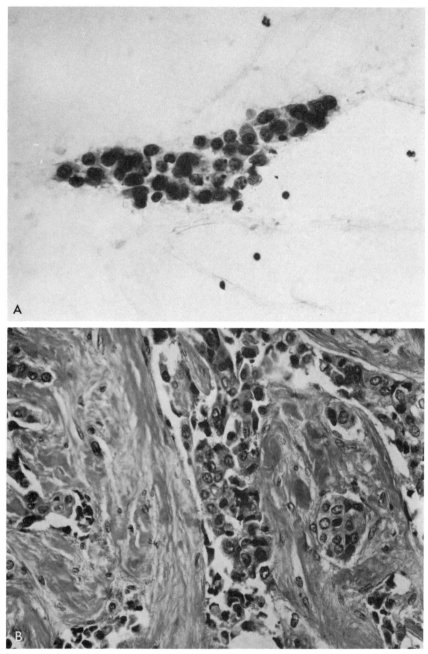

Figure 3–18 Infiltrating duct carcinoma, large-cell type. Compare the cell arrangement and nuclear structure of the aspiration smear with the tissue pattern of this invasive duct carcinoma. *A*, Papanicolaou × 375. *B*, Hematoxylin and eosin × 300.

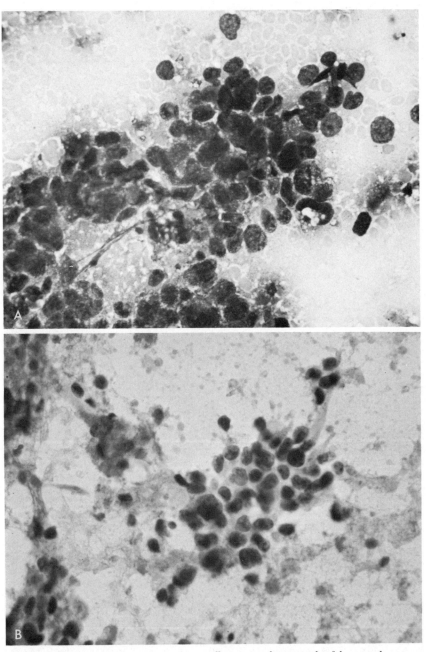

Figure 3–19   Infiltrating duct carcinoma, large-cell type. Another example of the typical smear patterns, both air-dried and alcohol-fixed, of large-cell type of infiltrating duct carcinoma. *A*, Diff-Quik × 375. *B*, Papanicolaou × 375.

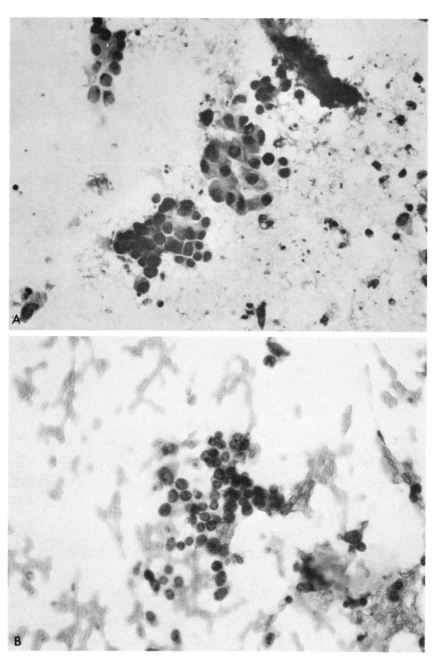

Figure 3–20. Infiltrating duct carcinoma, medium-cell type. Overall cellularity of these aspirates is somewhat diminished from that represented in Figure 3–17. Cells are also smaller but do show variation in size and shape, more evident in the air-dried preparation *(A)*. Nuclear chromatin is finely granular, and only small nucleoli are present in the malignant cells in *B*. Some variation and relatively loose arrangement of the cells support a diagnosis of carcinoma. *A*, metachrome B × 375. *B*, Papanicolaou × 375.

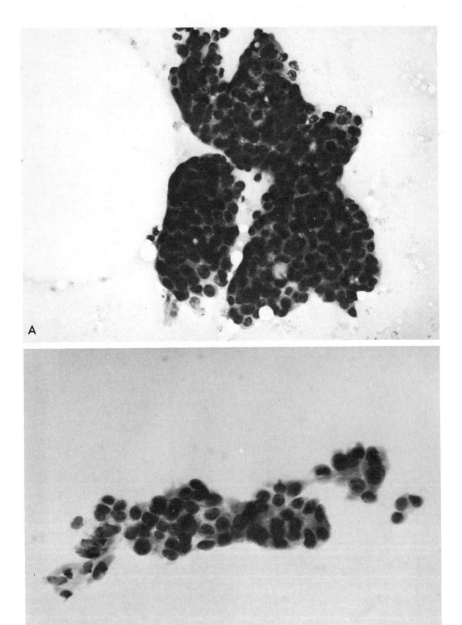

Figure 3–21 Infiltrating duct carcinoma, medium-cell type. A smear pattern with cells smaller than those of the usual infiltrating duct carcinoma and remarkably cohesive. There is also a branching pattern similar to that of fibroadenoma aspirates. Oval naked nuclei are not identified. In carcinoma smears, when Romanovsky stains are used, the chromatin pattern is much more metachromatic than in smears of fibroadenoma. Variation in nuclear size and shape as well as some nuclear chromatin granularity is more evident in *B*. Uniformity of this carcinoma smear pattern can be confusing. Clinical features of the mass and the "feel" on aspiration are important in making the differential diagnosis between carcinoma and fibroadenoma. *A*, Diff-Quik × 240. *B*, Papanicolaou × 375.

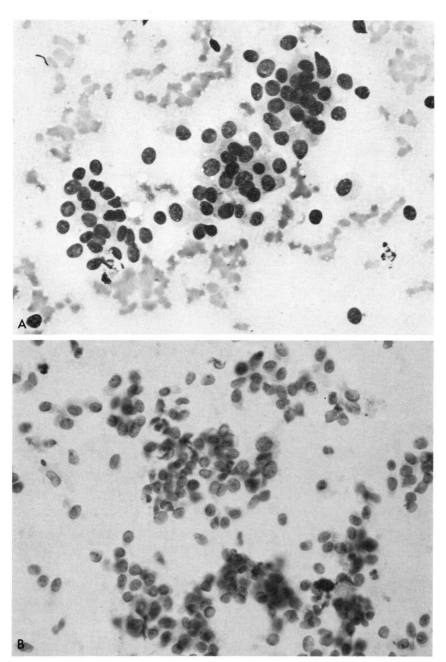

Figure 3–22 Infiltrating duct carcinoma, medium-cell type. A smear with high cellularity and with both sheets and single cells. Single cells in the fixed smear *(B)* suggest oval naked nuclei similar to those in the aspirates from fibroadenomas. However, the cellularity is too high to support a diagnosis of fibroadenoma, and even the sheets are poorly cohesive. *A*, Diff-Quik × 240. *B*, Papanicolaou × 240.

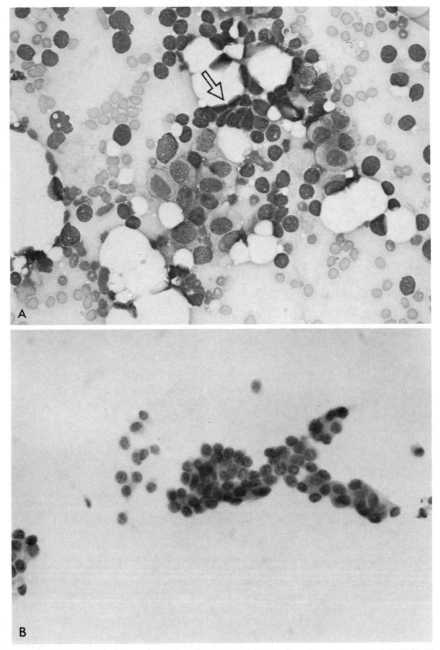

Figure 3–23 Infiltrating duct carcinoma, small-cell type. Smear pattern shows high cellularity, with both single cells and sheets, but the cells are relatively small for an air-dried preparation. Note the single-file arrangement (*A*, arrow). Marked uniformity of the cells is apparent in *B*. Diagnosis of the fixed, Papanicolaou-stained aspirate is quite difficult, but the air-dried preparation is relatively easy to diagnose. *A*, Diff-Quik × 375. *B*, Papanicolaou × 375.

DIFFERENTIAL DIAGNOSIS

Although some authors consider it impossible to differentiate among the various histologic types of breast cancer with aspiration biopsies,[44] experienced cytopathologists have made the attempt based on a thorough study of the smear patterns. Using the pathologic classification of Fisher,[52] this author has been able to recognize from aspiration biopsy the patterns of infiltrating duct carcinoma, including its comedo

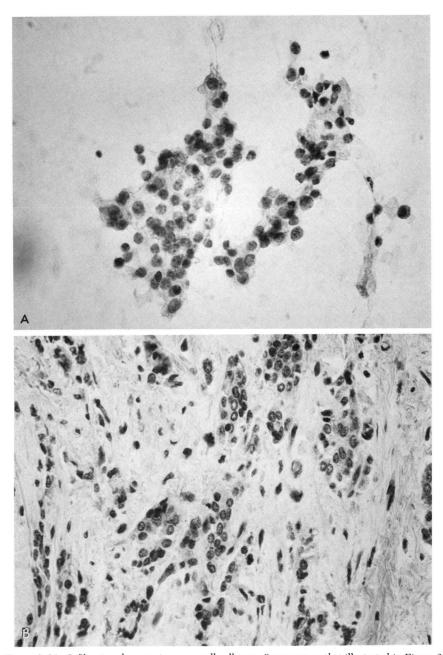

Figure 3–24 Infiltrating duct carcinoma, small cell type. Same case as that illustrated in Figure 3–23. Compare Papanicolaou-stained smear pattern with tissue pattern of small-cell infiltrating duct carcinoma. Note the bland character of the tumor cells and the few disassociated naked nuclei, which might suggest a diagnosis of fibroadenoma from this single field. *A*, Papanicolaou × 475. *B*, Hematoxylin and eosin × 240.

form, medullary carcinoma, mucinous (colloid) carcinoma, tubular carcinoma, squamous cell carcinoma, and lobular carcinoma, although the latter is not clearly distinguishable from the small-cell form of infiltrating duct carcinoma.[53]

Comedocarcinoma and Medullary Carcinoma. The comedo pattern of infiltrating duct carcinoma is illustrated in Figures 3–25 and 3–26. The aspirate is highly cellular with obviously malignant cells in clusters and clumps. The background reveals many histiocytes as well as necrosis noted from the granular debris between the cellular elements. A clinical clue is provided by the actual aspiration, since these tumors are

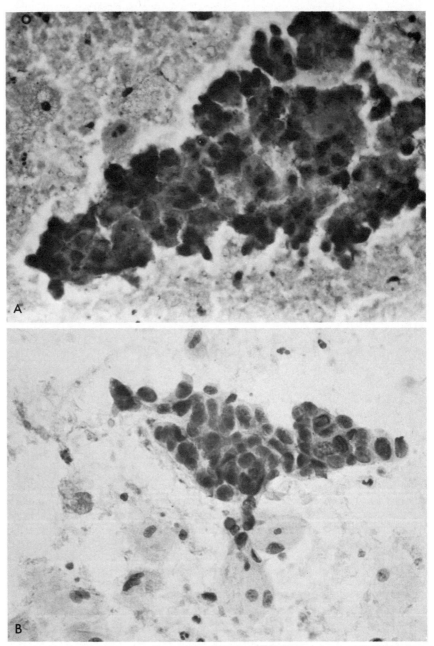

Figure 3–25   Comedocarcinoma of the breast. Large cells in sheets with abundant necrotic debris in the background and scattered histiocytic-appearing duct cells. *A*, Metachrome B × 375. *B*, Papanicolaou × 375.

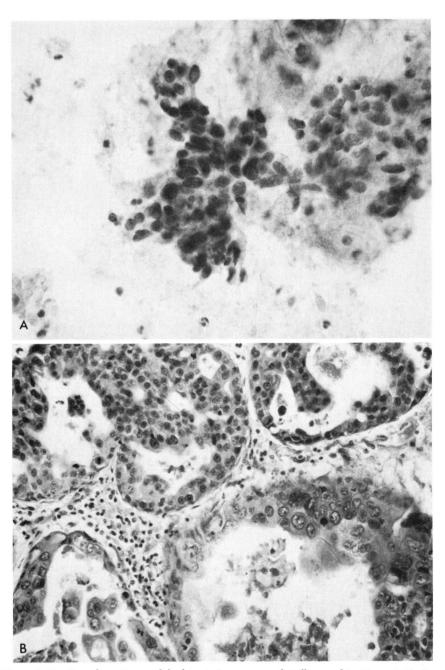

Figure 3–26 Comedocarcinoma of the breast. Same case as that illustrated in Figure 3–25. Compare cell pattern with tissue pattern in this case. *A*, Papanicolaou × 375. *B*, Hematoxylin and eosin × 240.

quite soft and yield abundant specimen, which may begin to fill up the syringe if the aspiration is too vigorous. A medullary carcinoma is also very soft, and aspiration of this lesion provides abundant, large, undifferentiated malignant cells. A case is illustrated in Figure 3–27. Visible as well are a scant number of lymphocytes. The diagnosis cannot be dependent upon them. The large, undifferentiated cells with their prominent nucleoli and very degenerated filmy cytoplasm, combined with the lack of resistance of the mass during the actual aspiration, indicate the correct diagnosis.

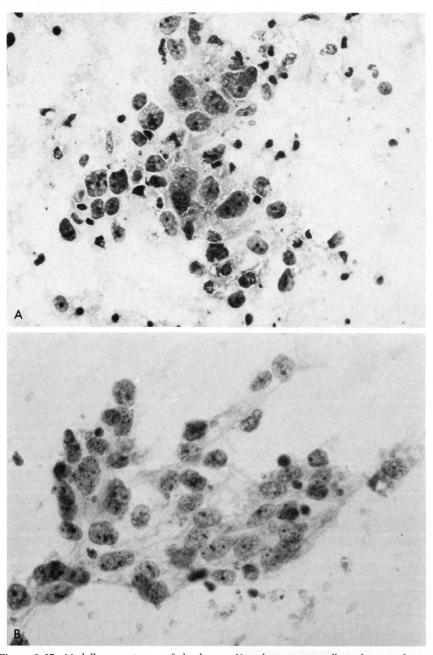

Figure 3–27 Medullary carcinoma of the breast. Very large tumor cells with scant degenerated cytoplasm are seen in both *A* and *B*. There are only a few lymphocytes in the background. Malignant nuclear features are evident. The smear pattern combined with the clinical features of a large, soft breast mass strongly suggests a diagnosis of medullary carcinoma. The presence of a pushing border or the amount of lymphocytic infiltrate cannot be predicted from the aspiration biopsy. *A*, Diff-Quik × 375. *B*, Papanicolaou × 375.

Mucinous (Colloid) Carcinoma.   Aspiration of a mucinous, or colloid, carcinoma also provides abundant cells, usually in clusters. The chromatin pattern, while distinct, is not as impressive as a typical poorly differentiated infiltrating duct cancer (Fig. 3–28). The clue to the diagnosis is the large abundant metachromatic stroma, which is best seen on Romanovsky stains. This mucin is not very apparent with the Papanicolaou stain (Fig. 3–28*B*).

Smears from the signet-cell type of mucinous carcinoma contain very little metachromatic stroma, but they are extremely cellular and have the general appearance

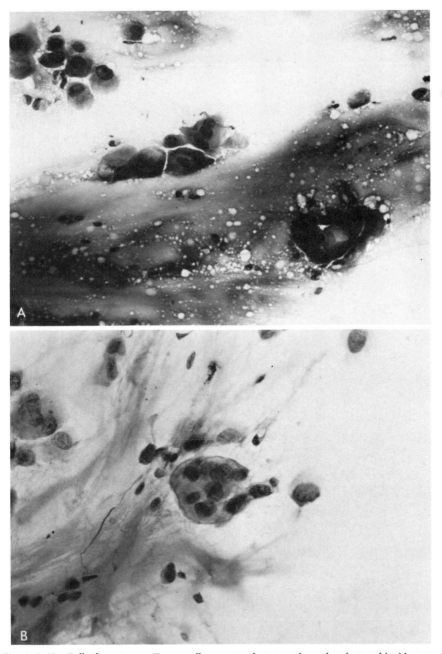

Figure 3–28   Colloid carcinoma. Tumor cells occur in clusters with an abundant and highly metachromatic stroma in the background. As in the tissue pattern of a typical colloid carcinoma, the tumor cells appear to float in the mucin. Variation in cell size is evident but not as striking as in typical infiltrating duct carcinoma. *A*, Diff-Quik × 240. *B*, Papanicolaou × 375.

of a nonspecific infiltrating duct carcinoma. Look carefully and note the number of cells with a slightly or completely eccentric nucleus (Fig. 3–29). With the Romanovsky stains, there will also be a very faint metachromasia to the cytoplasm adjacent to the eccentrically positioned nucleus. The overall pattern of these smears resembles that of a sheet of plasma cells, but the typical clockface chromatin pattern is absent. This is not an unimportant cytologic diagnosis, since this particular type of duct carcinoma is extremely aggressive.[54] The aspiration pattern of signet-cell carcinoma also confirms

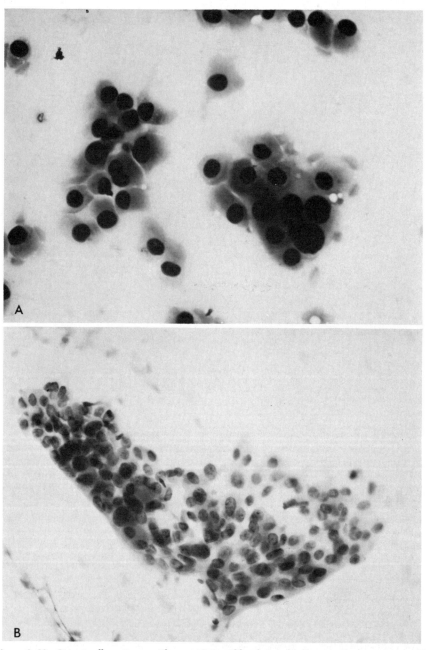

Figure 3–29   Signet cell carcinoma. These aspirates, like those of infiltrating duct carcinomas of large cell type, are highly cellular. The signet cell pattern is suggested by the eccentric position of the nuclei of many of the tumor cells and by a slight metachromasia of the cytoplasm seen with the Romanovsky stains. A distinctive pattern for this carcinoma is less obvious in the Papanicolaou preparation *(B)*. A, Diff-Quik × 375. *B* Papanicolaou × 375.

that the lesion is of duct origin, although at least one author reports that this tumor originates from cells of the mammary lobule.[55]

Aspiration for detecting mucin production can be remarkably sensitive. This author reports one case in which the aspiration was reported as infiltrating duct carcinoma with a colloid component. Excision of the lesion and histologic study revealed only typical infiltrating duct carcinoma. After additional material from the original biopsy was examined, areas of mucin production were readily identified.

Tubular Carcinoma.   Because of the unusually well-differentiated and uniform pattern of tubular carcinoma, it was thought impossible to diagnose this neoplasm from needle aspiration biopsy. This author has successfully used aspiration to diagnose two cases of tubular carcinoma seen in his personal series to date. Both cases presented a very uniform cellular pattern (Figs. 3–30 and 3–31). The peculiar angularity of the glandular structures was unlike that seen in mammary dysplasias or benign neoplasms. If one compares this pattern, which is essentially a microbiopsy, with the typical histologic appearance of infiltrating tubular carcinoma, the similarity (Fig. 3–31*B*) is obvious. It is conceivable that areas of sclerosing adenosis might yield similar cellular fragments. In this respect, it seems prudent to regard this type of smear pattern from tubular carcinoma as only suspect and to request a biopsy with frozen-section confirmation before initiating definitive therapy. Until one gains experience with aspiration specimens, it is best to report as unequivocally malignant only those cases with smear patterns typical of the infiltrating duct carcinoma.[57,58]

Lobular Carcinoma.   Infiltrating lobular carcinoma should also be reported cautiously as suspected carcinoma and a histologic confirmation should be requested. This author prefers this conservative diagnostic approach because the tumor cells are small and have a strikingly uniform appearance. Their most telling malignant characteristic is their single-file pattern (Figs. 3–32 and 3–33). This morphology is maintained with either the air-dried smears or the alcohol-fixed aspirates. The latter show a pale, uniform, but distinct nuclear chromatin structure with a very high nuclear-cytoplasmic ratio.

Comparison with Sclerosing Adenosis.   The similarity of the pattern of lobular carcinoma to that formed by isolated cell clusters and groups from aspirations of sclerosing adenosis or fibrocystic disease is fairly apparent, however (Fig. 3–34). The cells from an infiltrating lobular carcinoma demonstrate greater variation on the air-dried smears. When arranged in a single-file pattern, the cells are more obviously malignant. While this author has been cautious about the aspiration diagnosis of lobular carcinoma, other authors have had excellent success.[18,40]

Inflammatory Carcinoma.   Although it is a rare form of breast cancer, inflammatory carcinoma may bear considerable clinical resemblance to mastitis. Aspiration biopsy easily distinguishes inflammatory carcinoma because of the large number of obviously malignant tumor cells present in this condition. Inflammatory cells are found in the background, but there are fewer than in the usual case of mastitis. An example is illustrated in Figure 3–35. Tumor cells in this aspirate are fairly large, but it should be remembered that inflammatory carcinoma is a clinical as well as a histologic diagnosis. Therefore, it may occur with a variety of breast-cancer cell types of an undifferentiated nature. Aspiration biopsy is recommended in such cases, because the patient will in no way benefit from either an excisional biopsy or radical surgery. Also, radiation therapy is more easily applied to a field that has not been surgically violated.

Pleomorphism.   Breast carcinomas may be extremely pleomorphic, showing both very anaplastic and pseudosarcomatous patterns. These devious forms may be suspected from aspiration biopsy. Two examples are illustrated in Figures 3–36 to 3–38. Tumor cells may be spindle-shaped, extremely irregular in nuclear configuration, and

Text continued on page 60

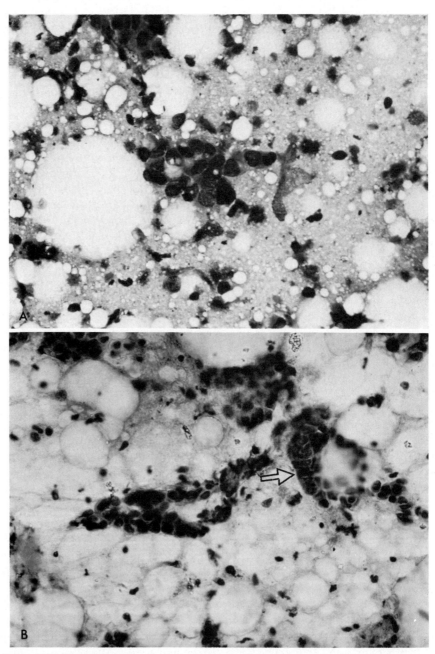

Figure 3–30 Well-differentiated tubular carcinoma of the breast. Cells in these smears are rather small and very bland. There is some single-file arrangement (*B*, arrow), but the clue to the correct diagnosis of tumor type is the peculiarly pointed nature of the glands. Note the relationship of these glands to the adipose tissue in the background of the smear *(B)*. *A*, Diff-Quik × 375. *B*, Papanicolaou × 375.

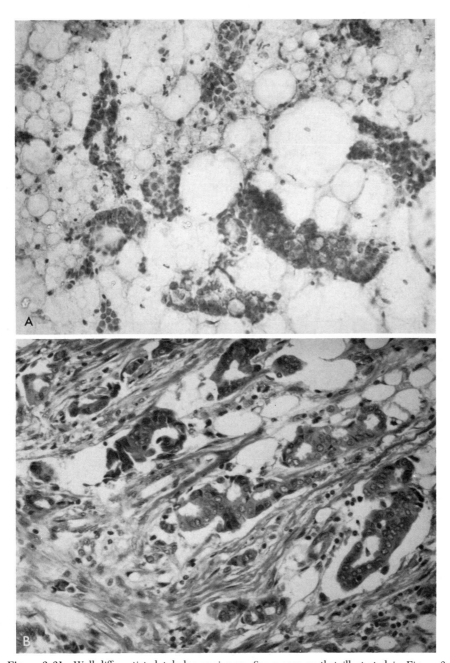

Figure 3–31 Well-differentiated tubular carcinoma. Same case as that illustrated in Figure 3–30. Compare smear pattern at low-power magnification with tissue pattern that is so distinctive for this type of breast carcinoma. Note the similar pointed infiltrating structure of the glands. *A,* Papanicolaou × 100. *B,* Hematoxylin and eosin × 240.

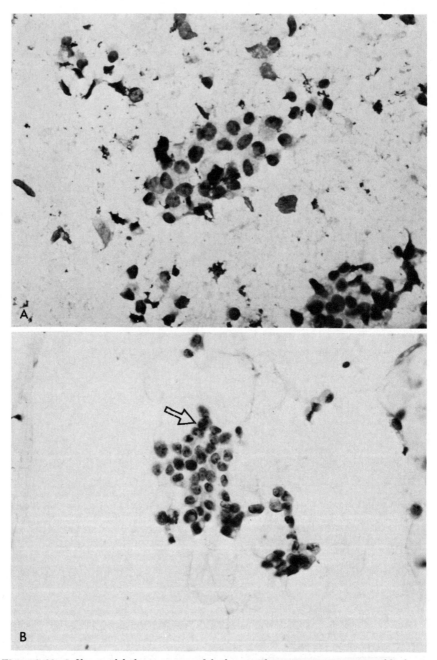

Figure 3–32   Infiltrating lobular carcinoma of the breast. These smears are quite variable, being either highly cellular or rather sparse in cells. The tumor cells are bland but do demonstrate some variation in size and shape that is more evident in air-dried smears. A single-file arrangement is often found (*B*, arrow), but it is also seen in duct carcinomas with small cells and in tubular carcinomas (Fig. 3–30). A consistently distinct chromatin structure can usually be found in well-fixed, Papanicolaou-stained aspirates. *A*, Diff-Quik × 375. *B*, Papanicolaou × 375.

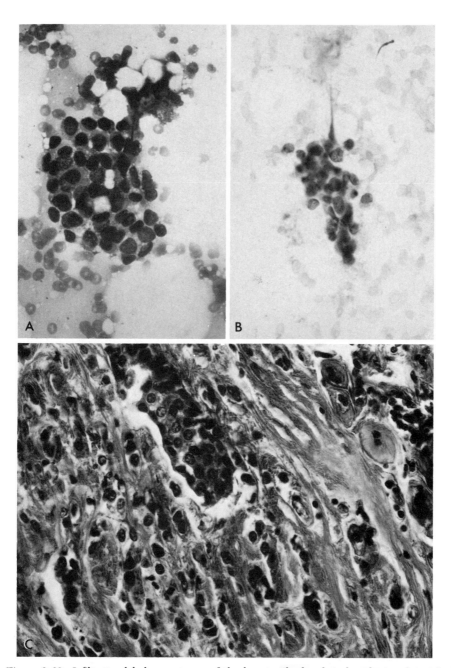

Figure 3–33 Infiltrating lobular carcinoma of the breast. Bland, relatively cohesive sheet of cells displaying some variation in size and shape. Note the similarity to cells of sclerosing adenosis (Fig. 3–34). Usually, smears from lobular carcinoma are more cellular than those from sclerosing adenosis, and the fixed smears have a greater proportion of cells with finely granular chromatin and small, irregular nucleoli. Caution is required in reporting this type of case. A confirmatory frozen section or other tissue biopsy is usually requested before definitive surgical therapy. A, Diff-Quik × 375. B, Papanicolaou × 375. C, Hematoxylin and eosin × 375.

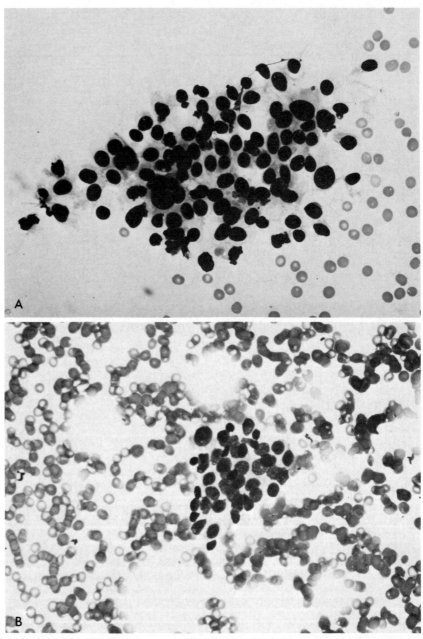

Figure 3–34   Sclerosing adenosis. Smear with cell sheets that are very similar to those from infiltrating lobular carcinoma. Greater variation in cell size and shape is present in this benign aspirate than in the examples of smears from lobular carcinoma. *A* and *B*, Diff-Quik × 375.

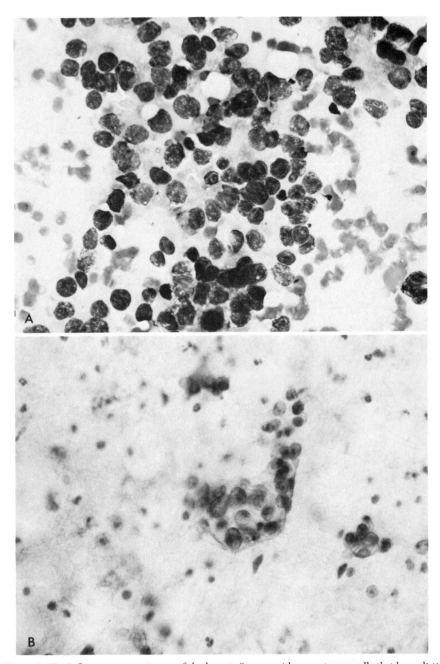

Figure 3–35   Inflammatory carcinoma of the breast. Smears with many tumor cells that have distinctly malignant features. The amount of inflammatory infiltrate is variable, but much less is present in this condition than in acute mastitis. The inflammatory cells are better seen in the Papanicolaou-stained smear, while the tumor cells in this smear are bland in appearance. Clinical features of inflammatory carcinoma should also be present before such a specific diagnosis is made from aspiration biopsy alone. In their absence, only a diagnosis of carcinoma should be reported. *A*, Diff-Quik × 375. *B*, Papanicolaou × 375.

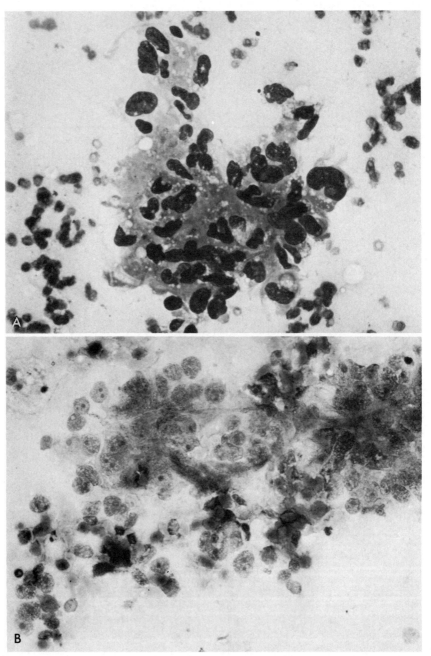

Figure 3–36   Pleomorphic breast carcinoma with chondroid stromal metaplasia. Malignant tumor cells are obviously present, but the pattern is not typical of the usual infiltrating duct carcinoma. The cells are spindle-shaped and surrounded in some foci with markedly metachromatic stroma, seen best with Romanovsky stains. Clustering of the cells in *B* supports a diagnosis of carcinoma. An unusual pattern should be expected, and a diagnosis of possible sarcoma cannot be excluded. *A*, Diff-Quik × 375. *B*, Papanicolaou × 375.

multinucleated, with the formation of giant cells. Adequate histologic sections from these tumors will also reveal pleomorphism that may include cartilaginous and osteoid tissue, which can be detected by similar patterns in aspiration biopsy. If pleomorphism is the predominant feature of the cytologic smear, a frank sarcoma diagnosis must be considered.

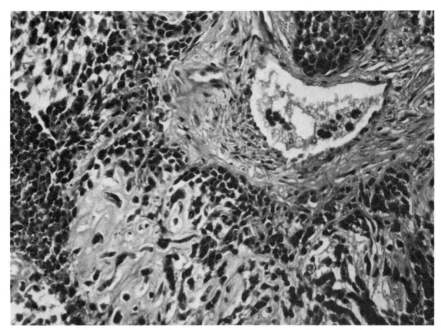

Figure 3–37 Pleomorphic breast carcinoma with chondroid stromal metaplasia. An area of infiltrating duct carcinoma is visible at the top of the illustration, and an area of malignant spindle cells and chondroid stroma, simulating immature cartilage, appears in the bottom half of the illustration. Smear patterns from this neoplasm are depicted in Figure 3–36. Hematoxylin and eosin × 240.

Granular Cell Myoblastoma and Sarcoidosis.   Two conditions clinically simulate breast cancer but can be diagnosed from aspiration biopsy: granular cell myoblastoma and sarcoidosis. One case of each rare condition has been reported.[59,60] Diagnosing the granular cell myoblastoma from the cytologic findings was relatively easy. This has been this author's experience with one case of a soft-tissue, granular-cell neoplasm (see Chapter 10). A diagnosis of carcinoma was excluded, but a specific diagnosis of sarcoid granulomas was not made in the other case.

MALIGNANT NONEPITHELIAL NEOPLASMS (SARCOMAS)

True sarcomas of the breast are extremely rare, even in large series of malignant neoplasms, including the malignant forms of cystosarcoma phyllodes. This author has not encountered a true sarcoma in his personal series of aspiration biopsies, but only pleomorphic breast cancers. In one very well-illustrated treatise and an additional extensive reference, true sarcomas are not mentioned, while in the monograph by Zajicek only the malignant cystosarcoma phyllodes is described.[8,31,40] Kreuzer and Boquoi reported a series of needle aspiration biopsies of breast sarcomas, including both lymphosarcoma and angiosarcoma. They used quantitative cytophotometry on Feulgen-stained aspirates to measure DNA values, which, in some sarcomas, ranged as high as 8N. DNA values failed to correlate with the type of the sarcoma. The more pleomorphic sarcomas did have a higher total DNA and a greater range of individual nuclear values.[61]

While not observing true sarcomas, the author has seen examples of mycosis fungoides involving the breast (Fig. 3–39) and a granulocytic leukemic infiltrate that presented clinically as a fibroadenoma in a 14-year-old girl (Fig. 3–40). The correct diagnosis was made from the needle aspiration biopsy in each case.

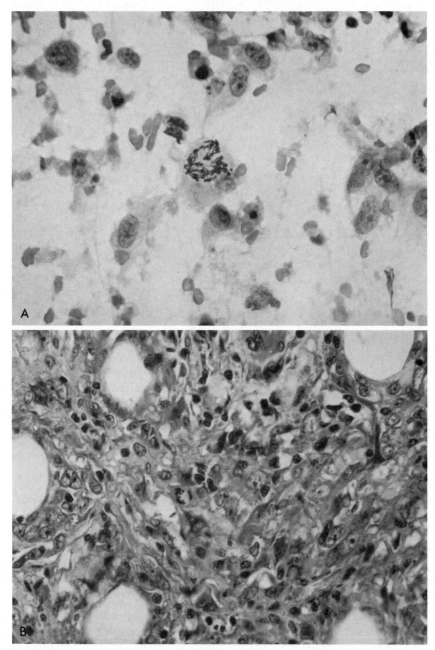

Figure 3–38   Pleomorphic breast carcinoma with malignant fibrous histiocytoma pattern. Smear with single pleomorphic spindle-shaped cells, some multinucleated and demonstrating bizarre mitotic figures. The tissue pattern *(B)* is not unlike that of malignant fibrous histiocytoma. This tumor in other areas resembled infiltrating duct carcinoma. A small duct is visible in the upper right-hand corner of the photomicrograph. *A,* Papanicolaou × 375. *B,* Hematoxylin and eosin × 375.

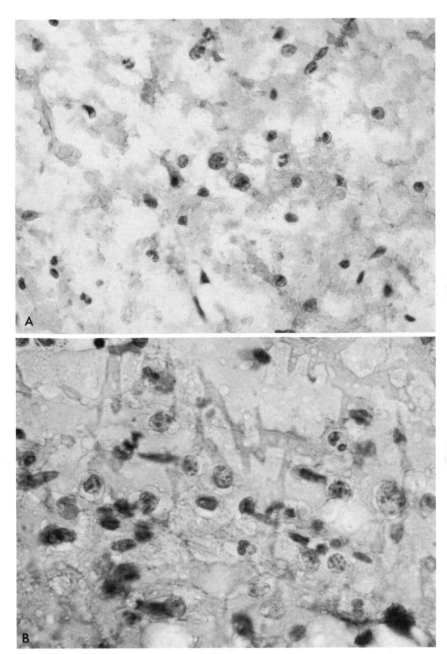

Figure 3–39 Mycosis fungoides involving the breast. Aspirate demonstrates single malignant-appearing lymphoid cells of variable size. This patient had a long history of mycosis fungoides at the time of appearance of the breast mass. Basic differential diagnosis is accomplished by ruling out breast cancer, an easy procedure with this aspiration smear pattern. A and B, Papanicolaou; A × 375, B × 600.

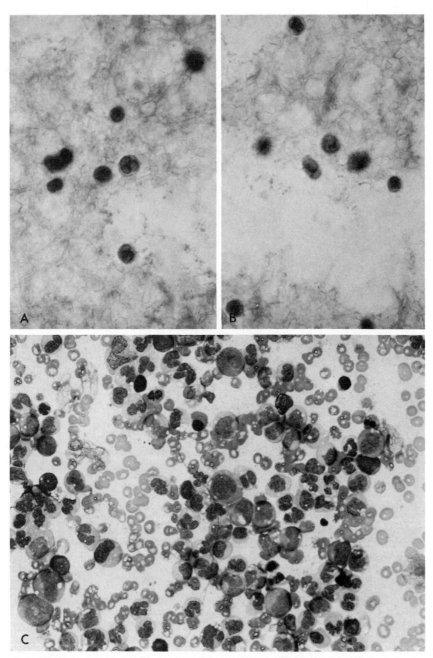

Figure 3–40.   Granulocytic leukemic infiltrate of the breast. This patient was admitted to the hospital for evaluation of anemia. A breast mass was palpated and thought to be a fibroadenoma. Aspiration revealed immature granulocytes, strongly suggestive of acute granulocytic leukemic infiltrate of the breast (*A* and *B*). Bone marrow examination (*C*) confirmed the diagnosis. Marked leukocytosis subsequently appeared. *A*, and *B*, Papanicolaou × 600. *C*, Wright's stain × 375.

Although rare, metastatic tumors may also present as breast lumps, particularly malignant melanoma. An example is illustrated in Figure 3–41, which depicts cells stained by both the Papanicolaou and Diff-Quik methods. Although superfluous, Fontana-staining was performed on one aspiration smear and proved many of the tumor cells positive.

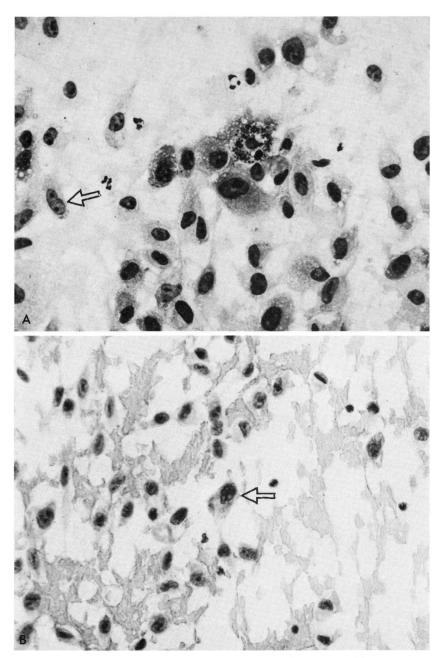

Figure 3–41. Metastatic malignant melanoma of the breast. This patient had a malignant melanoma removed from the cheek two years before the appearance of a breast mass. Spindle-cell pattern of the neoplastic cells is illustrated in both *A* and *B*. A few cells have two nuclei that are mirror images of each other (*A*, arrow). Pigment that stains dark bluish-purple with Diff-Quik stain is visible in the cell located just above the center of *A*. In *B* (arrow), note the intranuclear glassy inclusions, which can be found in cells from many different tumors. A Fontana stain was also positive for melanin. *A*, Diff-Quik × 375. *B*, Papanicolaou × 375.

COMPLICATIONS OF BREAST ASPIRATIONS

This author has encountered no complications with fine needle aspiration biopsy of the breast, and no serious problems have been reported in the literature. A small hematoma has developed as a rare occurrence at the puncture site. This is more likely to happen with breast cancers than with benign diseases.[31,43]

Critics of aspiration biopsy base their objections on their belief that the method causes needle-tract seeding and spread of tumor cells. Although it is theoretically possible, actual documentation of needle-tract seeding or dissemination is virtually lacking, except in a few cases in which large bore needles were used (see Chapters 7, 8, and 9 and Table 7–3).[40] The large series of Berg and Robbins showed no clinical effects of aspiration biopsy on breast-cancer patients staged and treated in the same manner as a control group. The follow-up period was 15 years.[62] Experimental evidence has also been provided that fails to substantiate any appreciable risk of dissemination of tumor cells following aspiration biopsy, even though a majority of the cells can be shown to be viable.[40,63-66]

RESULTS OF BREAST ASPIRATIONS

Table 3–1 summarizes this laboratory's experience with 600 fine-needle aspiration biopsies of breast masses. There has been histologic follow-up for almost all the lesions that were reported as benign but not cystic, and those cystic masses that did not disappear completely after aspiration of the fluid.

False-Positives.   Only one true false-positive case has occurred, although histologic follow-up proved that 6 of 26 aspirates considered suspect for carcinoma were benign. The single false-positive, only an atypical cystosarcoma phylloides, was reported as infiltrating duct carcinoma with a papillary component. This tumor also appeared clinically as a carcinoma: a firm mass in a 50-year-old female with some skin fixation and nipple retraction. Figures 3–42 and 3–43 illustrate cells from this neoplasm. With the Diff-Quik stain, the cells appear large and pleomorphic, lying in loose clusters. No oval naked nuclei were identified, and this was true even upon review of the smears. In contrast, the alcohol-fixed, Papanicolaou-stained aspirate shows rather uniform cells. Although there are no oval naked nuclei, the sheets are of uniform cellularity. Most of the cells have a small nucleolus and a finely dispersed chromatin. This contrast of abnormality between the air-dried and fixed smears is the feature that indicates the need for caution in reporting this case as unequivocal carcinoma. Reexamination failed to demonstrate metachromatic stroma, which might have helped

TABLE 3–1. THIN-NEEDLE ASPIRATION BIOPSY OF BREAST LESIONS

Malignant Tumor	Malignant Tumor Suspected	Benign Tumor	Inflammation or Other	False-Positive	False-Negative
191	26*	302	46	(1)†	(22)

Total aspirations	600
Unsatisfactory aspirations	35
Sensitivity for breast cancer	90%
Specificity for absence of breast cancer	99%

*Six cases in the suspect group were proved not to be carcinoma after excisional biopsy.
†A single case of benign cystosarcoma phylloides diagnosed as carcinoma, infiltrating duct type, from aspiration biopsy.

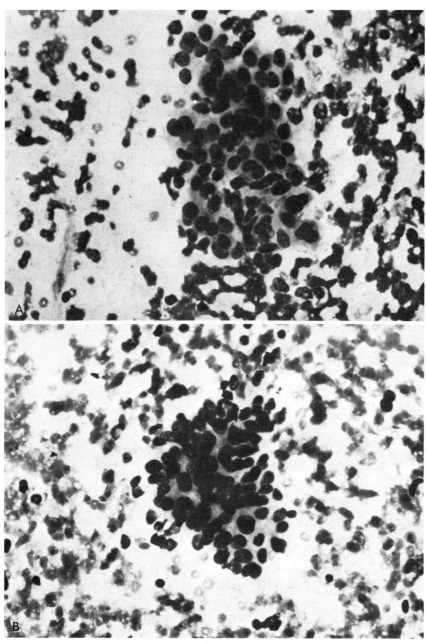

Figure 3–42 Cystosarcoma phylloides. False-positive aspiration from breast mass, with skin fixation and nipple retraction in a middle-aged female. Note variation in cell pattern and similarity to cases of breast carcinoma (Figs. 3–21, 3–22, 3–23). No metachromatic stroma was present in these smears, and the single cells were considered malignant tumor cells rather than oval naked nuclei. Metachromasia of the nuclear chromatin was not as prominent as in the usual breast cancer. *A* and *B*, Diff-Quik × 375.

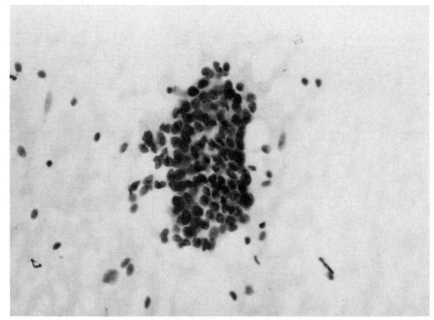

Figure 3–43 Cystosarcoma phylloides. Same case as that illustrated in Figure 3–42. The fixed, Papanicolaou-stained smear demonstrates bland cells. The oval naked nuclei were not found in the Diff-Quik smears, but they are visible in this smear. Papanicolaou × 375.

identify the true nature of this neoplasm. The histopathology of this tumor is illustrated in Figure 3–44. Although the stroma is somewhat active, the neoplasm appears to belong to the so-called benign group of cystosarcoma phylloides cases. A contrast between the patterns of atypia for the air-dried smears and the alcohol-fixed aspiration preparations was also demonstrated for comedomastitis (Figs. 3–7 and 3–8). These findings should serve to caution against enthusiastic unequivocal diagnosis of breast cancer in similar cases. This author has not encountered a second cystosarcoma, although one correctly diagnosed from fine-needle aspiration has been reported by Stawicki and Hsiu.[67]

Sensitivity and Specificity. A small number of false-positives have occurred in virtually every series reported, 15 of which are summarized in Table 3–2.[8, 10, 11, 15, 20, 21, 26, 31, 32, 37, 42, 47, 57, 68, 69] The data have been reorganized to document the true-negative, true-positive, false-positive, and false-negative results. Sensitivity for the diagnosis of carcinoma and specificity for the absence of carcinoma have then been calculated, including the values for the present series.

Suspicious Cases. Most authors used a "suspicious" category for a small number of cases. To simplify reporting, the suspicious group was divided into those subsequently found to be carcinoma and those diagnosed as benign after tissue biopsy examination. Those cases that proved to be carcinoma were added to the true-positive category, while those found to be actually negative but with a suspicious aspiration diagnosis were added to the false-positive category. For example, in this author's own series, this raises the number of false-positive cases to seven and accounts for a specificity of 98 per cent for the absence of carcinoma versus 99 per cent as reported in Table 3–1 on the basis of a single actual false-positive diagnosis. In Table 3–2, sensitivity for carcinoma is as low as 83 per cent and as high as 100 per cent. The latter series contains a substantial number of false-positive cases, more than one third of the total true-positives. While that series obviously indicates very high sensitivity, it demonstrates a relatively low specificity.[20]

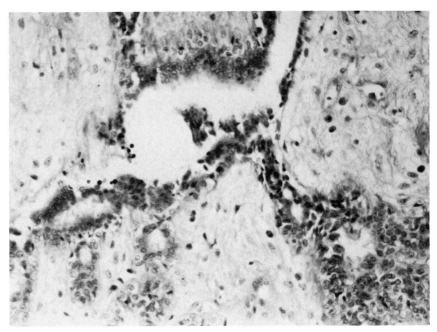

Figure 3–44 Cystosarcoma phylloides, benign form. Tissue from the patient whose aspirate is depicted in Figures 3–42 and 3–43. Definite benign form of cystosarcoma with minimal stromal atypia. Gross features of this lesion were unusual in that there was skin fixation and nipple retraction, and, when cut, the consistency of the tumor resembled that of the usual breast carcinoma. Hematoxylin and eosin × 240.

Not all authors reported the number of unsatisfactory aspirates, that is, those that were essentially acellular or of poor quality and not truly reflective of the lesion present. This is unfortunate because, in some series, these aspirates may account for a significant number of cases. It then becomes necessary to perform either additional aspirations or an open biopsy.[47] Overuse of the "suspicious" category may lead to numerous unnecessary biopsies, as seen in the series reported by Kline. The results of her study also emphasize, in this author's opinion, the need for the pathologist to examine the patient and actually perform the aspiration.[70] Chu and Hoye reported a 70 per cent accuracy for breast tumors in a series in which the cytologist read the material with no clinical information and without having examined the patient.[71] The report of Furnival and colleagues did demonstrate a 95 per cent accuracy in the diagnosis of both benign and malignant lesions in 237 patients. This series was also one in which the cytopathologist read the smears without foreknowledge of the case. While overall accuracy was high, there were two false-positives and five false-negatives. Twenty-four per cent of the aspirations were unsatisfactory. This may have been due either to a variation in technique, that is, holding suction on the needle as the syringe is withdrawn, or to the insecurity of the cytopathologist reading aspirates obtained by others without clinical information.[72]

SUMMARY

If fine-needle aspiration biopsy of the breast were to replace the frozen-section diagnosis as a definitive preoperative or pretherapy method, what then would be the standard by which to compare these results? Rosen has published a study of 556 consecutive breast specimens evaluated by frozen-section diagnosis. Of these, 145 were carcinomas. There were no false-positives in his group of carcinomas. Of 381 cases diagnosed negative by frozen section, eight contained carcinomas. A diagnosis

TABLE 3–2. RESULTS OF SELECTED SERIES OF FINE-NEEDLE ASPIRATION BIOPSIES OF THE BREAST

Reference	True-Positive	True-Negative	False-Positive*	False-Negative*	Sensitivity for Cancer (%)	Specificity No Cancer Present (%)	Unsatisfactory Aspirations
Franzen and Zajicek[8]	796	782	26	48	94	96	29
Kiovuniemi[10]	161	307	4	31	83	98	10
Kruezer and Boquoi[11]	284	305	50	33	86	86	NR‡
Stavric et al.[15]	103	133	9	5	95	93	NR
Sartorius et al.[20]	41	204	15	0	100	93	NR
Moller and Mikkelsen[21]	75	95	11	1	98	89	NR
Bjurstam et al.[26]	157	787	8	18	89	98	30
Schondorf[31]	323	193	19	10	97	98	NR
Russ et al.[32]	41	158	19	21	66	88	18
Kline and Neal[37]	114	1007	4	13	89	99	NR
Rosen et al.[42]	179	0	0	32	84	†	NR
Oatham and Randall[47]	70	130	2	12	85	98	60
Bodo et al.[57]	80	32	5	7	91	86	NR
Duguid et al.[68]	56	79	0	2	96	100	27
Deschenes et al.[69]	105	237	50	9	92	82	NR
Present series	211	348	7	22	90	98	35

*Suspicious cases counted as false-positive when histologic findings were negative and false-negative when histologic findings were positive.
†No true-negatives in this series; therefore, specificity can not be calculated.
‡NR = Not recorded.

was deferred in 30 of the 381 cases. Excluding the deferred cases, the findings represent a false-negative rate of 2 per cent; including the deferred cases, this rate is 7.4 per cent.[73] The figures for several of the series of fine-needle aspiration biopsies summarized in Table 3–2 compare favorably with this number of false-negatives seen with frozen section. In terms of hospitalization, operating time, and anesthesia time, needle aspiration biopsy is less expensive than the frozen-section method. Thus, if acceptable accuracy can be obtained, needle aspiration biopsy is a valuable and efficient procedure.

REFERENCES

1. Martin, H. E., and Ellis, E. B.: Aspiration biopsy. Surg. Gynecol. Obstet. *59*:578–589, 1934.
2. Stewart, F. W.: The diagnosis of tumors by aspiration biopsy. Am. J. Pathol. *9*:801–812, 1933.
3. Davies, C. J., Elston, C. W., Cotton, R. E., et al.: Preoperative diagnosis in carcinoma of the breast. Br. J. Surg. *64*:326–328, 1977.
4. Devitt, J. E., and Curry, R. H.: Role of aspiration breast biopsy. Can. J. Surg. *20*:450–451, 1977.
5. Gibson, A., and Smith, G.: Aspiration biopsy of breast tumours. Br. J. Surg. *45*:236–239, 1957.
6. Glassman, J. A.: Aspiration biopsy for detection of carcinoma of the breast. A critique. J. Int. Coll. Surg. *36*:195–202, 1961.
7. Elston, C. W., Cotton, R. E., Davies, C. J., et al.: A comparison of the use of the "Tru-cut" needle and fine needle aspiration cytology in the pre-operative diagnosis of carcinoma of the breast. Histopathology *2*:239–254, 1978.
8. Franzen, S., and Zajicek, J.: Aspiration biopsy in diagnosis of palpable lesions of the breast. Acta Radiol. *7*:241–262, 1968.
9. Hogbin, B. M., Melcher, D. H., Smith, R., et al.: The value of breast aspiration to the general surgeon. Acta Cytol. *21*:711, 1977.
10. Kiovuniemi, A. P.: Fine needle-aspiration cytology of the breast. Ann. Clin. Res. *8*:272–283, 1976.
11. Kreuzer, G., and Boquoi, E.: Aspiration biopsy cytology, mammography and clinical exploration: A modern set up in diagnosis of tumors of the breast. Acta Cytol. *20*:319–322, 1976.
12. Lange, M., Brebner, D., and Klempman, S.: Cytology and mammography in the diagnosis of breast cancer. S. Afr. Med. J., *50*:2132–2133, 1976.
13. Manheimer, L. H., and Rywlin, A. M.: Fine needle aspiration cytology. South. Med. J. *70*:923–925, 1977.
14. Murad, T. M., and Snyder, M. E.: The diagnosis of breast lesions from cytologic material. Acta Cytol. *17*:418–422, 1973.
15. Stavric, G. D., Tevcev, D. T., Kaftandjiev, D. R., et al.: Aspiration biopsy cytologic method in diagnosis of breast lesions. A critical review of 250 cases. Acta Cytol. *17*:188–190, 1973.
16. Vilaplana, E. V., and Jiminez-Ayala, M.: The cytologic diagnosis of breast lesions. Acta Cytol. *19*:519–526, 1975.
17. Wilson, S. L., and Ehrmann, R. L.: The cytologic diagnosis of breast aspirations. Acta Ctyol. *22*:470–475, 1978.
18. Zajicek, J., Franzen, S., Jakobsson, P., et al.: Aspiration biopsy of mammary tumors in diagnosis and research. A critical review of 2200 cases. Acta Cytol. *11*:169–175, 1967.
19. Olsen, T. S., Egedorf, J., Ibsen, J., et al.: Use of fine-needle aspiration biopsy in the diagnosis and therapy of tumors of the breast. A review of the literature. Ugeskr. Laeger. *140*:2973–2975, 1978.
20. Sartorius, O. W., Morris, P. L., and Benedict, D. L.: Fine needle aspiration for the cytologic diagnosis of benign and malignant breast lesions. Proc. Am. Assoc. Cancer Res. *20*:275, 1979.
21. Mooler, J. C., et al.: Fine needle biopsy of the breast. A 5-year series. Ugeskr. Laeger. *140*:1847–1848, 1978.
22. Degrell, I.: The significance of aspiration biopsy cytology of diseases of the mammary gland. Langenbecks Arch. Chir. *348*:147–155, 1979.
23. Manheimer, L. H., and Rywlin, A. M.: Fine needle aspiration cytology. South. Med. J. *70*:923–925, 1977.
24. Borek, E., Pedio G., and Ruttner, J. R.: The significance of fine needle puncture in the investigation of breast nodules: Results of 617 cytological rapid diagnoses. Praxis *66*:1543–1546, 1977.
25. Talukder, B. C., Ray, J. C., and Talukder, G.: Thin needle aspiration biopsy as a diagnostic aid for breast tumours. Indian J. Cancer. *15*:1–5, 1978.
26. Bjurstam, N., Hedberg, K., Hultborn, K. A., et al.: Diagnosis of breast carcinoma: Evaluation of clinical examination, mammography, thermography and aspiration biopsy in breast disease. Progr. Surg. *13*:1–65, 1974.
27. Boquoi, E., and Kreuzer, G.: The importance of fine needle biopsy in modern breast diagnosis. Arch. Geschwulstforsch. *47*:616–623, 1977.
28. Cornillot, M., Cappelaere, P., Granier, A.-M., et al.: La cyto-ponction des tumeurs du sein (2260 confrontations histo-cytologiques). Arch. Anat. Cytol. Path. *25*:333–339, 1977.

29. Thomas, J. M., Fitzharris, B. M., Redding, W. H., et al.: Clinical examination, xeromammography, and fine-needle aspiration cytology in diagnosis of breast tumours. Br. Med. J. 2:1139–1141, 1978.

30. Reinisch, H., and Schneider, G.: Mammary diagnostics: Mammography—punction cytology, completion and comparison. Arch. Geschwulstforsch. 47:595–610, 1977.

31. Schöndorf, H. translated by Schneider, V.: *Aspiration Cytology of the Breast*. Philadelphia, W. B. Saunders Co., 1978, p. 17.

32. Russ, J. E., Winchester, D. P., Scanlon, E. F., et al.: Cytologic findings of aspiration of tumors of the breast. Surg. Gynecol. Obstet. 146:407–411, 1978.

33. Vassilakos, P.: Tuberculosis of the breast: Cytologic findings with fine-needle aspiration. Acta Cytol. 17:160–165, 1973.

34. Haagensen, C. D.: The relationship of gross cystic disease of the breast and carcinoma. Ann. Surg. 185:375–376, 1977.

35. Haagensen, C. D.: *Diseases of Breast*. 2nd Ed. Philadelphia, W. B. Saunders Co., 1971, pp. 172–175.

36. Johnston, J. H., Jr.: Aspiration as diagnostic and therapeutic procedure in cystic disease of the breast. Ann. Surg. 139:635–643, 1954.

37. Kline, T. S., and Neal, H. S.: Needle aspiration of the breast—Why bother? Acta Cytol. 20:327, 1976.

38. Rosemond, G. P.: Differentiation between the cystic and solid breast mass by needle aspiration. Surg. Clin. N. Amer. 43:1433–1437, 1963.

39. McSwain, G. R., Valicenti, J. F. Jr., and O'Brien, P. H.: Cytologic evaluation of breast cysts. Surg. Gynecol. Obstet. 146:921–925, 1978.

40. Zajicek, J.: Monograph I. *Aspiration Biopsy Cytology Part I. Cytology of Supradiaphragmatic Organs*. Monographs in Clinical Cytology. Basle, S. Karger, 1974, pp. 20–21, 151, 164, 171–178, 185–190.

41. Linsk, J., Kreuzer, G., and Zajicek, J.: Cytologic diagnosis of mammary tumors from aspiration biopsy smears. II. Studies on 210 fibroadenomas and 210 cases of benign dysplasia. Acta Cytol. 16:130–138, 1972.

42. Rosen, P., Hajdu, S. I., Robbins, G., et al.: Diagnosis of carcinoma of the breast by aspiration biopsy. Surg. Gynecol. Obstet. 134:837–838, 1972.

43. Budd, J. W.: Evaluation of needle aspiration technique in breast lesions. Radiology 52:502–505, 1949.

44. Geier, G. R., Kornen, B. H., and Schuhmann, R.: Differential cytology of breast cancer. Exp. Cell Biol. 45:167–175, 1977.

45. Ide, P.: Thin needle aspiration cytology of the breast. J. Belge Radiol. 60:197–199, 1977.

46. Magarey, C. J., and Watson, W. J.: The outpatient diagnosis of breast lumps. Aust. N. Z. J. Surg. 46:344–349, 1976.

47. Oatham, S. A., and Randall, K. J.: Problems in cytologic diagnosis of breast aspirates. Acta Cytol. 21:711, 1977.

48. Takeda, T., Takaso, K., Isono, S., et al.: Studies on cytologic characteristics of mammary aspiration smears based on histologic types. Acta Cytol. 21:424–428, 1977.

49. Kreuzer, G., and Zajicek, J.: Cytologic diagnosis of mammary tumors from aspiration biopsy smears. III. Studies on 200 carcinomas with false negative or doubtful cytologic reports. Acta Cytol. 16:249–252, 1972.

50. Fisher, E. R.: Ultrastructure of the human breast and its disorders. Am. J. Clin. Pathol. 66:291–375, 1976.

51. Murad, T. M.: A proposed histochemical and electron microscopic classification of human breast cancer according to cell of origin. Cancer 27:288–299, 1971.

52. Fisher, E. R., Gregorio, R. M., and Fisher, B.: The pathology of invasive breast cancer. A syllabus derived from findings of the National Surgical Adjuvant Breast Project (Protocol No. 4). Cancer 36:1–85, 1975.

53. Fisher, E. R.: The pathologist's role in the diagnosis and treatment of invasive breast cancer. Surg. Clin. N. Am. 58:705–721, 1978.

54. Hull, M. T., Seo, I. S., Battersby, J. S., et al.: Signet-ring cell carcinoma of the breast. A clinicopathologic study of 24 cases. Am. J. Clin. Pathol. 73:31–35, 1980.

55. Steinbrecher, J. S., and Silverberg, S. G.: Signet-ring cell carcinoma of the breast. The mucinous variant of infiltrating lobular carcinoma? Cancer 37:828–840, 1976.

56. Leiman, G.: Squamous carcinoma in breast aspiration cytology. Acta Cytol 26:201–209, 1982.

57. Bodo, M., Dobrossy, L., Rahoty, P., et al.: Diagnosis of carcinoma of the breast by aspiration biopsy cytology. Arch. Geschwulstforsch. 47:624–626, 1977.

58. Kern, W. H.: The diagnosis of breast cancer by fine-needle aspiration smears. J.A.M.A. 241:1125–1127, 1979.

59. Lowhagen, T., and Rubio, C. A.: The cytology of granular cell myoblastoma of the breast. Report of a case. Acta Cytol. 21:314–315, 1977.

60. Bodo, M., Dobrossy, L., and Sugar, J.: Boeck's sarcoidosis of the breast: Cytologic findings with aspiration biopsy cytology. A case clinically mimicking carcinoma. Acta Cytol. 22:1, 1978.

61. Kreuzer, G., and Boquoi, E.: Die Feinnadelpunktion von Sarkomen der Mamma: Zytomorphologie und DNA-Zytophotometrie. Geburtshilfe Frauenheilkd. 37:416–422, 1977.

62. Berg, J. W., and Robbins, G. F.: A late look at the safety of aspiration biopsy. Cancer 15:826–827, 1962.

63. Engzell, U., Esposti, P. L., Rubio, C., et al.: Investigation of tumour spread in connection with aspiration biopsy. Acta Radiol. *10*:385–398, 1971.
64. Zajicek, J., Engzell, U., Plesnicar, S., et al.: Studies on cell viability in aspirates from human lymph nodes. Eur. J. Cancer *4*:23–26, 1968.
65. Plesnicar, S., Rubio, C., Sigurdson, A., et al.: Cell viability studies on the effect of aspiration biopsy on aspirated cells. Acta Cytol. *12*:454–461, 1968.
66. Criborn, C. O., Franzen, S., Unsgaard, B., et al.: Studies on the effect of aspiration biopsy on the viability of aspirated cells. 1. Registration of pressure differences during aspiration. Scand. J. Haematol. *1*:272–279, 1964.
67. Stawicki, M. E., and Hsiu, J.: Malignant cystosarcoma phyllodes. A case report with cytologic presentation. Acta Cytol. *23*:61–64, 1979.
68. Duguid, H. L., Wood, R. A., Irving, A. D., et al.: Needle aspiration of the breast with immediate reporting of material. Br. Med. J. *2*:185–187, 1979.
69. Deschenes, L., Fabia, J., Meisels, A., et al.: Fine needle aspiration biopsy in the management of palpable breast lesions. Can. J. Surg. *21*:417–419, 1978.
70. Kline, T. S.: Breast lesions. Diagnosis by fine-needle aspiration biopsy. Am. J. Gynecol. Obstet. *1*:11–16, 1979.
71. Chu, E. W., and Hoye, R. C.: The clinician and the cytopathologist evaluate fine-needle aspiration cytology. Acta Cytol. *17*:413–417, 1973.
72. Furnival, C. M., Hocking, M. A., Hughes, H. E., et al.: Aspiration cytology in breast cancer. Its relevance to diagnosis. Lancet *2*:446–449, 1975.
73. Rosen, P. P.: Frozen section diagnosis of breast lesions. Recent experience with 556 consecutive biopsies. Ann. Surg. *187*:17–19, 1978.

Chapter Four

Lymph Nodes

ASPIRATION OF LYMPH NODES

TECHNIQUES

In 1904, Grieg and Gray performed what is believed to be the first needle aspiration biopsy of lymph nodes, identifying trypanosomes to confirm the diagnosis of sleeping sickness.[1] It was not until ten years later that Ward commented on the application of needle aspiration biopsy to the diagnosis of tropical disease involving lymph nodes and wondered why it was not used for the study of tumors, particularly for cases of Hodgkin's disease. This author did report one case in which aspiration biopsy was used to diagnose "lymphaemia" (lymphatic leukemia).[2] Guthrie did not tabulate his results in the diagnosis of Hodgkin's disease, but the technique of aspiration biopsy that he described is quite similar to that used today, except that the specimen was pulled into the syringe, and a vacuum was applied continuously while withdrawing the needle. Despite these variations, Guthrie's method led to successful diagnoses of syphilis, tuberculosis, Hodgkin's disease, acute and chronic myeloid leukemia, trypanosomias, and metastatic tumors. He does not, however, comment on false-positive or false-negative results.[3]

After the report of Martin and Ellis, a number of monographs specifically about needle aspiration biopsy diagnosis of lymph node disease appeared in the European and South American literature from the 1930's through the 1960's, but during that time there was little interest in this type of biopsy in the United States.[4-14] Most of these early works are out of print and unavailable, making it impossible to detail the procedures used by the various authors or to determine their success. Lukas reviewed the subject and commented on it favorably. In his own series involving 85 pathologic nodes, he found a good correlation for the diagnosis of lymphomas and leukemias from aspiration smears. Even with no clinical information, the examination of a single smear resulted in a diagnosis of a specific lymph node disease in 52 of 85 aspirated nodes, and the only known error in follow-up was a diagnosis of monocytic leukemia in a case of reticulum cell sarcoma. That certainly would not be a significant error, since clearly a malignant lymphomatous process was recognized.[15]

Variations of the biopsy technique have been employed, including use of the tissue-type needle biopsy as reported by Meatheringham and Ackerman. They used local anesthesia, which is required with a 15- to 17-gauge needle and an obturator. Because of their bias toward surgical pathology, these authors thought the aspiration smears were worthless. However, they did find core needle biopsy of value.[16] Forkner preferred using a 17- or 18-gauge needle for biopsy but also injected local anesthesia.

He used a dental broach passed through the needle to obtain bits of tissue on its spurs. The tissue fragments, however, were processed as smears. Results were excellent, with a diagnosis in 22 of 23 cases, including ten of Hodgkin's disease, five of metastatic carcinoma, two of sarcoma, one of tuberculosis, and one of hyperplasia.[17]

CLINICAL DATA

Fine-needle aspiration biopsy of lymph nodes accounts for the largest single group of cases in this author's personal experience through 1980: 787 aspirations. Of these aspirates, 554 have been performed on lymph nodes of the head and neck and include cervical, supraclavicular, submaxillary, submental, and postauricular areas, while the remaining 233 have been inguinal, axillary, epitrochlear, and mammary nodes. As in most series, unless specifically directed toward certain types of lesions, metastatic tumors are the conditions most frequently discovered by aspiration of lymph nodes. The diagnosis of metastatic neoplasm is usually quite easy, since there are abundant tumor cells that bear no relationship to normal lymph node constituents. Lymph nodes are often extensively replaced by metastatic tumor before they become clinically apparent, and therefore the chance of making a diagnosis of tumor is extremely likely if the node is actually punctured. These general principles have been confirmed several times by large series of cases reported in the literature. A number of these are summarized in Table 4–1 with a calculation of their sensitivity and specificity.[18-22]

Good results have not always been reported. Betsill and Hajdu reported a series of 361 patients from whom aspirates of superficial lymph nodes were obtained. Of these specimens, 55 were considered unsatisfactory and 23 were excluded because of inadequate follow-up. Of the remaining cases, 78 per cent were positive for malignant cells and 18 per cent were considered negative. While there were no false-positive cases, 31 of the 52 negative aspirations subsequently revealed neoplasm on excisional biopsy. The high number of false-negatives might be attributed to one or both of the following factors: (1) the technique was faulty, and (2) the authors did not actually perform the aspiration biopsies themselves and thus did not have the opportunity to examine the patients.[23] This author has found that performance of the aspiration by the one who reads the smear is extremely valuable both to obtain a complete clinical history and to ensure that adequate material is taken. The importance of this is reflected in Tables 4–2 and 4–3, which reveal that only 45 of the 787 aspirations of lymph nodes were considered unsatisfactory and that the specificity for the absence of tumor among both node groups is near or at 100 per cent.

In a much larger series with high specificity and sensitivity, few false-positives or false-negatives were reported when attempts were not made to read unsatisfactory aspirates.[19]

METASTATIC CARCINOMA

Squamous Cell Carcinoma. It is apparent from review of both clinical material and reported series of cases that specific diagnoses of tumor type metastatic to lymph nodes can frequently be made from the aspiration smear. Most of the cases that this author has seen have been squamous cell carcinomas from either the oral cavity or the lung. Aspiration biopsy smear from the metastatic sites reflects the degree of differentiation that may be seen in the primary. Hence, there are large, irregular, keratinized cells with abundant eosinophilic cytoplasm or relatively undifferentiated cells occurring in sheets with "windows," or spaces, between individual cells and sharply outlined cell borders. Since the cells are clearly epithelial and obviously foreign to a lymph node, the diagnosis of metastatic tumor is immediately evident. Two examples of

TABLE 4–1.   RESULTS OF SELECTED SERIES OF ASPIRATION BIOPSIES OF LYMPH NODES

References	True-*Positive	True-Negative	False-Positive	False-Negative	Sensitivity for Tumor (%)	Specificity for No Tumor (%)	Unsatisfactory Aspirations
Engzell et al.[18]	240	0	0	17	93	—	0
Lopes Cardozo[19]	701	594	2	0	100	99	229
Russ et al.[20]	48	39	2	1	97	95	0
Zajdela et al.[21]	1258	410	53	35	97	88	—
Block[22]	27	10	1	4	87	90	3

*Positive and negative refer to the presence of a malignant tumor.

**TABLE 4–2. RESULTS OF ASPIRATION BIOPSY OF
LYMPH NODES IN HEAD AND NECK**

Site	Malignant Tumors	Lymphomas	Benign Tumors	False-Positive*	False-Negative
Cervical	168	22	133	(2)	(10)
Supraclavicular	123	2	35	(1)	(3)
Submaxillary	16	3	31	(1)	(2)
Submental	6	1	12	—	—
Postauricular	1	—	1	—	—
TOTALS	314	28	212	(4)	(15)

Total head and neck nodes aspirated	554
Unsatisfactory aspirations	29
Sensitivity for tumor	96%
Specificity for the *absence* of tumor	98%

*False-positives are all cases of suspected malignant lymphoma proved by biopsy to be reactive and atypical reactive hyperplasia.

aspirations from lymph nodes demonstrating different patterns of metastatic squamous cell carcinoma are illustrated in Figures 4–1 and 4–2.

Lymphoepithelioma. A specific pattern of squamous or epidermoid carcinoma, lymphoepithelioma, can also be recognized in aspiration smears. This is an important diagnosis because the clinical presentation of this neoplasm as an occult nasopharyngeal primary may be that of enlarged cervical nodes, not infrequently bilateral. The aspirate demonstrates very large undifferentiated tumor cells that frequently occur either singly or together in a very loose arrangement, particularly in the air-dried Giemsa stained smears (Fig. 4–3A). In the air-dried smear, the pattern may suggest a malignant lymphoma, but the alcohol-fixed, Papanicolaou-stained preparation more clearly demonstrates the aggregates of undifferentiated cells with very prominent nucleoli and the surrounding lymphoid elements that constitute the typical histologic pattern of lymphoepithelioma (Fig. 4–3B). Compare these cells with those of the biopsy from the small nasopharyngeal primary (Fig. 4–4).

Occasionally, the pattern of lymphoepithelioma may present in the Papanicolaou-stained, fixed smears as single cells. Those tumor cells have definite squamoid characteristics with thick cell boundaries. Many lymphocytes are also found (Fig. 4–5). Metastatic lymphoepithelioma is an important pattern to recognize because it directs the clinician's attention immediately to the nasopharynx for examination and biopsy of any suspicious primary sites. Several cases of this type have been identified.

Small-Cell (Oat Cell) Carcinoma. Small-cell carcinomas, regardless of their site of origin, show anaplastic, small malignant cells that usually demonstrate good nuclear

TABLE 4–3. RESULTS OF ASPIRATION BIOPSY OF OTHER LYMPH NODES

Site	Malignant Tumors	Lymphomas	Benign Tumors	False-Positive	False-Negative
Inguinal	71	5	58	—	(3)
Axillary	42	10	44	—	(1)
Epitrochlear	—	1	1	—	—
Mammary	1	—	—	—	—
TOTALS	114	16	103	—	(4)

Total aspirations of other nodes	233
Unsatisfactory aspirations	16
Sensitivity for tumor	98%
Specificity for the *absence* of tumor	100%

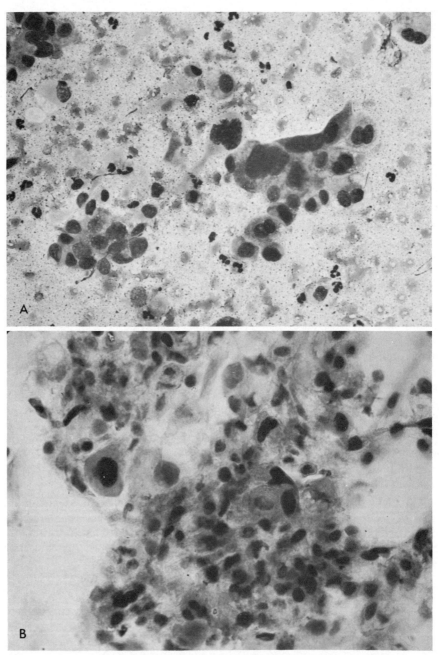

Figure 4–1 Keratinizing squamous cell carcinoma metastatic to cervical lymph node. Cells occur in sheets and demonstrate marked pleomorphism. The cytoplasm stains deeply and intensely blue with Romanovsky dyes. Papanicolaou-stained smear depicts the same features, with the keratinized cells staining brightly eosinophilic. *A*, Diff-Quik × 375. *B*, Papanicolaou × 375.

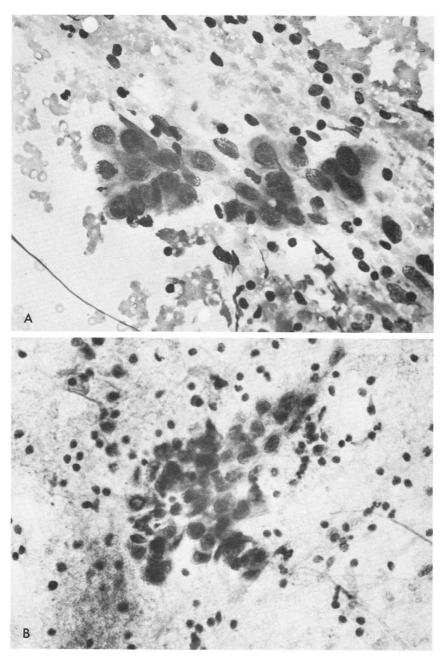

Figure 4–2 Squamous cell carcinoma, poorly differentiated, metastatic to supraclavicular lymph node. Cells also occur in sheets with a high nuclear-cytoplasmic ratio and prominent nucleoli. The sheet-like arrangement, relatively dense, non-vacuolated cytoplasm, and well-defined cell boundaries are the cytologic features that suggest squamous cell carcinoma. *A,* Diff-Quik × 375. *B,* Papanicolaou × 375.

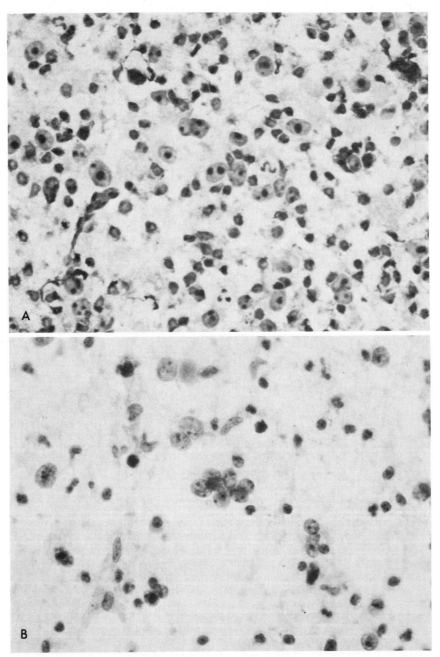

Figure 4–3 Lymphoepithelioma metastatic to cervical lymph node. The pattern visible with air-dried, Romanovsky-stained smears is one of individual undifferentiated cells, having particularly large nucleoli and occurring singly in a background of many lymphocytes. With alcohol fixation (B), the tumor cells appear in aggregates, a pattern that is more diagnostic of an epithelial neoplasm than of a malignant lymphoma. Numerous lymphocytes are also present. A, Diff-Quik × 375. B, Papanicolaou × 375.

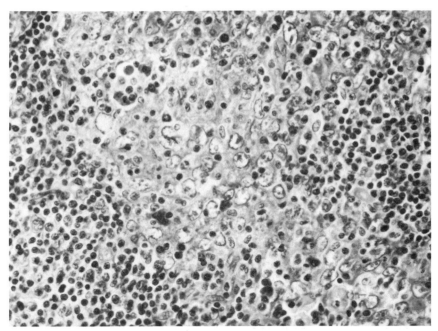

Figure 4–4 Lymphoepithelioma of nasopharynx. Tissue from the small nasopharyngeal primary diagnosed from metastases to the cervical lymph nodes by aspiration biopsy (Fig. 4–3). Compare the nuclear features of the undifferentiated tumor cells of the biopsy with those of the cells in the aspiration. Hematoxylin and eosin × 375.

molding. These aspirates tend to be bloody but also contain numerous tumor cells. The neoplastic cells appear larger than one might expect when viewed on air-dried, Giemsa-stained smears. That pattern must be seen several times before it may be specifically recognized as small-cell, or oat cell, carcinoma (Fig. 4–6). Fixed specimens more accurately reflect the same cytomorphologic features as those seen in sputum or bronchial washings from a case of oat cell carcinoma of the lung. The particular example demonstrated (Fig. 4–7) is from an aspiration of a supraclavicular lymph node, the primary tumor having originated as a small-cell carcinoma of the cervix.

Giant-Cell Carcinoma. Special stains such as mucicarmine, alcian blue, or periodic acid–Schiff reaction (PAS) with or without diastase for determination of mucopolysaccharide and glycogen may be important in the diagnosis of some of the gastrointestinal and lung carcinomas metastatic to lymph nodes. A rather specific morphologic pattern that does not require special stains is evident in Figure 4–8, which depicts a giant-cell carcinoma of the lung metastatic to a cervical lymph node. There is a large-tumor giant cell that contains not only multiple nuclei but also many phagocytized polymorphonuclear leukocytes. Surrounding the giant cell are undifferentiated tumor cells. Some of these, owing to their clear or finely vacuolated cytoplasm, might be mucicarmine positive, reflecting a basic adenocarcinoma pattern that has evolved into giant-cell carcinoma of the lung. This morphology has been very consistent for the diagnosis of giant-cell carcinoma found metastatic to supraclavicular, cervical, and other lymph nodes.

Malignant Melanoma. Malignant melanoma has several features other than pigmented cells that may identify it in metastatic sites.[24] In Figure 4–9, double, mirror-image nuclei that face each other but do not touch are illustrated in several cells from both the Giemsa-stained and the Papanicolaou-stained smears. Some melanomas also have large intranuclear inclusions. These should not be confused with the same finding in papillary carcinoma of the thyroid, since the melanoma cells appear much more anaplastic and also occur in sheet-like arrangements on aspiration smears.

Text continued on page 87

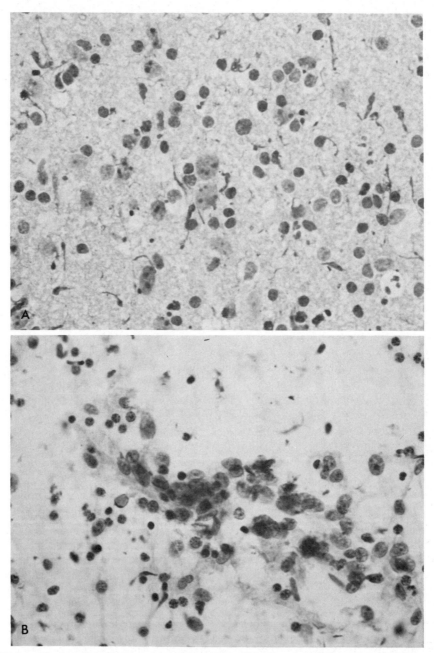

Figure 4–5 Lymphoepithelioma metastatic to cervical lymph node. Another example, with scattered pale tumor cells that could be mistaken for reactive histiocytes (A). In the Papanicolaou-stained preparation, the tumor cells are found in sheets and aggregates. The nuclear chromatin pattern of the individual cells is more easily diagnosed as malignant. Because of the contrast between the patterns of the two smears and the presence of many lymphocytes, metastatic lymphoepithelioma should be the first consideration. A, Metachrome B × 375. B, Papanicolaou × 375.

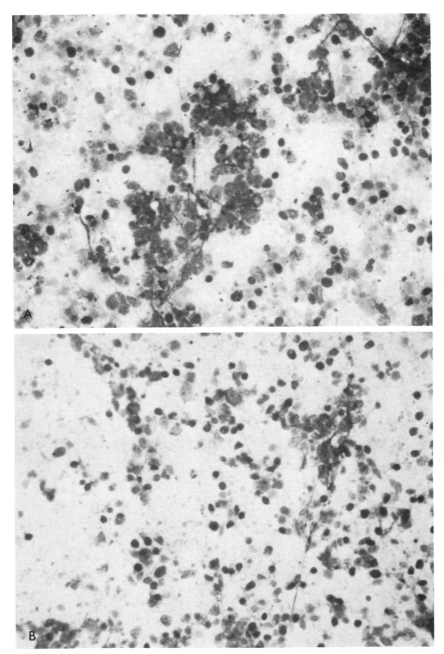

Figure 4–6 Oat cell carcinoma of the lung, metastatic to supraclavicular lymph node. Masses of tumor cells, largely degenerated and necrotic, are found in both fields. The pattern and degenerative changes are similar to those of oat cell carcinoma in bronchial washings and sputum, except that there are many more cells. Compare the air-dried preparation (A) with the wet-fixed smear (B) and note the difference in the size of the cells. A, Diff-Quik × 375. B, Papanicolaou × 375.

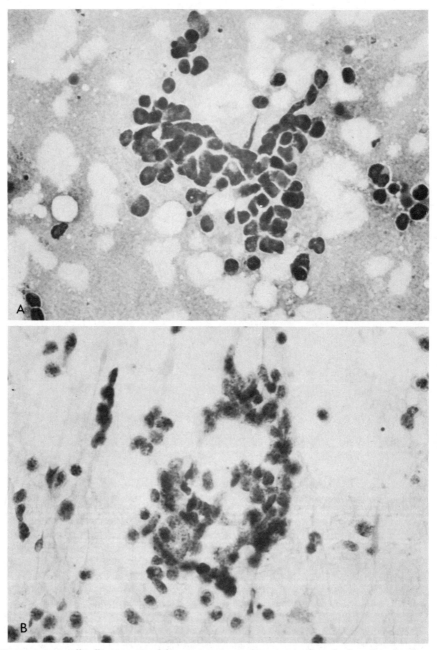

Figure 4–7   Small-cell carcinoma of the cervix, metastatic to a supraclavicular lymph node. This smear has better-preserved tumor cells with good nuclear molding. The pattern is reminiscent of that of small-cell carcinoma in bronchial washings or brushings prepared fresh and alcohol-fixed. *A*, Diff-Quik × 375. *B*, Papanicolaou × 375.

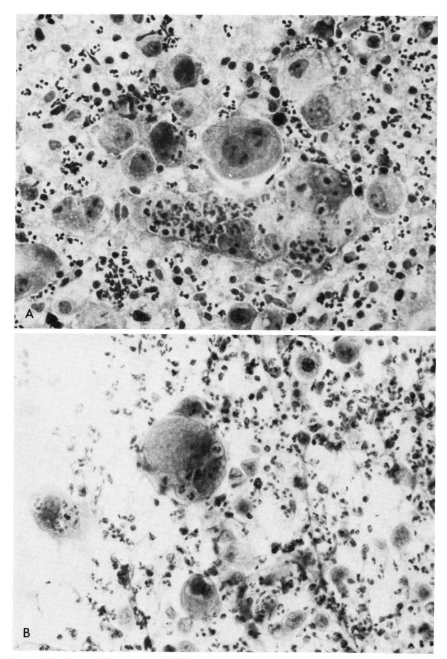

Figure 4–8   Giant-cell carcinoma of the lung, metastatic to supraclavicular lymph node. Both smears contain undifferentiated and tumor giant cells. Note the phagocytosis of polymorphonuclear leukocytes, indicated by the tumor giant cells, a characteristic feature of this neoplasm. *A*, Diff-Quik × 375. *B*, Papanicolaou × 375.

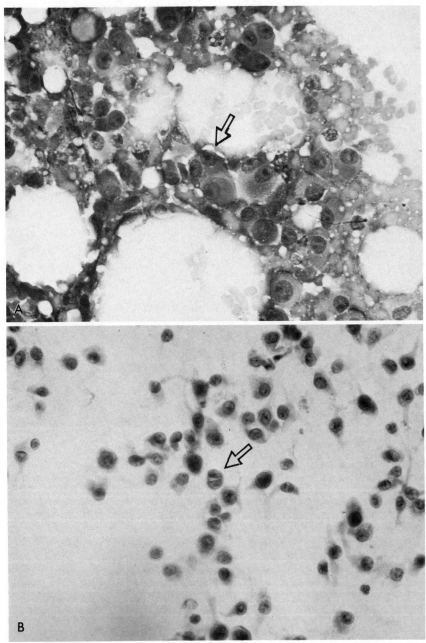

Figure 4–9 Malignant melanoma metastatic to lymph node. Several examples of the double mirror-image nuclei, relatively common in melanomas, are depicted (arrows). Pigment may or may not be present to identify the tumor cells as melanin producing. *A*, Diff-Quik × 375. *B*, Papanicolaou × 375.

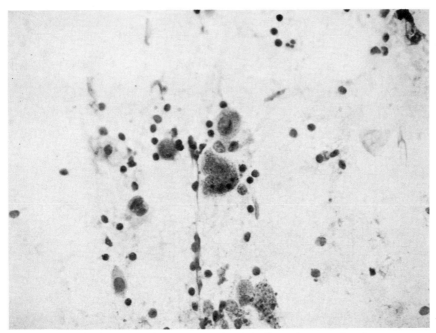

Figure 4–10 Malignant melanoma metastatic to lymph node. Malignant cell with prominent nucleoli in the center of the field contains granular brown pigment in the cytoplasm. Papanicolaou × 375.

Of course, the presence of pigment in melanoma cells is a very helpful clue, as seen in Figure 4–10. With the Romanovsky techniques, the pigment stains dark bluish-purple; with Papanicolaou stains, the pigment appears brown. In some cases of suspected melanoma, in the absence of visible pigment, a Fontana stain may reveal cells that are positive. An ultrastructural examination of the aspirate may demonstrate pre-melanosomes.

Prostatic Carcinoma. Special immunologic tests, which are gaining in importance in surgical pathology, may also be used to evaluate aspiration smears. This author, with the help of his colleagues, has identified several cases of metastatic prostatic carcinoma through the use of a specific immuno-diffusion test for prostatic acid phosphatase. An example of such an aspirate with the small uniform acinar pattern of malignant tumor cells is represented in Figure 4–11. The immunodiffusion test, which was highly positive for prostatic acid phosphatase, is depicted in Figure 4–12A. In this particular case, the clinical presentation was a palpable supraclavicular lymph node, and essentially no urinary tract symptoms were present. However, observation of the well-delineated acinar pattern, which is reminiscent of well-differentiated prostatic carcinomas, and detection of an enlarged, somewhat suspicious prostate led to a transrectal needle biopsy that confirmed the presence of prostatic carcinoma. Note how well the histologic pattern matches the aspiration smear (Fig. 4–12B, inset).

Occult Papillary Carcinoma. Occasionally, a specific morphologic feature revealed by the aspiration smear will give an immediate clue to the identity of an unknown primary site in the case of metastatic tumor in a lymph node. Figure 4–13 depicts a papillary fragment aspirated from an enlarged cervical lymph node that demonstrates some cells with intranuclear inclusions. Since this was a cervical node, the immediate primary site of concern would be an occult papillary carcinoma of the thyroid. A thyroid lobectomy revealed a 3 mm occult papillary carcinoma (Fig. 4–14).

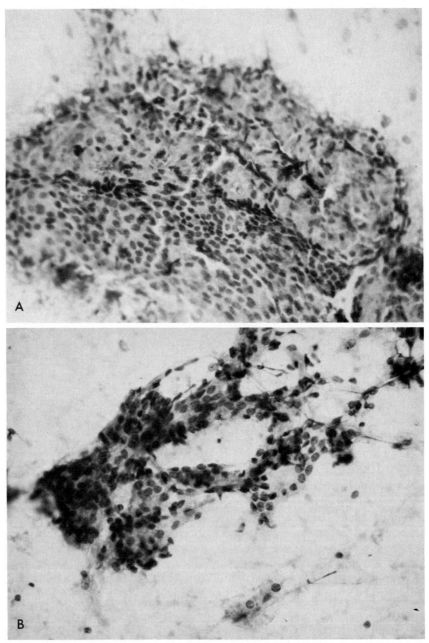

Figure 4–11   Carcinoma of the prostate, metastatic to a supraclavicular lymph node. Sheets of small uniform epithelial cells with a definite acinar arrangement are visible in *A* and *B*. Symptoms suggesting a primary site were minimal. The prostate was enlarged and somewhat suspect for cancer. *A*, Diff-Quik × 375. *B*, Papanicolaou × 375.

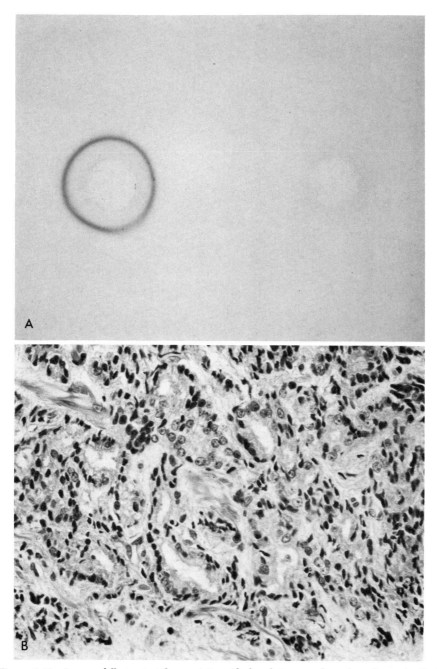

Figure 4–12 Immunodiffusion test for prostatic acid phosphatase, performed on digested cells from aspirate. Compare the positive ring on the left with the control on the right in *A*. Transperineal needle biopsy reveals carcinoma of the prostate in this patient. Compare the acinar pattern of the tissue with the same pattern in the aspiration biopsy (Fig. 4–11). *B*, Hematoxylin and eosin × 375.

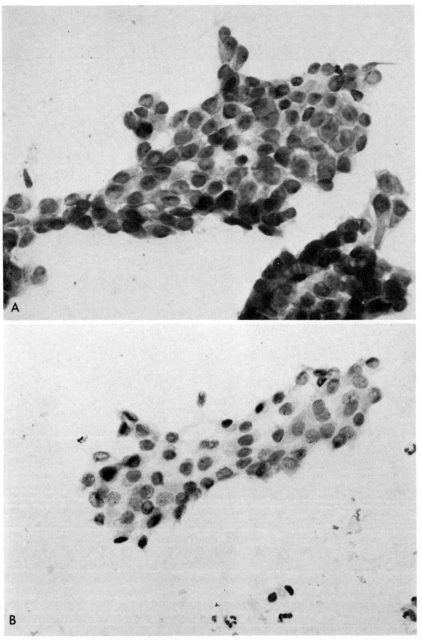

Figure 4–13 Occult papillary carcinoma of the thyroid, metastatic to cervical lymph node. In both *A* and *B*, the cluster of epithelial cells demonstrates some examples of glassy intranuclear inclusions. This finding as well as the papillary appearance of the cell aggregates suggests that the thyroid is the primary site. *A*, Diff-Quik × 375. *B*, Papanicolaou × 375.

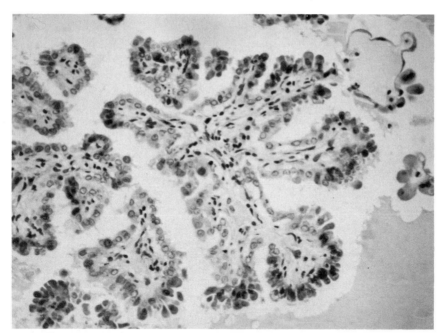

Figure 4–14 Occult papillary carcinoma of the thyroid, same case as that illustrated in Figure 4–13. The tumor was discovered after aspiration biopsy of the cervical node and removal of the thyroid lobe on the same side. Hematoxylin and eosin × 240.

COMPARING ASPIRATION SMEARS WITH TISSUE SECTIONS

Paramount in recognition of the primary site of metastatic carcinoma in aspirates of lymph nodes is familiarity with tumor patterns. These are not modified greatly because of the aspiration biopsy method and smear preparation. Several examples are documented in Figures 4–15 to 4–18: cases of signet cell carcinoma of the rectum metastatic to an inguinal node, clear cell carcinoma of the ovary metastatic to inguinal nodes, adenocarcinoma of the cervix metastatic to a cervical node, and transitional cell carcinoma of the urinary bladder metastatic to an inguinal node. In each of these cases, compare closely the arrangement and nuclear structure of the tumor cells with the tissue pattern. Note the remarkable similarities, even for relatively undifferentiated malignancies. These similarities become the foundation in diagnosis of primary sites of metastatic tumors and in determining if one is dealing with a recurrent neoplasm or a new primary. It cannot be overemphasized that comparison of the aspiration smears with prior tissue samples is absolutely mandatory for accurate and useful diagnoses.

LYMPHOMAS AND LEUKEMIAS

Fine-needle aspiration has generally not been considered a suitable technique for the primary diagnosis of malignant lymphomas, although historically this has been a major area of interest.[3, 15, 25-28] Generally, the diagnostic accuracy has been less than with metastatic tumor.[20-22, 25, 27] For example, the rate of accuracy for a small series of cases of Hodgkin's disease reported by Loseke and Craver was only 56 per cent.[28]

This author's experience with lymphoma cases has been quite successful, particularly with Hodgkin's disease. In an initial report, 22 cases were correctly diagnosed, and the evaluations were corroborated by clinical findings or subsequent histopathology. Two thirds of these cases involved patients with known lymphoma and clinical

Text continued on page 97

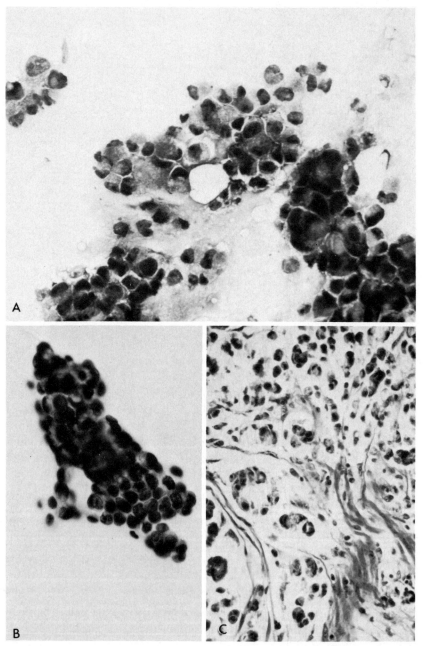

Figure 4–15 Signet cell carcinoma of the rectum, metastatic to inguinal lymph node. Compare the smear patterns in *A* and *B* with the tissue sections from the original primary tumor. The eccentric position of the nucleus is more apparent in the air-dried preparation *(A)*. The cytoplasm of the Romanovsky-stained cells is slightly metachromatic, suggesting the presence of mucin. *A*, Diff-Quik × 375. *B*, Papanicolaou × 375. *C*, Hematoxylin and eosin × 240.

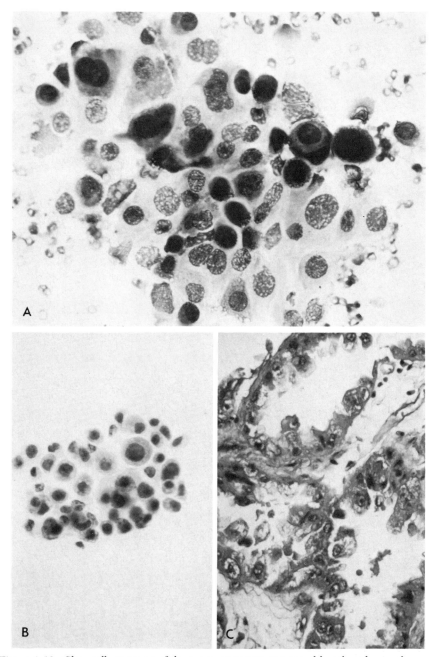

Figure 4–16 Clear cell carcinoma of the ovary, metastatic to inguinal lymph node. Another example in which the variations among cells seen on the aspirate are also reflected in the original tissue section of the clear cell ovarian carcinoma. Compare the smears with the surgical specimen and note particularly the light- and dark-cell pattern and the variation in nuclear size. *A*, Diff-Quik × 375. *B*, Papanicolaou × 375. *C*, Hematoxylin and eosin × 240.

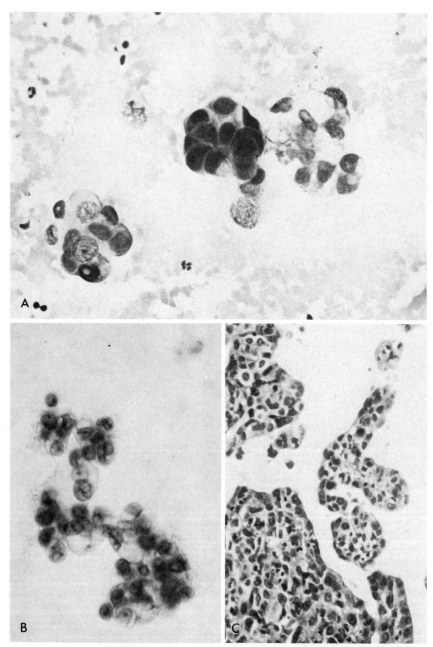

Figure 4–17   Adenocarcinoma of the cervix, metastatic to cervical node. Metastasis appeared several years after treatment of Stage IIB carcinoma of the cervix. Note the similarity of the papillary clusters in both the smear and the original biopsy of the cervix. The superimposition of the dark cells over the lighter-staining cells is most apparent in the air-dried smear (A). A, Diff-Quik × 375. B, Papanicolaou × 375. C, Hematoxylin and eosin × 240.

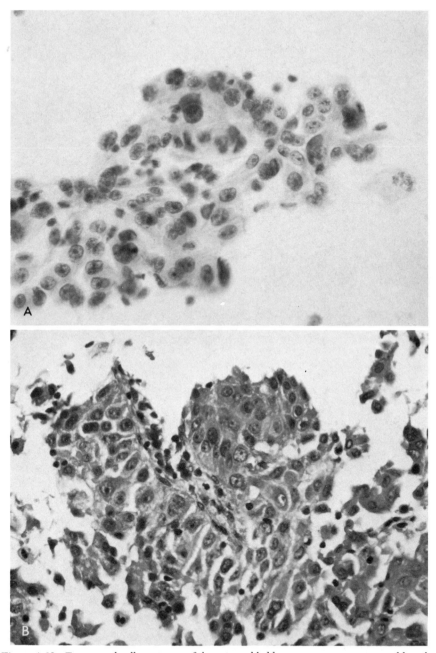

Figure 4–18 Transitional cell carcinoma of the urinary bladder, metastatic to an inguinal lymph node. Compare the cell pattern of the aspiration smear with the tissue section of the bladder tumor, noting similarity in nuclear structure and arrangement of the cells. *A*, Papanicolaou × 375. *B*, Hematoxylin and eosin × 375.

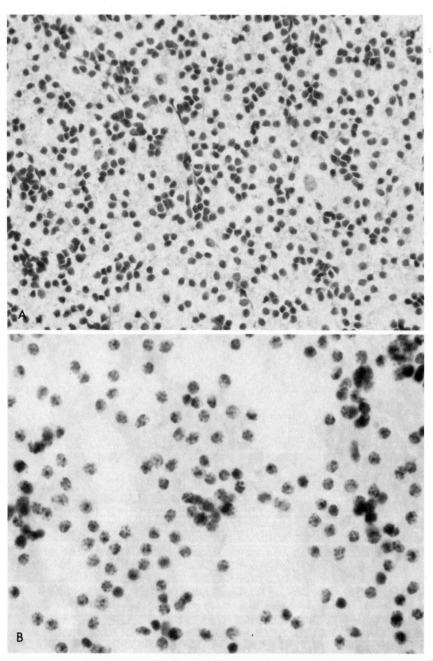

Figure 4–19 Non-Hodgkin's lymphoma, well-differentiated lymphocytic. Aspirate reveals a uniform cell population of lymphocytes but shows an open and distinct chromatin pattern that is more visible in the wet-fixed smear (B). Only an occasional histiocytic or germinal center cell disrupts the uniformity of the smear pattern. A, Diff-Quik × 375. B, Papanicolaou × 500.

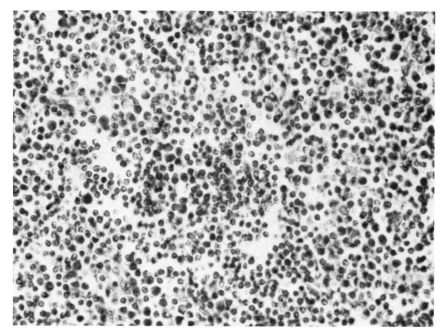

Figure 4–20 Non-Hodgkin's lymphoma, well-differentiated lymphocytic. Illustrated is a lymph node biopsy obtained after aspiration diagnosis of non-Hodgkin's lymphoma (Fig. 4–19) for comparison. Hematoxylin and eosin × 375.

evidence of recurrent disease.[29] From all node groups, this author has made the correct diagnosis in a total of 44 cases with four false-positive diagnoses for lymphoma. All these latter nodes, which were clinically quite large, revealed severe atypical reactive hyperplasia and were difficult to classify when subsequently examined histologically. Friedman and colleagues and Desmet and coworkers also confirmed the usefulness of needle aspiration biopsy in the diagnosis of recurrent Hodgkin's disease in a series of 228 patients who had been treated.[30, 31]

Non-Hodgkin's Lymphoma. Clinically, the nodes of malignant lymphoma are usually larger than those of metastatic carcinoma, so the target for aspiration biopsy is not easily missed. Except in Hodgkin's disease, the smear patterns are monomorphic and reflect quite accurately the cell type, whether it is a well differentiated or poorly differentiated lymphocyte, cleaved or non-cleaved. The May-Grünwald-Giemsa stain or other variants of the Romanovsky stain are quite useful in identifying the specific cell type of malignant lymphoma. Several examples with the corresponding Papanicolaou smears are demonstrated in Figures 4–19, 4–21, 4–23, and 4–25. Histologic sections from either the prior lymph node biopsy or the excision of the lymph node following a needle aspiration biopsy diagnosis of malignant lymphoma in primary cases are illustrated in Figures 4–20, 4–22, 4–24, and 4–26.

Obviously, it is difficult to differentiate between the nodular pattern and the diffuse pattern of malignant lymphomas with a needle aspiration biopsy. In primary cases, this author believes that the lymph node should be excised for an exact histopathologic classification. In addition to complementing the aspiration diagnosis of cell type in malignant lymphomas, the cells obtained can be used for determination of surface markers and for a number of the other immunologic tests for specific cell classification. Acid phosphatase: T-cells

More than 12 years ago, Rubio and Zajicek reported that the lymphocytes from either normal lymph nodes or malignant lymphomas were more than 80 per cent viable in the aspiration material, as determined by dye permeability tests. They also

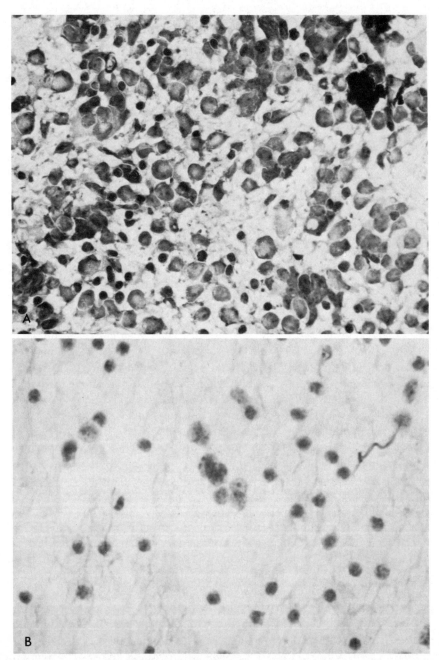

Figure 4–21 Non-Hodgkin's lymphoma, poorly differentiated lymphocytic. Smears composed of a uniform population of immature lymphocytes, with both a visible chromatin pattern and nucleoli. Note the numerous cells in the air-dried smear (A) and their pale nuclear centers. A, Diff-Quik × 375. B, Papanicolaou × 600.

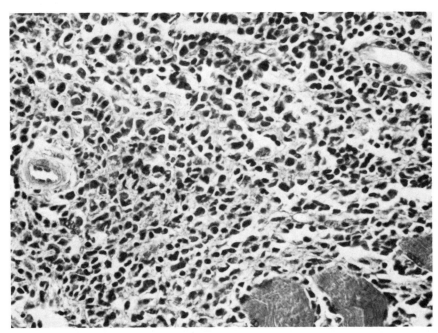

Figure 4–22 Non-Hodgkin's lymphoma, poorly differentiated lymphocytic. Section of the original neoplasm that arose in the mandible and invaded the adjacent muscles in an 18-year-old male. Figure 4–21 depicts the aspirate obtained from the enlarged cervical lymph node that developed after radiation therapy to this jaw tumor. Note the similarity between the cell configuration of the tissue and that of the air-dried smear (Fig. 4–21, *A*).

demonstrated that these same cells, including pyronophilic blast-type cells, could be stimulated into blastic transformation in approximately 80 per cent of cases.[32] Scanning electromicroscopy of aspirate specimens will also demonstrate the surface structure of the cell for identification purposes.

Hodgkin's Disease.   The diagnosis of Hodgkin's disease from aspiration smears depends on the identification of Reed-Sternberg cells. These cells may demonstrate either the typical double, mirror-image, overlapping nuclei illustrated in Figure 4–27A or the type of pleomorphism that is seen particularly in the nodular sclerotic variety of Hodgkin's disease (Fig. 4–27B). An attempt has been made to subclassify Hodgkin's disease from the aspirate, but this has usually been unsuccessful. The basic usefulness of aspiration is in patients who have been treated for and who have developed evidence of recurrent Hodgkin's disease, although this author has made the primary diagnosis in several cases. One of these diagnoses was particularly important because it led to a correct interpretation of a previous limited mediastinal biopsy that had been classified as a germinoma. Subsequent aspiration of an enlarged axillary lymph node in that case demonstrated a pattern completely inconsistent with a malignant epithelial tumor but one quite typical of Hodgkin's disease (Fig. 4–28). Subsequent excision of the node confirmed that diagnosis, and review of the mediastinal biopsy also revealed a pattern that was thought to be consistent with Hodgkin's disease of nodular sclerotic type.

Chronic Leukemia.   Leukemic involvement of lymph nodes or organs can be confirmed easily by aspiration biopsy. The battery of histochemical stains used for more precise classification of leukemic cells, particularly in the monocytic and granulocytic series, can easily be applied to the aspiration biopsy material. Examples of leukemic infiltrate from lymph nodes are depicted in Figures 4–29 and 4–30.

Lymphadenitis-Hyperplasia.   Enlargement of lymph nodes on a reactive or

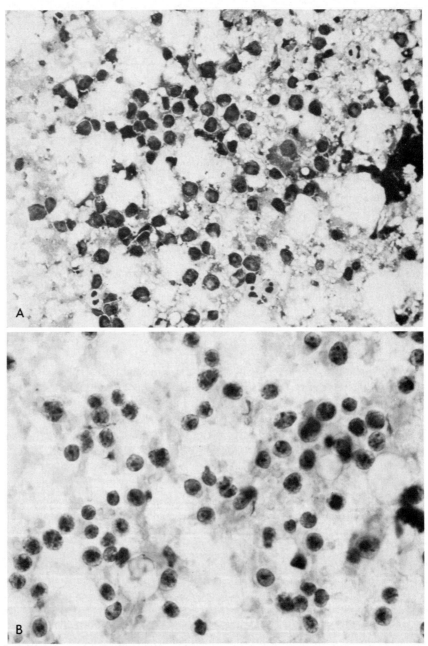

Figure 4–23 Non-Hodgkin's lymphoma, poorly differentiated lymphocytic. Aspirate from a cervical node occurring in an elderly male in whom non-Hodgkin's lymphoma was previously diagnosed. This node enlarged while the patient was under chemotherapy. The smears indicate a homogeneous population of immature lymphocytic cells. Prominent nucleoli are evident in both the air-dried and fixed smears. A, Diff-Quik × 375. B, Papanicolaou × 600.

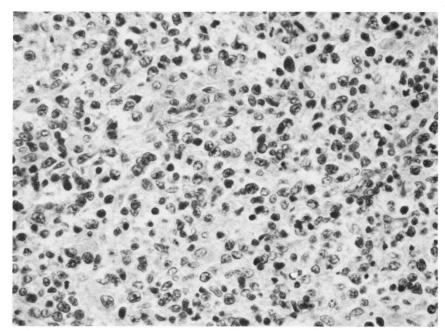

Figure 4–24 Non-Hodgkin's lymphoma, poorly differentiated lymphocytic. Original node biopsy from the patient whose aspirate is illustrated in Figure 4–23. Hematoxylin and eosin × 375.

inflammatory basis accounts for the largest number of benign cases for which fine-needle aspiration biopsy is requested. Lymphadenitis-hyperplasia must obviously be differentiated from metastatic malignant tumor and malignant lymphoma. Many of these cases occur in children, and a careful clinical history will reveal one or several bouts of pharyngitis and tonsillitis with subsequent enlargement of cervical lymph nodes, either bilaterally or unilaterally. This author's personal experience shows that aspiration biopsy in these cases, which cause great concern, provides an added measure of reassurance that the process is reactive and not malignant.[29]

The smear pattern of reactive lymphadenitis is one of a mixture of cell types, with lymphocytes of various degrees of differentiation and stimulation, plasma cells, and enlarged histiocytic phagocytes, some of which contain nuclear debris. The mixed cell pattern and the presence of phagocytic cells quite reliably indicate the diagnosis of lymphadenitis-hyperplasia.

No false-negatives with respect to lymphoma have been encountered in the lymphadenitis-hyperplasia group; however, there have been 19 false-negatives with respect to metastatic carcinoma. Two thirds of the false-negative cases have probably not been actual tumor in lymph nodes but neoplastic deposits in scar tissue at the site of previous radical surgery, specifically radical neck dissection. This type of aspiration in the presence of a thick scar is technically difficult to perform. The yield of cells, of any type, tends to be scant. This author has recommended open biopsy in such cases if there is any clinical doubt about the nature of the process. In the patient who has had a radical neck dissection, other masses that may simulate lymph nodes in the low cervical area are attributable to enlargement or increased prominence of the thyroid gland that occurs after removal of the sternocleidomastoid muscle, residual lymph nodes, and adipose tissue. Proof that a mass is thyroid is quite easily documented by aspiration.

Specimens of cells from cases of reactive hyperplasia and lymphadenitis are illustrated in Figures 4–31 through 4–33. Note particularly the mixed cell pattern and the evidence of phagocytosis. Another feature that is helpful but not absolutely reliable

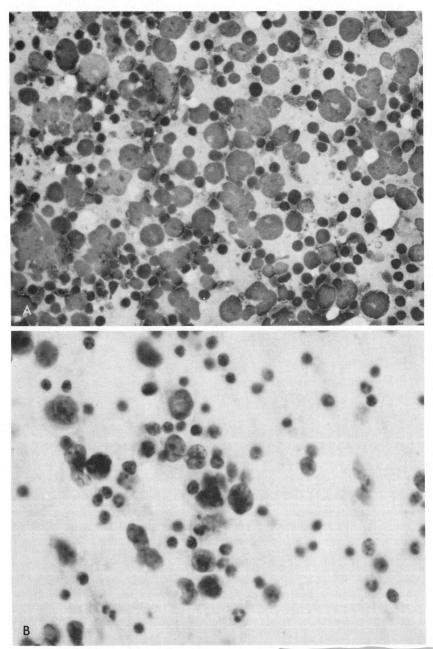

Figure 4–25   Non-Hodgkin's lymphoma, poorly differentiated, large-cleaved follicular center cell type. Aspirates from recurrent non-Hodgkin's lymphoma within the cervical area, demonstrating large undifferentiated lymphoid cells. The cleaved character of the nucleus is more apparent in the fixed smears. *A*, Diff-Quik × 375. *B*, Papanicolaou × 600.

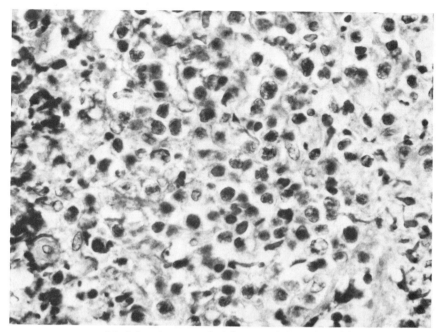

Figure 4–26 Non-Hodgkin's lymphoma, poorly differentiated, large-cleaved follicular center cell type. Compare this original node section with the aspiration pattern of the recurrent non-Hodgkin's lymphoma illustrated in Figure 4–25. Hemotoxylin and eosin × 600.

in differentiating between lymphadenitis-reactive hyperplasia and non-Hodgkin's lymphoma is the presence of numerous lymphoid cells with pale nuclear centers (Fig. 4–21A). These cells definitely indicate non-Hodgkin's lymphoma. The peculiar paleness appears to be an artefact of drying, but the reason that it occurs much more frequently in non-Hodgkin's lymphoma cells than in lymphocytes from reactive hyperplasia is completely unknown.[29] The air-dried smear stained with Diff-Quik or other Romanovsky stains is quite valuable in differentiating non-Hodgkin's lymphoma from reactive hyperplasia. The Papanicolaou stain on alcohol-fixed material is much less useful, unless the surface of the smear is allowed to dry very slightly before the cells are fixed. Otherwise, the artefact is completely eliminated by the immediate fixation of the aspiration smear. It also seems that this artefact occurs more frequently in the lymphoid cells associated with Hodgkin's disease than in cells from reactive lymph node hyperplasia aspirates, although this phenomenon is not documented by cell counts.

ASPIRATION FOR DIAGNOSIS OF INFECTIOUS DISEASES

While the emphasis in recent years has been on the aspiration biopsy diagnosis of tumors and lymphomas involving lymph nodes, infectious diseases may also be specifically identified. The aspiration biopsy is readily usable for culture techniques. Several methods of diagnosing actinomycosis have been reported recently, including the application of immunofluorescence for specific identification of the organism *Actinomyces israelii*[33,34] (Fig. 4–34). The "sulfur" granules are readily visible but are more easily seen on Papanicolaou-stained material than on an air-dried smear stained with May-Grünwald-Giemsa. Heavy, acute inflammatory exudate should be the first clue that suggests the presence of actinomycosis in an aspirate from a cervical lymph

Text continued on page 114

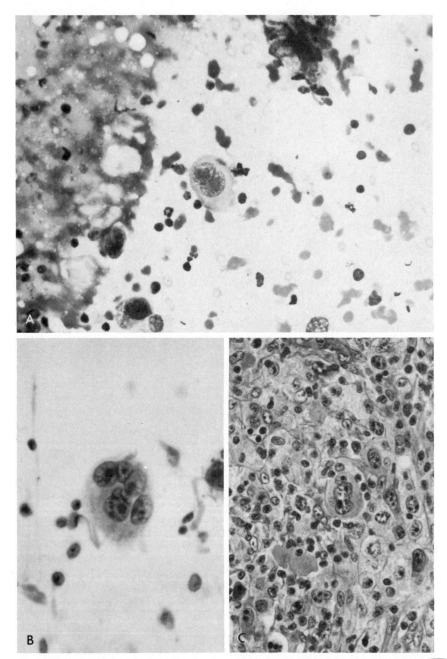

Figure 4–27 Hodgkin's disease. Example of a Reed-Sternberg cell with classic double overlapping nuclei and large nucleoli *(A)*. With Romanovsky stains, these nucleoli are a vivid blue. Compare the pleomorphic Reed-Sternberg cell depicted in *B* with similar cells found in the tissue sections of the lymph node illustrated in *C. A*, Diff-Quik × 375. *B*, Papanicolaou × 600. *C*, Hematoxylin and eosin × 375.

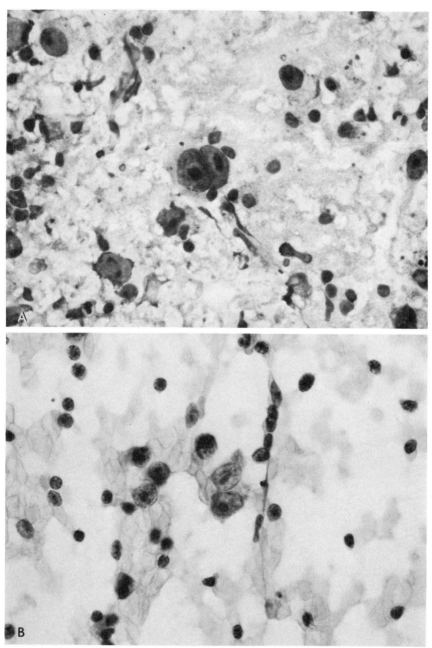

Figure 4–28 Hodgkin's disease. Aspirate of an axillary lymph node from a patient with a previous diagnosis of germinoma of the anterior mediastinum. Reed-Sternberg cells are evident in both *A* and *B*. Aspiration indicated that a diagnosis of metastatic germinoma was unlikely. Excision of the axillary node and review of the original biopsy from the mediastinum led to the correct diagnosis of Hodgkin's disease, nodular sclerotic type. *A*, Diff-Quik × 425. *B*, Papanicolaou × 600.

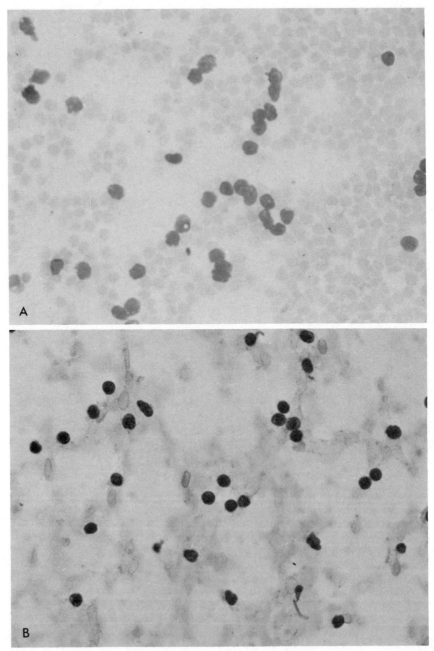

Figure 4–29 Chronic lymphocytic leukemia. Enlarged lymph nodes in patient with chronic lymphocytic leukemia were aspirated. A monomorphic pattern of lymphocytes is present, with many smudge cells in the air-dried preparation. *A*, Diff-Quik × 425. *B*, Papanicolaou × 600.

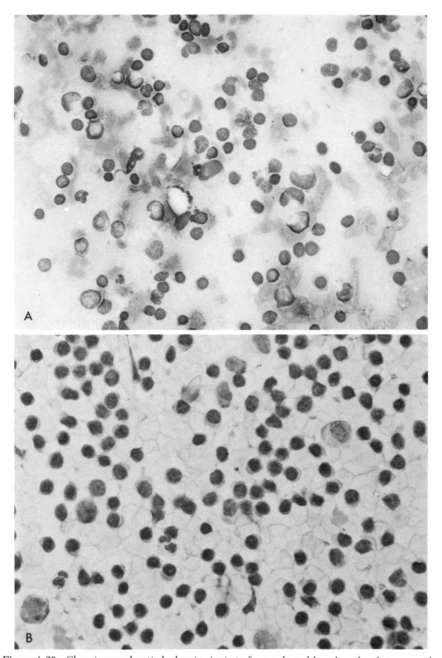

Figure 4–30 Chronic granulocytic leukemia. Aspirate from enlarged lymph nodes that occurred with recurrent chronic granulocytic leukemia. The monomorphic pattern of immature cells is evident in both *A* and *B*. A morphology suggesting that the cells are granulocytic in type is more evident in the air-dried smear (*A*). *A*, Diff-Quik × 375. *B*, Papanicolaou × 600.

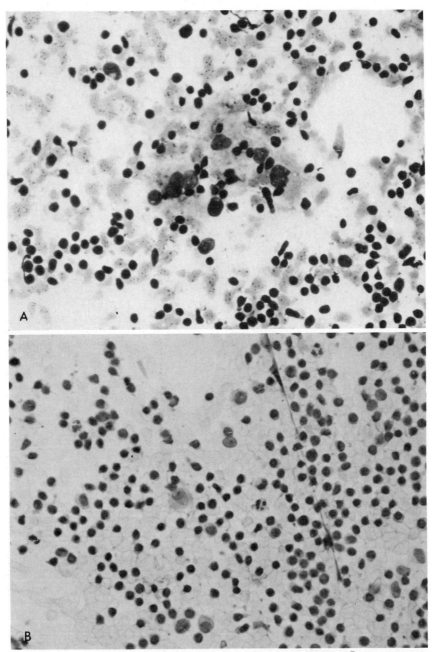

Figure 4–31 Lymphadenitis-hyperplasia. Aspirate from reactive lymph node depicting multiple cell types, including phagocytic cells with some nuclear debris in the cytoplasm (A). Selected fields from such aspirates can present a uniform cell population. The entire smear must be examined carefully before a malignant lymphoma diagnosis is considered. Some polymorphonuclear leukocytes can be detected in B. A, Diff-Quik × 375. B, Papanicolaou × 375.

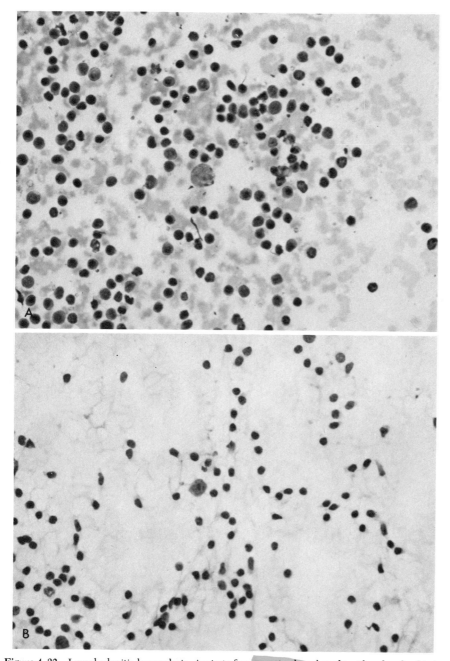

Figure 4–32   Lymphadenitis-hyperplasia. Aspirate from reactive lymph node with only a few histiocytic cells. Diagnosis of this case as only reactive is more difficult than for the smears illustrated in Figure 4–31. The lymphoid cells are extremely uniform and have a spindle shape, best seen in *B*. This feature is more common in benign lymph node aspirates. *A*, Diff-Quik × 375. *B*, Papanicolaou × 375.

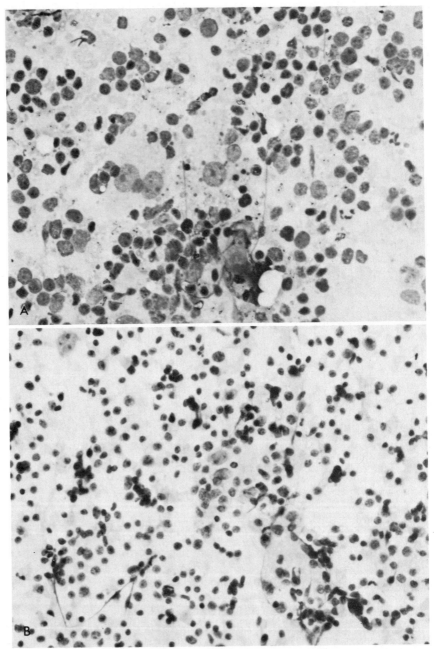

Figure 4–33   Lymphadenitis-hyperplasia. Aspirate from an enlarged cervical node in a child. The mixed cell pattern is a prominent feature, with phagocytes having nuclear debris in their cytoplasm. Aggregation of the lymphoid cells seen in the alcohol-fixed smear (A), is much more commonly seen in benign lymph node aspirates than in lymphoma aspirates. A, Diff-Quik × 375. B, Papanicolaou × 375.

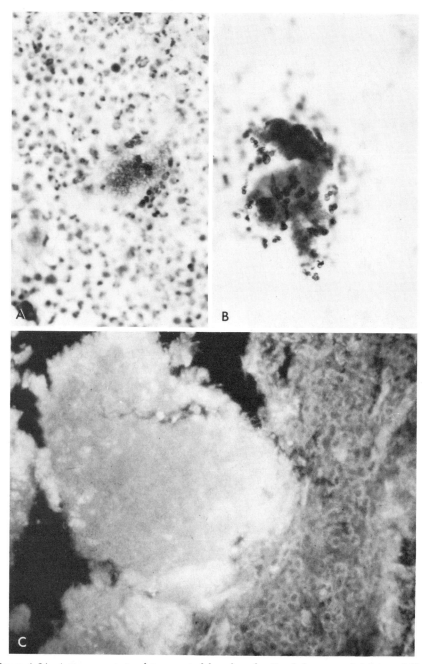

Figure 4–34   Actinomycosis involving cervical lymph node. Tangled masses of debris and filaments that make up the "sulfur" granules are visible in *A* and *B*, surrounded by many acute inflammatory cells. The organism may be mistaken for necrotic debris if the observer is not familiar with this presentation. *C* illustrates immunofluorescence of the organism *Actinomycosis israelii*, performed on one of the aspiration smears using specific antiserum. *A*, Diff-Quik × 375. *B*, Papanicolaou × 375. *C*, Immunofluorescence × 1000. (Courtesy of Dr. J. F. Valicenti, Jr.)

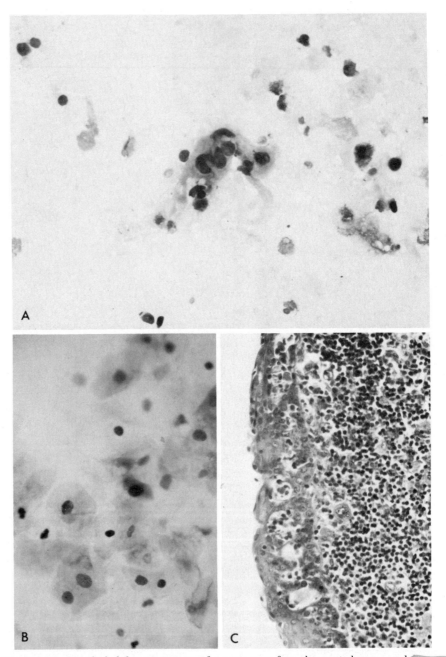

Figure 4–35 Branchial cleft cyst. Aspirate of a cystic mass from the cervical area reveals squamous cells that demonstrate some atypia in the air-dried preparation (A). The Papanicolaou-stained, alcohol-fixed smear reveals well-differentiated squamous cells with only a single small dark nucleus suggesting atypia. The lining of the branchial cleft cyst, which required surgical excision in this case, is illustrated in C. A, Diff-Quik × 375. B, Papanicolaou × 375. C, Hematoxylin and eosin × 240.

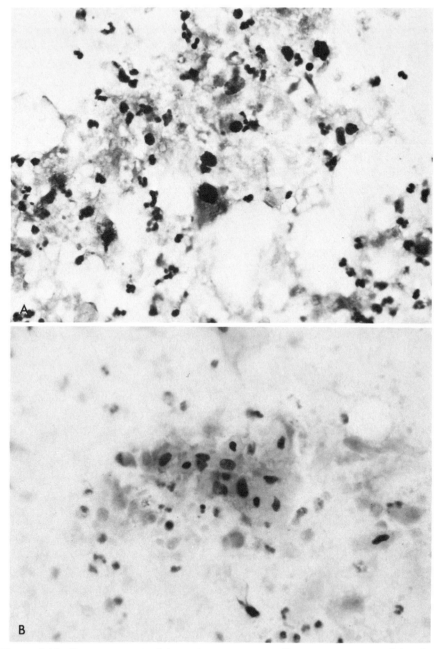

Figure 4–36 Cystic metastasis of keratinizing squamous cell carcinoma to cervical lymph node. Compare the pattern of atypical and degenerated squamous cancer cells in this cystic metastasis with the smear pattern from the branchial cleft cyst (Fig. 4–35). Such cases can be confusing, but any consistent degree of dysplasia of squamous cells should be considered suspect for metastatic keratinizing squamous cell carcinoma rather than for branchial cleft cyst. Sometimes, only a small primary in the tonsil may be found with this type of metastasis. A, Diff-Quik × 375. B, Papanicolaou × 375.

node. Theoretically, it should be possible to identify the inclusion bodies in an aspirate from the lymph nodes involved by lymphopathia venereum; however, the disease is rare in the United States, and this author has neither personally encountered this type of case nor found a report of it in the literature. Aspiration has been used recently in the diagnosis of lymph nodes or skin nodules involved with leprosy and has proved quite satisfactory in those forms in which the acid-fast organisms are prevalent.[35]

ASPIRATION OF MASSES SIMULATING LYMPH NODES

Cysts.   Almost all tumors simulating enlarged lymph nodes are confined to the head and neck area, where the complex anatomy and the presence of numerous structures may potentially give rise to masses that must be differentiated from enlarged lymph nodes. The lesion most commonly found in this area is a congenital cyst. Engzell and Zajicek have reported aspiration biopsy cytologic findings in 100 cases of cystic masses.[36] These cysts may be found in the midline or laterally; those in the former location are generally the thyroglossal duct type, and those in the latter site are of so-called branchial cleft origin. Theoretical considerations about development of the branchial cleft cysts lead to a conclusion that many of them are probably attributable to cystic degeneration of salivary gland epithelium found in lymph nodes.[37] Engzell and Zajicek correctly identified all their cases as cysts, except one in which the aspirate disclosed only inflammatory cells.

These authors do comment on the potential pitfall, in the laterally located cysts, of overdiagnosing or underdiagnosing a very well-differentiated keratinizing squamous cell carcinoma metastatic to a cervical node. Some of these metastases may occur with very small, intraoral, essentially occult primary carcinomas. Careful review of the aspiration smear is required to ensure that there are no dysplastic or pleomorphic squamous cells present.[36] An additional feature emphasized by Engzell and Zajicek and seen personally by this author is that true cystic lesions should completely disappear after aspiration. This author has performed aspirations in cases in which no recurrence or residual mass appeared after the aspiration. One cyst refilled. It was subsequently excised and proved to be a branchial cleft cyst. These cysts are usually lined with squamous epithelium accompanied by a variable amount of lymphoid tissue in the cyst wall. The aspirate from a branchial cleft cyst is illustrated in Figure 4–35, which also depicts the lining of the cyst in the case that was subsequently excised.

In keeping with the general principles of aspiration, if the cyst is not completely evacuated and if there then is a residual mass, aspiration should be repeated. There are cases of metastatic squamous cell carcinoma, particularly those of heavily keratinized tumors in which cystic degeneration may occur, that both clinically and cytologically may simulate branchial cleft cysts (Fig. 4–36).

Cysts located in the midline may be lined by either squamous or columnar epithelium or by a mixture of both. The aspiration will reflect one or both cell types and the cyst wall usually contains lymphoid tissue. Metastatic tumors rarely occur directly in the midline, so the differential diagnosis is quite limited. The principle of evacuating the cyst completely so that there is no residual mass applies to this type of case as well.

Carotid Body Tumors.   Carotid body tumor is the other neoplasm that is of real concern in aspiration biopsy of neck masses that might simulate lymph nodes. From a recent small series, Engzell and colleagues concluded that aspiration biopsy of at least large carotid body tumors is contraindicated. One of 13 patients in his series developed thrombosis of the internal carotid artery and a fatal cerebral infarction after fine-needle aspiration biopsy of a carotid body tumor. The biopsy itself yielded only blood. While the other 12 aspirations were successfully performed, two of the masses were reported as suspected metastatic carcinoma from the thyroid, two as possible neurofibrosarcomas, and one as a neurofibroma. Hence, the diagnostic accuracy was poor. The tumor cells obtained from aspiration of carotid body tumors are quite pleomorphic, with giant nuclei in some fields and a remarkable spindle-cell pattern in others. Specific relationships between the tumor cells and blood vessels are not seen on aspiration smears. Despite the conclusion that aspiration biopsy is unwarranted in cases of suspected carotid body tumor, the authors did cite seven references in which this type of diagnostic procedure was recommended.[38]

One case of carotid body tumor was encountered in the present series. The aspiration was unsatisfactory, yielding only blood. In retrospect, that result may well have been fortunate, since no complications ensued. The diagnosis was correctly made at subsequent surgery. No bruit was heard in this case. When an enlarged suspected lymph node is encountered in the area consistent with the carotid bifurcation, it is probably wise for one to listen for the bruit of a possible carotid body tumor and hence avoid potential complications of aspiration biopsy of such a neoplasm.

SPECIAL TECHNIQUES

Lymphangiography using fluoroscopy or ultrasound or both combined with fine-needle aspiration has allowed the confirmation of metastatic involvement of retroperitoneal, deep pelvic, and mediastinal lymph nodes.[39-47] This procedure seems particularly valuable in diagnosing metastatic malignancies of the female genital tract, specifically carcinoma of the cervix, endometrium, and ovary, where the clinical evaluation alone is limited in providing accurate staging.[40] Bonfiglio and colleagues reported 47 cases in which aspiration was performed after lymphangiography and in which a rapid Papanicolaou stain was used for immediate evaluation. These authors as most others feel that biplane fluoroscopy is required for accurate placement of the needle. They reported a positive diagnosis of metastatic carcinoma in 11 patients and unsatisfactory results in two patients.[39] Gothlin reported multiple aspirations in 29 patients and divided the successful and unsuccessful cases according to the size of the lymph node as measured on the films. He believed that the node had been hit if it moved on fluoroscopy when the needle was moved. Difficulty was encountered with nodular sclerotic Hodgkin's disease because of the marked amount of fibrosis thought to be present in the nodes. Other failures in this series most commonly occurred in patients who had been treated previously with radiation therapy or who were markedly obese.[41]

A large series is reported by Rupp and colleagues in which 23 patients, subsequent to lymphangiography, underwent three to nine node aspirations per examination. About two thirds of the punctures were cytologically successful. In three cases that demonstrated metastasis on the aspiration smear, the same lymph node radiographically was considered negative. In seven other cases, both the cytologic material and the lymphangiographic examination indicated metastatic disease. In an additional 14 cases, aspiration biopsy suggested that the masses were negative for metastatic tumor, but eight of these were considered to have a suspicious lymphangiogram. Five of these masses, subsequently operated upon, demonstrated no metastatic tumor in the lymph nodes during histologic examination.[43]

This author's current experience includes a few instances of performing this type of aspiration after lymphangiography. CAT scans and ultrasonography have been used to guide the needle to the node in a few cases and have yielded a positive diagnosis, as demonstrated in a case of carcinoma of the cervix metastatic to a periaortic lymph node (Fig. 4–37). In some patients, nodes of this type were so large that they were palpable abdominally, and a direct aspiration of the mass was successfully performed. In all the reported series of retroperitoneal and deep pelvic lymph node aspirations,

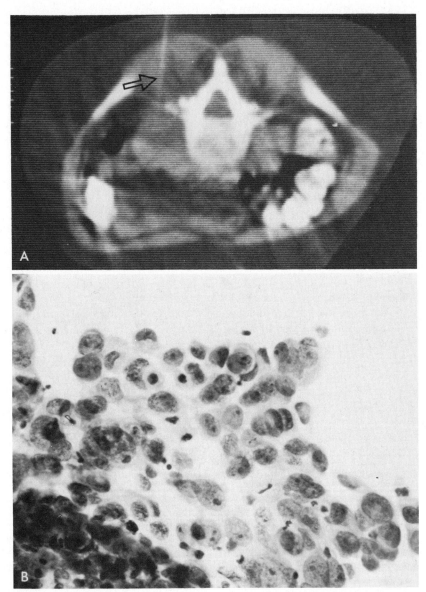

Figure 4–37 Aspiration of periaortic lymph node with metastatic squamous cell carcinoma of the cervix, performed with the aid of a CAT scan. The track of the needle is seen (arrow) passing toward the mass, adjacent to the vertebral body. *B* demonstrates sheets of poorly differentiated tumor cells obtained from this aspiration. *A*, CAT scan image. *B*, Papanicolaou × 375.

the difficulty is in confirming that negative results are actually negative. The correlation of long-term clinical evaluation of these patients and histologic studies of lymph node dissection specimens with the results of prior aspiration is necessary in a larger number of cases to confirm the utility of this procedure. When the aspirate is positive, however, it is of great value in more accurately determining the stage of a neoplasm, particularly female genital tract cancers, and hence in selecting appropriate therapy more effectively.

COMPLICATIONS OF LYMPH NODE ASPIRATIONS

A single complication has occurred in this series, a small immediate 1.0 cm hematoma that appeared after aspiration of a submaxillary lymph node. The hematoma disappeared quickly, leaving no residual. The aspiration showed only reactive lymphoid hyperplasia, and the node later shrank and also disappeared. Complications of lymph node aspiration, including those of transabdominal aspiration of retroperitoneal and pelvic nodes, have not been reported in the literature. Not even puncture of the bowel has produced either hemorrhage or peritonitis.[41, 48]

REFERENCES

1. Grieg, E. D. W., and Gray, A. C. H.: Note on lymphatic glands in sleeping sickness. Lancet 1:1570, 1904.
2. Ward, G. R.: *Bedside Hematology.* Philadelphia, W. B. Saunders Co., 1914, p. 129.
3. Guthrie, C. G.: Gland puncture as a diagnostic measure. Bull. Johns Hopkins Hosp. 32:266–269, 1921.
4. Andre, R., and Dreyfus, B.: *La Ponction Ganglionnaire.* Paris, L'expansion scientifique française, 1954.
5. Leiber, B.: *Der menschliche Lymphknoten.* Munich, Urban & Schwarzenberg, 1961.
6. Lennerth, K.: Lymphknoten. Bandteil A: Cytologie und Lymphadenitis; *in Handbuch der speziellen pathologischen Anatomie und Histologie.* Berlin, Springer, 1961.
7. Lopes Cardozo, P.: *Clinical Cytology.* Leiden, Stafleu, 1954.
8. Pavlovsky, A.: *La puncion ganglionar. Su contribucion al diagnostico clinico-quirurgico des las afecciones ganglionares.* Buenos Aires, Tesis, 1934.
9. Stahel, R.: *Diagnostische Drusenpunktion.* Leipzig, Thieme, 1939.
10. Streicher, H. J., and Sandkühler, S.: *Klinische Zytologie.* Stuttgart, Thieme, 1953.
11. Strunge, T.: *La Ponction des ganglions lymphatiques. Une description cytologique controlé par la clinique.* Copenhagen, Munksgaard, 1944.
12. Tischendorf, W.: *Cytodiagnostik des Lymphknotenpunktates.* Vol. 2. Ergebn. Inn. Med. Kinderh. Berlin, Springer, 1951, p. 183.
13. Weil, P. E., Isch-Wall, P., and Perles S.: Le diagnostic de la maladie de Hodgkin par la ponction des ganglions. Presse Med. 44:1540–1543, 1936.
14. Zajicke, J., Engzell, U., and Franzen, S.: Aspiration biopsy of lymph nodes in diagnosis and research; *in* Ruettimann, A. (Ed): Progress in Lymphology. Stuttgart, Thieme, 1967, pp. 262–264.
15. Lukas, P. F.: Lymph node smears in the diagnosis of lymphadenopathie: A review. Blood 10:1030–1054, 1955.
16. Meatheringham, R. E., and Ackerman, L. V.: Aspiration biopsy of lymph nodes. Surg. Gynecol. Obstet. 84:1071–1076, 1947.
17. Forkner, P. E.: Material from lymph node of man: Studies in living and fixed cells withdrawn from lymph nodes of man. Arch. Inn. Med. 40:532–537; 647–660, 1927.
18. Engzell, U., Jakobsson, P. A., Sigurdson, A., et al.: Aspiration biopsy of metastatic carcinoma in lymph nodes of the neck. Acta Otolaryngol. 72:138–147, 1971.
19. Lopes Cardozo, P.: The cytologic diagnosis of lymph node punctures. Acta Cytol. 8:194–202, 1964.
20. Russ, J. E., Scanlon, E. F., and Christ, M. A.: Aspiration cytology of head and neck masses. Am. J. Surg. 136:342–347, 1978.
21. Zajdela, A., Ennuyer, A., Bataini, P., et al.: Valeur du diagnostic cytologique des adenopathies par ponction aspiration. Bull. Cancer (Paris) 63:327–340, 1976.
22. Bloch, M.: Comparative study of lymph node cytology by puncture and histopathology. Acta Cytol. 11:139–144, 1967.
23. Betsill, W. L. Jr., and Hajdu, S. I.: Percutaneous aspiration biopsy of lymph nodes. Acta Cytol. (Abstr.) 22:601, 1978.
24. Friedman, M., Forgione, H., and Shanbhag, V.: Needle aspiration of metastatic melanoma. Acta Cytol. 24:7–15, 1980.

25. Morrison, M., Samwick, H. A., Rubinstein, J., et al.: Lymph node aspiration. Am. J. Clin. Pathol. 22:255–262, 1952.
26. Soderstrom, N.: *Fine-needle Aspiration Biopsy.* Stockholm, Almqvist and Wiksell, 1966, pp. 62–82.
27. Zajicek, J.: *Aspiration Biopsy Cytology. Part I. Cytology of Supradiaphragmatic Organs.* Monographs in Clinical Cytology. New York, S. Karger, 1974, pp. 97–107.
28. Loseke, L., and Craver, L. F.: The diagnosis of Hodgkin's disease by aspiration biopsy. Blood 1:76–82, 1946.
29. Frable, W. J., and Frable, M. A. S.: Thin-needle aspiration biopsy. The diagnosis of head and neck tumors revisited. Cancer 43:1541–1548, 1979.
30. Friedman, M., Kim, U., Shimaoka, K., et al.: Appraisal of aspiration cytology in management of Hodgkin's disease. Cancer 45:1653–1663, 1980.
31. Desmet, V., Beert, J., and Reybrouck, G.: Value of the cytological diagnosis of Hodgkin's disease in comparison with histological findings. Sangre 9:73–76, 1964.
32. Rubio, C. A., and Zajicek, J.: Human lymph node cell transformation. Lancet 1:579, 1967.
33. Pollock, P. G., Meyers, D. S., Frable, W. J., et al.: Rapid diagnosis of actinomycosis by thin-needle aspiration biopsy. Am. J. Clin. Pathol. 70:27–30, 1978.
34. Pollock, P. G., Koontz, F. P., Viner, T. F., et al.: Cervicofacial actinomycosis. Rapid diagnosis by thin-needle aspiration. Arch. Otolaryngol. 104:491–494, 1978.
35. Kaur, S.: Fine needle aspiration of lymph nodes in leprosy. A study of bacteriologic and morphologic indices. Int. J. Lepr. 45:369–372, 1977.
36. Engzell, U., and Zajicek, J.: Aspiration biopsy of tumors of the neck. I. Aspiration biopsy and cytologic findings in 100 cases of congenital cysts. Acta Cytol. 14:51–57, 1970.
37. Bhaskar, S. N., and Bernier, J. L.: Histogenesis of branchial cysts. A report of 468 cases. Am. J. Pathol. 35:407–424, 1959.
38. Engzell, U., Franzen, S., and Zajicek, J.: Aspiration biopsy of tumors of the neck. II. Cytologic findings in 13 cases of carotid body tumor. Acta Cytol. 15:25–30, 1971.
39. Bonfiglio, T. A., MacIntosh, P. K., Patten, S. F., Jr., et al.: Fine needle aspiration cytopathology of retroperitoneal lymph nodes in evaluation of metastatic disease. Acta Cytol. 23:126–130, 1979.
40. Berkowitz, R. S., Leavitt, T. Jr., and Knapp, R. C.: Ultrasound-directed percutaneous aspiration biopsy of periaortic lymph nodes in recurrence of cervical carcinoma. Am. J. Obstet. Gynecol. 131:906–908, 1978.
41. Gothlin, J. H.: Post-lymphographic percutaneous fine needle biopsy of lymph nodes guided by fluoroscopy. Radiology 120:205–207, 1976.
42. Kidd, C. R., and Mennemeyer, R. P.: Diagnostic cytology and electron microscopy of fine needle aspirates of retroperitoneal lymph nodes in the diagnosis of metastatic pelvic neoplasms. Acta Cytol. (Abstr.) 22:597, 1978.
43. Rupp, N., Rothenberger, K., Bayer-Pietsch, E., et al.: Percutaneous fine needle aspiration biopsy of lymph nodes. ROEFO 130:328–331, 1979.
44. Zornoza, J., Wallace, S., Goldstein, H. M., et al.: Transperitoneal percutaneous retroperitoneal lymph node aspiration biopsy. Radiology 122:111–115, 1977.
45. Zornoza, J., Lukeman, J. M., Jang, B. S., et al.: Percutaneous retroperitoneal lymph node biopsy in carcinoma of the cervix. Gynecol. Oncol. 5:43–51, 1977.
46. Zajicek, J.: *Aspiration Biopsy Cytology, Part 2. Cytology of Infradiaphragmatic Organs.* Monographs in Clinical Cytology. New York, S. Karger, 1979, pp. 212–223.
47. Zornoza, J., Jonsson, K., Wallace, S., et al.: Fine needle aspiration biopsy of retroperitoneal lymph nodes and abdominal masses: An updated report. Radiology 125:87–88, 1977.
48. Lagergren, C., and Friberg, S.: Aspirationsbiopsi av lymfkortlar efter lymfografi. Swed. Soc. Med. Radiol. Forhandl 5:14–15, 1976.

Chapter Five

Salivary Glands

Salivary gland swellings are readily accessible to fine-needle aspiration biopsy. Even intraoral neoplasms arising from minor salivary glands in the palate and the base of the tongue are accessible to needle aspiration biopsy in which the 22-gauge, 8.8 cm (3-1/2 in) spinal needle and a direct transoral route are used. The procedure is virtually painless, but topical oral mucosal anesthesia can be easily administered if required.

DIFFERENTIAL DIAGNOSIS

The principal differential diagnosis from aspiration biopsy smears of major salivary gland swellings involves distinguishing between tumor and inflammation. The latter condition seldom produces a discrete mass but is often unilateral and without demonstrable duct obstruction, at least that caused by calculi. Pre-aspiration clinical evaluation is important. A history of episodic swelling is usually encountered only with sialadenitis. This author's own experience suggests that if a good history of salivary gland inflammation can be obtained and correlated with the clinical findings of a somewhat tender gland without a discrete mass, then aspiration biopsy should probably not be undertaken, as it can be a somewhat painful procedure in this type of case. If there is any doubt concerning the nature of the lesion of a major salivary gland, a fine-needle aspiration biopsy can rather easily differentiate tumor from inflammation. Aspiration is particularly useful in those cases in which there appears to be a fixed mass, a finding seen in cases of both severe chronic sialadenitis and malignant tumors.

The first reported experience with fine-needle aspiration biopsy of salivary gland tumors demonstrates a somewhat greater number of false-negative results than might have been expected. Problems were also encountered in accurately classifying the various diverse tumors, both benign and malignant, that occur in the salivary glands. While the most common lesion is benign mixed tumor, the variable cellular patterns that may be encountered in the presence of this neoplasm lead to greater false-positive rates for malignancy than is probably acceptable.[1-6] Included in some of these series are a substantial number of unsatisfactory aspirations, partly composed of cases in which only cyst contents were sampled and in which no second aspiration was performed on a residual mass. The same concept of reexamining for a clinical tumor after aspiration of cystic content is as important in salivary gland lesions as it is in other areas where aspiration biopsy is attempted.[2, 3, 4]

Aspirations of true neoplasms yield abundant specimen in the vast majority of cases. Gross examination of the aspirate reveals a granular character. With available quick stains of the Romanovsky type, it is quite easy to make a preliminary diagnosis.

At least the fact that adequate material has been obtained is appreciated. In contrast, inflammatory lesions frequently yield somewhat bloody aspirates with relatively low cellularity. Certainly, as indicated by this author's personal experience, aspiration should be repeated in the case of a gross tumor mass when there is any doubt that an adequate sampling has been obtained. These principles are emphasized in the literature in later reports that document much better results in terms of both accurate differentiation of tumor from non-neoplastic conditions and accurate prediction of the histopathology from the cytologic smear.[1, 5, 7-10] Increased accuracy has been particularly noted in the diagnosis of specific malignant tumor types. This may in part reflect changing classifications of salivary gland neoplasms from a heterogenous group of tumors all considered of mixed cell type into specific categories, such as acinic cell carcinoma and cylindroma.[1, 2, 5, 10]

BENIGN TUMORS

Mixed Tumors (Pleomorphic Adenomas).   The majority of neoplasms in this author's personal series of aspiration biopsies have been benign mixed tumors, 30 in the parotid gland and 10 in the submaxillary gland. Diagnosis in these cases has so far been easy because the aspiration smears of the tumors demonstrate an almost histologic pattern that represents both the benign epithelial component and the chondroid myxoid stroma. The latter is highly metachromatic with the Giemsa stains (Figs. 5–1 to 5–4). The epithelial cells have a very bland appearance with a smooth chromatin structure and a very uniform nuclear shape, somewhat bipolar. They occur in large sheets and in well-prepared aspirates interdigitate with the myxoid chondroid stroma, which actually has spindle cells within it. This stroma stains only lightly with the Papanicolaou method, so the individual stromal cells are more visible. It is important to see these stromal cells to make the differential diagnosis between benign mixed tumor and low-grade mucoepidermoid carcinoma. The latter tumor has abundant metachromatic mucinous material, but no identifiable stromal cells are visible (Fig. 5–5).

Some of the aspirates from benign mixed tumors have been highly cellular, with very scant stroma that is difficult to identify. This has been true of two accessory salivary gland lesions in the palate and two neoplasms of this type in the major salivary glands (Fig. 5–6). The epithelial cells, however, appeared extremely uniform with no pleomorphism. The neoplasm would have to be either a benign mixed tumor with scant stroma, which the author reports as cellular but benign mixed tumor, or the true monomorphic adenoma of salivary-gland type described by Batsakis.[11]

It is well known that some pleomorphism may occur in benign mixed tumors. Observation of this feature might result in a diagnosis of malignancy (Figs. 5–7 and 5–8). Such neoplasms generally behave as benign mixed tumors, but, obviously, aspiration biopsy could provide a difficult diagnostic problem and has led to a few false-positive reports.[2, 5] For example, in one series of 204 cases of aspiration biopsy of benign mixed salivary gland tumors, 10 revealed pronounced atypia that suggested malignancy. These 10 cases were histologically classified as benign. Two other tumors were histologically classified as benign mixed tumor but cytologically identified as carcinoma. One patient died of metastatic carcinoma. Both patients had received extensive preoperative radiation therapy prior to histologic examination. As the authors point out, this may account for some of the diagnostic discrepancy.[2] In the present series, some pleomorphism of mixed tumor aspirates has so far not been confusing.

Papillary Cystadenoma Lymphomatosum (Warthin's Tumor).   The present series contains five examples of Warthin's tumor: three in the parotid gland and two in the submaxillary salivary gland. Whether this neoplasm is actually in the salivary gland or

Text continued on page 128

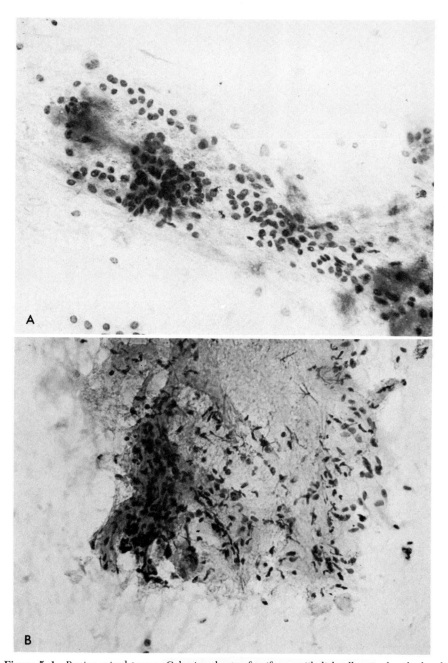

Figure 5–1 Benign mixed tumor. Cohesive sheets of uniform epithelial cells mixed with chondroid myxoid stroma. The stroma is markedly metachromatic with Romanovsky stains. In this example, the spindle-shaped stromal cells are easily seen in the Papanicolaou stain *(B)*. A, Diff-Quik × 240. B, Papanicolaou × 240.

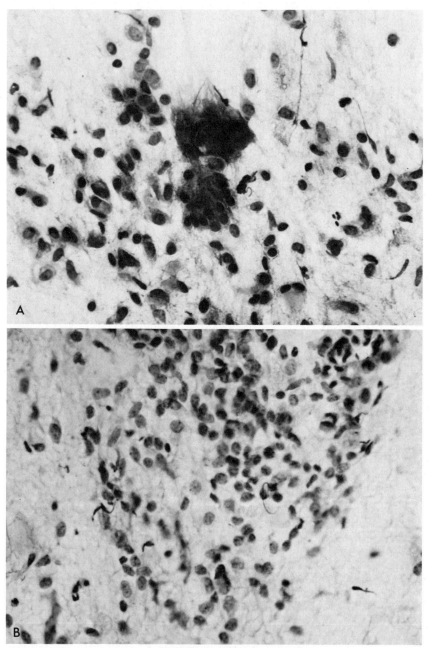

Figure 5–2   Benign mixed tumor. Sheets of uniform epithelial cells from benign mixed tumor at higher magnification. Dense stroma can be seen in the center of *A*. Spindle-shaped stromal cells are mingled with round to oval epithelial cells in *B*. *A*, Diff-Quik × 375. *B*, Papanicolaou × 375.

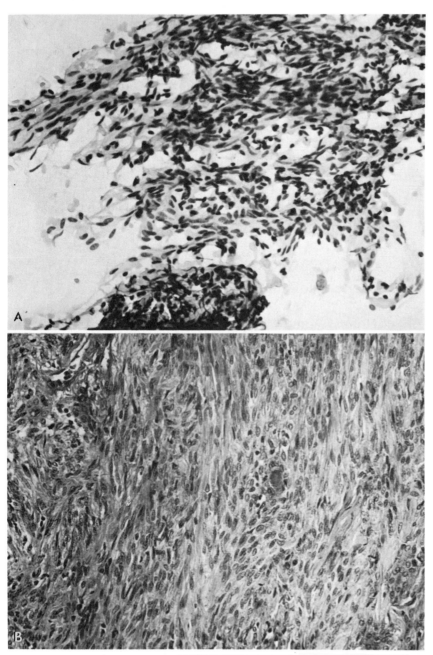

Figure 5–3   Benign mixed tumor with predominant spindle-cell, neurilemoma-like pattern. Although the spindle-cell pattern predominated throughout the smear, there were some metachromatic stromal foci and clusters of oval epithelial cells. B depicts the tissue with the same spindle-cell pattern but with a small duct identifiable in the center of the photograph. A, Papanicolaou × 240. B, Hematoxylin and eosin × 240.

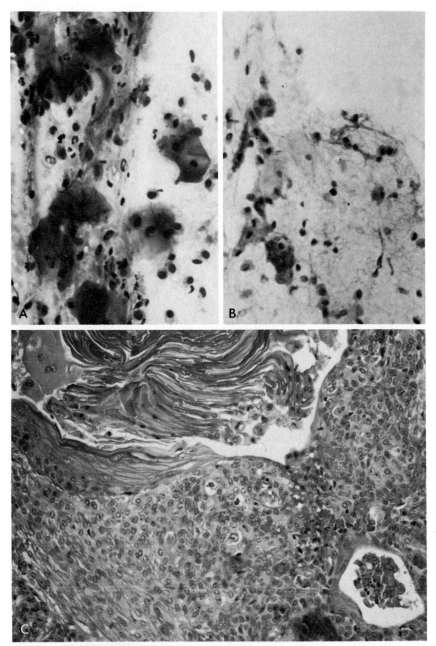

Figure 5–4   Benign mixed tumor with mature squamous metaplasia. Smear pattern demonstrates not only the pattern of a benign mixed tumor but also mature metaplastic squamous cells. Histologic sections also revealed a typical benign mixed tumor with multiple areas of squamous metaplasia and keratinization. A, Diff-Quik × 240. B, Papanicolaou × 375. C, Hematoxylin and eosin × 240.

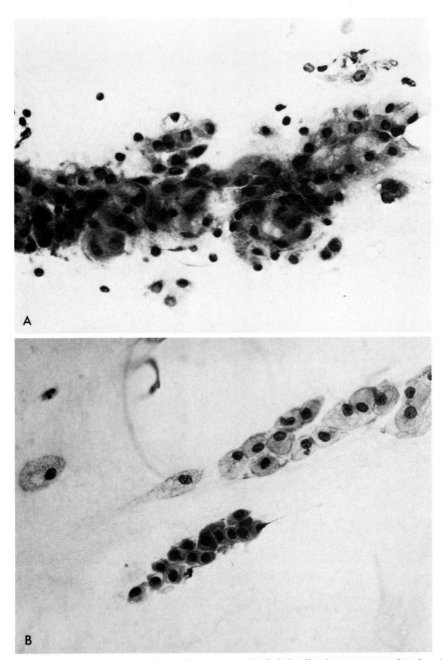

Figure 5–5 Low-grade mucoepidermoid carcinoma. Epithelial cells of two types are found in these aspirates: one with finely vacuolated metachromatic cytoplasm, the other with dense cytoplasm and well-defined cell borders. The contrast between the two cell types is more obvious in the Papanicolaou-stained smear, but the contrast between the color of the cytoplasm and that of the background metachromasia is more easily appreciated with the Romanovsky-stained smears. Note the absence of clearly definable spindle-shaped stromal cells, the only feature useful for differentiating these smears from those of benign mixed tumor. Also compare this smear with an aspiration smear from a mucocele (Fig. 5–18) and note the similarity between the two. A, Diff-Quik × 375. B, Papanicolaou × 375.

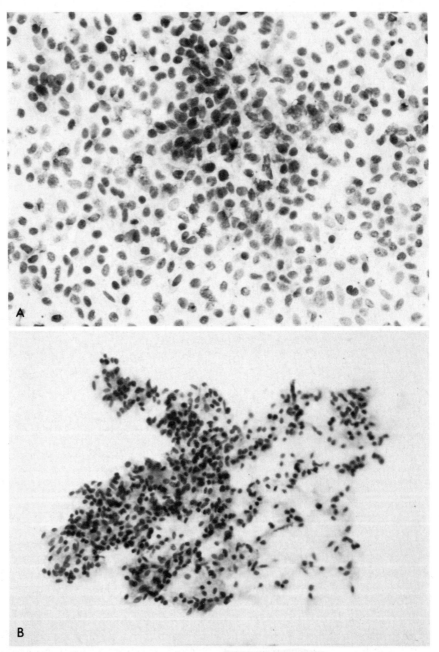

Figure 5–6 Cellular but benign mixed tumor. Abundant uniform cells are present in these smears, while typical stroma is scant. Note the tissue-like pattern of the aspirate in *B. A,* Diff-Quik × 375. *B,* Papanicolaou × 240.

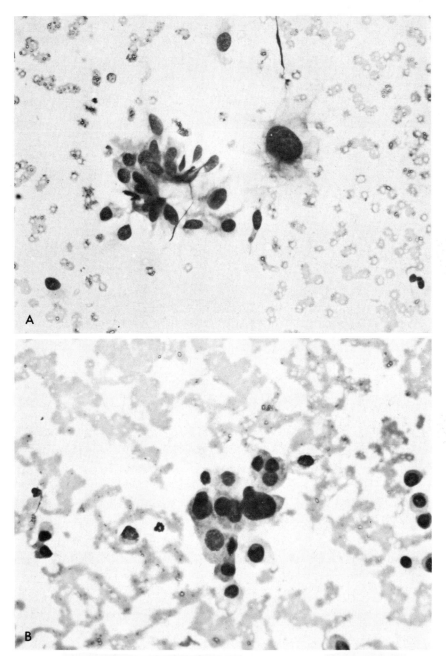

Figure 5–7   Pleomorphism in benign mixed tumor. Cell clusters with an occasional large and irregular nucleus in an otherwise typical smear pattern of benign mixed tumor. A and B, Diff-Quik × 375.

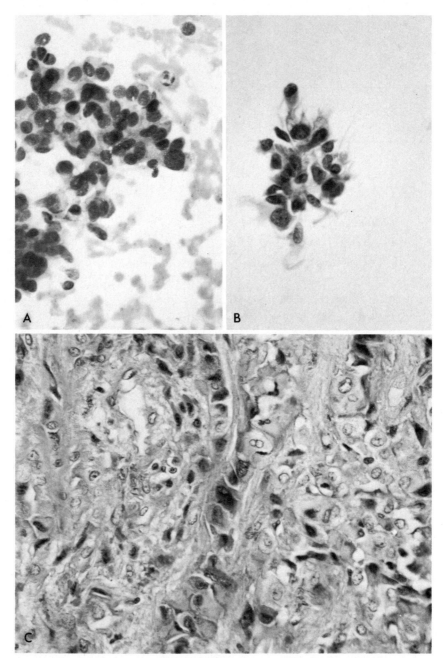

Figure 5–8 Pleomorphism in benign mixed tumor. Same case as that illustrated in Figure 5–7. This smear also contains rare cells with enlarged and irregular nuclei. Cells of this type do not indicate malignancy in an otherwise typical mixed tumor. Histologic section of this tumor contained scattered pleomorphic cells similar to those in the aspirate. Clinical follow-up after excision has shown no recurrence of tumor. *A* and *B*, Papanicolaou × 375. *C*, Hematoxylin and eosin × 375.

arises from salivary gland epithelium in adjacent lymph nodes is difficult to determine.[11] In any event, the diagnosis from the aspiration smear has been fairly easy in the present series, although it has caused some problems in several previous reports.[2, 3, 12]

  Differentiation from Oncocytoma. There were 33 cases of cystadenolymphoma included among the series of aspiration biopsies reported by Mavec and colleagues; however, only eight of these diagnoses are recognized cytologically. In 11 cases, the aspirate consisted only of discolored cyst fluid and an admixture of inflammatory cells.

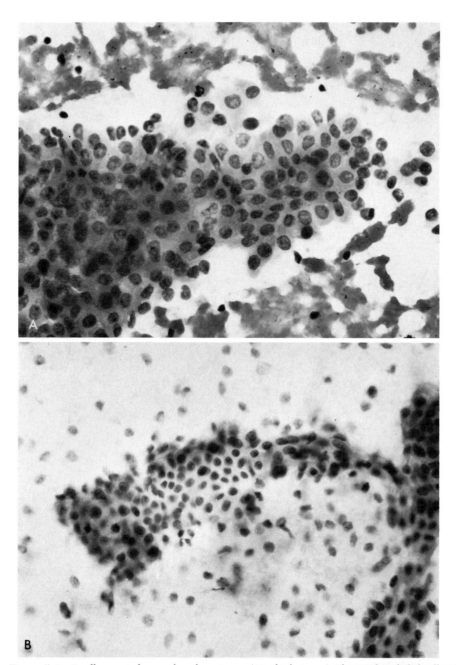

Figure 5–9 Papillary cystadenoma lymphomatosum (Warthin's tumor). Sheets of epithelial cells with abundant, finely granular cytoplasm. Scattered lymphocytes surround these epithelial cells. It is unlikely for both the lymphoid cells and the epithelial cells to appear together in the same arrangement as the histologic features of this tumor. The branching pattern visible in *B* suggests the interposition of the lymphocytes. *A*, Diff-Quik × 375. *B*, Papanicolaou × 375.

In five cases, only oncocytic cells were identified, and oncocytoma was diagnosed. In four cases, the aspirate demonstrated only cell detritus and inflammatory cells. With practice and review of the slides, the authors were able to make a diagnosis of Warthin's tumor based on their observation of <u>oncocytic epithelium</u> present on the aspirate in 22 of the 33 cases.

A typical example of papillary cystadenoma lymphomatosum is illustrated in Figures 5–9 and 5–10. There is often a variable pattern of oncocytic epithelium and

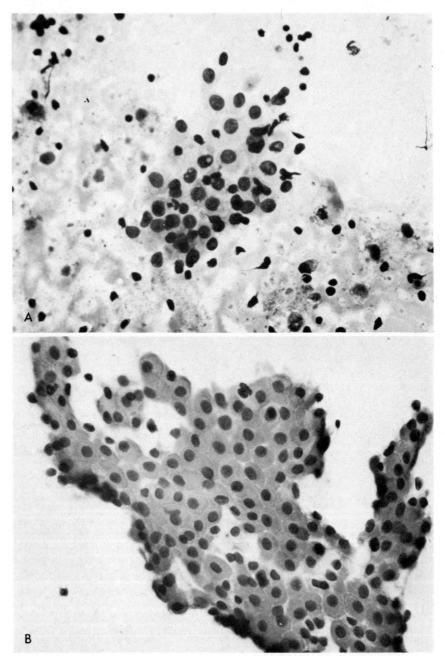

Figure 5–10   Papillary cystadenoma lymphomatosum (Warthin's tumor). An example of a smear with dissociation between the lymphoid elements, (A) and the oncocytic cells (B). The lymphoid cells mimic a germinal center, while the oncocytes occur in a flat sheet in this smear. A, Diff-Quik × 375. B, Papanicolaou × 375.

lymphocytes. In three of the five cases, the typical double-layered, brightly eosinophilic epithelium was seen in conjunction with lymphoid elements, making the diagnosis obvious. In the two other cases, the oncocytic cells predominated, with only a few scattered lymphocytes. The diagnosis in these cases is based solely on the observation of the oncocytic epithelium. It may not necessarily occur in the double-layer cellular arrangement; in fact, it is more likely to occur in sheets. Obviously, oncocytoma cannot be completely ruled out. Since oncocytoma is such a rare lesion, with essentially no clinical difference between it and Warthin's tumor, the distinction is not important.

Eneroth and Zajicek also noted the same differential diagnostic difficulty in a review of 45 cases of papillary cystadenoma lymphomatosum and four cases of oncocytoma. During a nine-year period extending from 1953 to 1962, the authors recognized only eight of 33 cases, but in the subsequent period from 1963 to 1964, 10 of 12 were diagnosed. Upon review of the original group of cases, they did find oncocytic epithelium in 24 of 33 cases. Nineteen of 45 cases in this series demonstrated no tumor cells in the specimen.[12]

There were no tumors diagnosed as oncocytoma in this author's experience. This neoplasm is very rare, accounting for less than 1 per cent of all parotid tumors. There were four cases in the series reported by Eneroth and Zajicek, and all four yielded abundant solid plugs of oncocytic cells similar to those seen in Warthin's tumor. Eneroth and Zajicek noted that the cytoplasmic granulation was much more intense in the oncocytoma than in the papillary cystadenoma lymphomatosum cases. In one of their patients, there was considerable nuclear pleomorphism among the oncocytes, but no statement was made as to whether this tumor behaved in an aggressive manner.[12] This author has not seen a malignant salivary gland oncocytoma.

MALIGNANT TUMORS

In the present series, carcinoma metastatic to the parotid salivary gland accounted for almost one third of the malignant epithelial tumors seen on aspiration biopsies. Metastatic melanoma and oat cell carcinoma represented two thirds of these metastases (Figs. 5–11 and 5–12). There were an equal number of primary anaplastic carcinomas and mucoepidermoid malignancies plus three recognizable squamous cell carcinomas, all of the latter occurring in the parotid salivary gland. This series is similar to that of Mavec and colleagues in terms of the number of metastatic carcinomas identified (13 of 32). Mavec observed a greater distribution of primary sites, but the majority of his cases were from primary salivary gland carcinomas that had grown into or metastasized to adjacent lymph nodes from which the aspirate was actually obtained.[2]

Mixed Tumors. Two malignant mixed tumors examined have been quite easy to diagnose, as they were very cellular aspirates that demonstrated obviously malignant features: large nucleoli and an irregular nuclear chromatin structure (Figs. 5–13 and 5–14). These neoplasms were clinically aggressive, as is typical of frankly malignant mixed tumors. In the short follow-up period to date, one tumor has already recurred twice and metastasized to regional lymph nodes and to the lung. In neither case was there evidence of any benign mixed tumor component in the aspirate or definitive myxoid or chondroid stroma. The aspirates were simply classified as carcinomas. A scant metachromatic background to the smear and a few spindle cells as well as cells with malignant features indicated a possible diagnosis of malignant mixed tumor. The number of cases in one reported series suggests that malignant mixed tumor has probably been overdiagnosed.[3] In another report, the carcinomas have been grouped with malignant mixed tumors; from a practical point of view, this classification is more realistic.[2]

Text continued on page 136

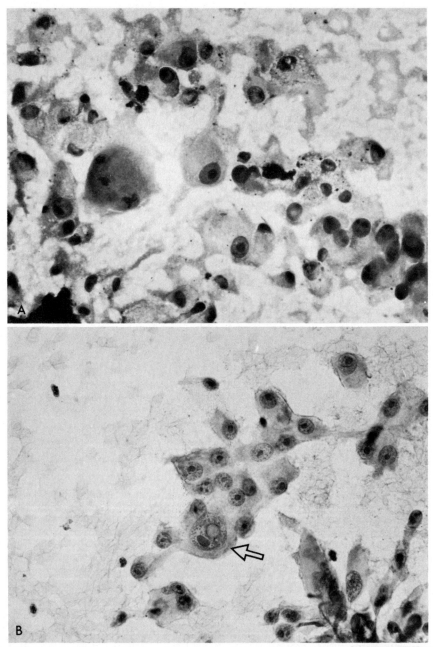

Figure 5–11 Malignant melanoma metastatic to the parotid gland. Some examples of the double-nucleus cell with prominent nucleoli. A bit of granular melanin pigment is present in a few cells in A. A very large intranuclear inclusion appears next to a large nucleolus in B (arrow). A, Diff-Quik × 375. B, Papanicolaou × 375.

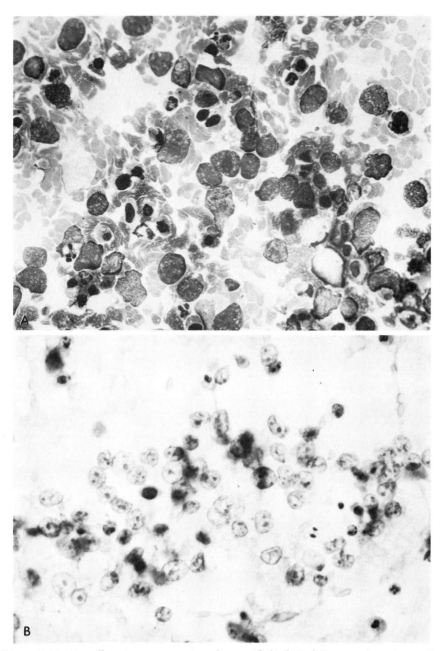

Figure 5–12   Oat cell carcinoma metastatic to the parotid gland. Undifferentiated neoplastic cells with some nuclear molding are seen in both smears. Clinical history of concurrent or prior oat cell carcinoma of the lung would be necessary to differentiate this tumor from an anaplastic salivary gland carcinoma. *A*, Diff-Quik × 375. *B*, Papanicolaou × 375.

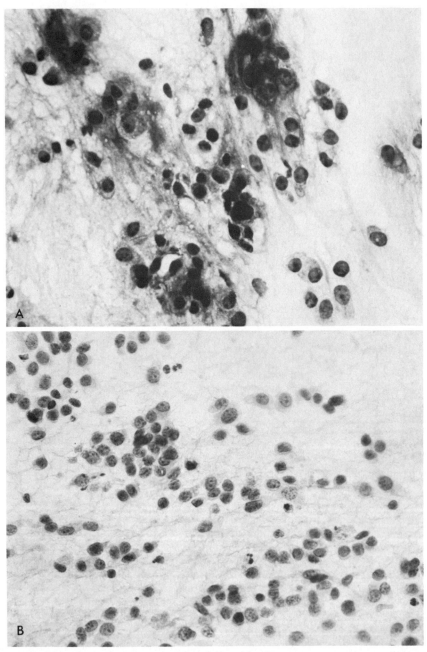

Figure 5–13   Malignant mixed tumor. Smears from a clinically aggressive parotid tumor demonstrating round epithelial cells, most of which have nucleoli. Some spindle-shaped cells and metachromasia of the background (A) suggest that this might be a malignant mixed tumor. A, Diff-Quik × 375. B, Papanicolaou × 375.

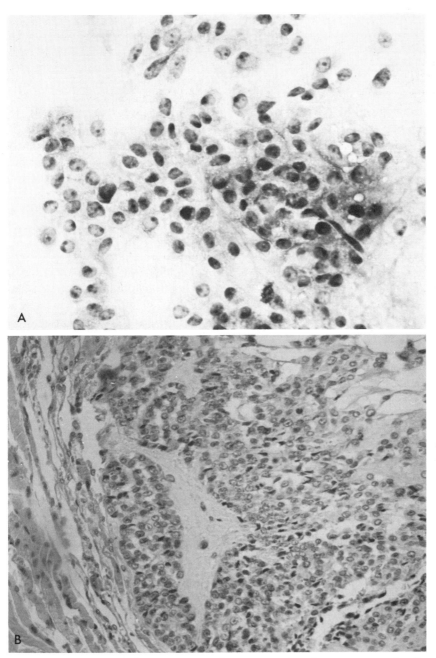

Figure 5–14 Malignant mixed tumor. Smear and comparative tissue from same case as that illustrated in Figure 5–13. In this particular field of the smear, nucleoli are more prominent. No features of this smear indicate that this neoplasm is specifically a malignant mixed tumor. An aspiration diagnosis of carcinoma is adequate. *A*, Diff-Quik × 375. *B*, Hematoxylin and eosin × 240.

Acinic-Cell Carcinoma.   In Mavec's series, the most common primary salivary gland carcinoma was the acinic cell variety, as was also true in several other series.[1-4] This is an uncommonly reported salivary gland tumor in the United States. This author has seen a single consultation case of acinic cell carcinoma in aspiration biopsy (Fig. 5–15). Noteworthy in that smear was the large number of cells with glassy intranuclear inclusions, a feature that is reminiscent of papillary carcinoma of the thyroid. Differentiating between the two would be difficult if the lesion were near the thyroid gland or in the upper cervical area, where it might be considered a metastatic papillary carcinoma from an occult thyroid primary. Acinic cell neoplasms, however, have PAS-positive granules that are not diastase resistant, indicating the presence of large amounts of glycogen.

Eneroth and colleagues have described in detail the cytomorphologic pattern of acinic cell carcinoma in a review of their 34 cases. Classification was somewhat difficult, since this tumor was originally considered benign in many instances. It is now believed to be a low-grade carcinoma. There appear to be no completely benign forms. The aspirates were described as semisolid and can be grouped into two categories: (1) those that demonstrated some cellular atypia but no obvious features of malignancy, and (2) those that demonstrated distinctly malignant features. The cytoplasm had a foamy appearance, strongly resembling that of normal acinic cells. They did not stain quite as brightly as oncocytes but had more of a blueish-gray hue. The clearly malignant features were pleomorphism of the nucleus and enlarged nucleoli.[10]

Woyke and colleagues have demonstrated that electronmicroscopy can be performed on the aspirate to identify multiple secretory granules in the neoplastic cells of acinic cell carcinoma. Woyke also found neoplastic cells without granules corresponding to the intercalated duct epithelium that can be found as a part of this neoplasm.[13] Another report has indicated the usefulness of transmission electronmicroscopy in differentiating acinic cell cancers from oncocytomas.[14]

Adenoid Cystic Carcinoma.   The present series contained only one case of adenoid cystic carcinoma, which arose in a parotid salivary gland. The aspirate demonstrated the expected cytomorphologic appearance, which was identical with the tissue pattern: uniform epithelial cells surrounding cylindrical masses of metachromatic and mucicarmine-positive mucopolysaccharide material (Fig. 5–16). This cytology was also found to be consistent for other sites. In one case, aspiration biopsy of a tumor of Bartholin's gland demonstrated the same typical pattern of adenoid cystic carcinoma, a very rare neoplasm for that site (Fig. 5–17).[15]

Eneroth and Zajicek reviewed the aspiration biopsy material from 45 cases of adenoid cystic carcinoma. Thirty-one of these aspirates were from primary lesions, three were from regional lymph nodes containing metastatic carcinoma, and 11 were from locally recurrent neoplasms. The difficulty in classification is evident in the division of the report into two series: (1) that conducted prior to reclassification of the adenoid cystic and acinic cell carcinomas as separate entities from variants of mixed salivary gland tumors, and (2) a second, later series.[16] Reclassification has also affected the overall results reported by Mavec and colleagues.[2] In Eneroth and Zajicek's series, for example, none of the adenoid cystic carcinomas was recognized specifically in the period extending from 1953 to 1965. Eight were regarded as carcinoma and 13 as pleomorphic adenomas, while one was thought to be only a cyst. In the subsequent period ranging from 1966 to 1967, eight were correctly diagnosed as primary lesions, 11 as recurrences, and three as metastatic masses. Only one lesion was incorrectly classified as pleomorphic adenoma. A review of the case in which the mass was classified as a cyst did reveal that there were cylinders of homogenous mucoid material as well as epithelial tumor cells. In this report, globules of mucus were seen in only 18 of 31 primary adenoid cystic carcinomas. Eight cases had only uniform tumor cells,

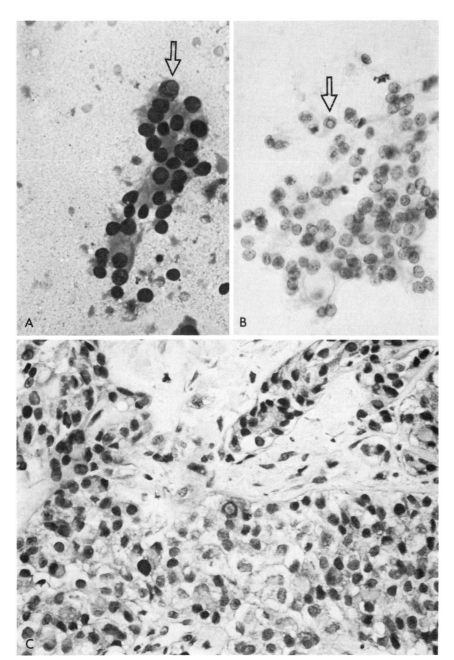

Figure 5–15   Acinic cell carcinoma. Aspirate from a carcinoma that recurred two years after excision of the original primary tumor. Note the uniform cells with their finely granular, lacy cytoplasm. No typical mixed tumor stroma is present. The cells themselves appear rather bland. Apparent in *A* and *B* are cells with glassy intranuclear inclusions (arrows). An intranuclear inclusion is also demonstrated in *C*, which illustrates a section of the original acinic cell carcinoma. Primary diagnosis of this tumor is difficult. *A*, Diff-Quik × 375. *B*, Papanicolaou × 375. *C*, Hematoxylin and eosin × 375. (Courtesy of Dr. L. Mohanty.)

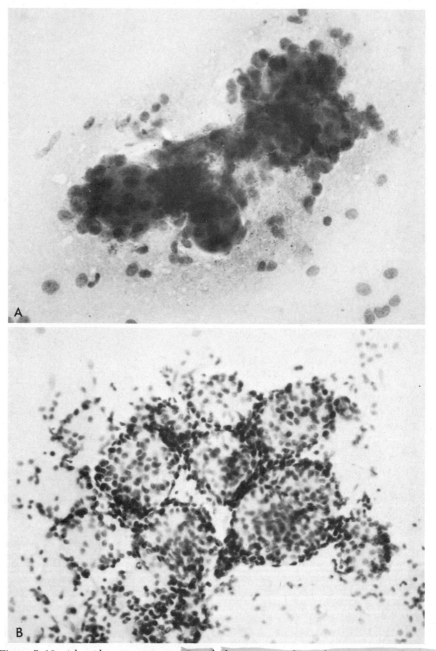

Figure 5–16   Adenoid cystic carcinoma. Round, dense masses of metachromatic mucopolysaccharide ground substance are covered by uniform small epithelial cells. Note the several ball-like masses of stroma and tumor cells in B. The diagnosis is based on the pattern of the smear and not on cytologic criteria for malignancy. A, Diff-Quik × 375. B, Papanicolaou × 240.

a finding that would make an exact classification difficult. The authors felt that the morphologic appearance of the cells, which demonstrated very scant cytoplasm and which were uniform and tightly packed in clusters, was diagnostic in itself.[16]

Mucoepidermoid Carcinoma.   Mucoepidermoid carcinomas, particularly low-grade tumors, may also present some problem in forming a diagnosis exclusively from aspiration biopsy. Sometimes, only cystic contents may be aspirated; other aspirations may extract cells that appear completely benign with histiocytic or benign squamous

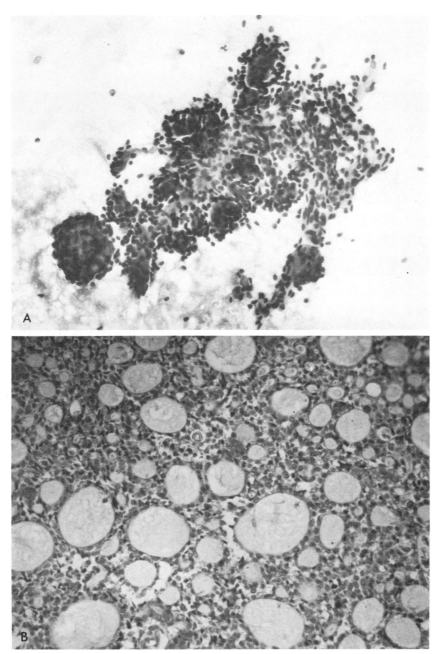

Figure 5–17   Adenoid cystic carcinoma of Bartholin's gland. Both the smear pattern and the histologic section show that the ball-like pattern of stroma and epithelial cells is consistent, regardless of the site at which this tumor originates. A, Diff-Quik × 310. B, Hematoxylin and eosin, × 240.

features. Differentiating this tumor from a mucocele or a ranula would be virtually impossible (Fig. 5–18). For comparison, a case of low-grade mucoepidermoid carcinoma is illustrated in Figure 5–5. The difficulty of differential diagnosis is documented in the series reported by Zajicek and colleagues, in which six of 11 cases of mucoepidermoid carcinoma encountered during the period ranging from 1953 to 1962 were diagnosed as cystic contents only, a false-negative rate of 55 per cent.[9] This author's four cases presented no problem except for one low-grade lesion that might easily

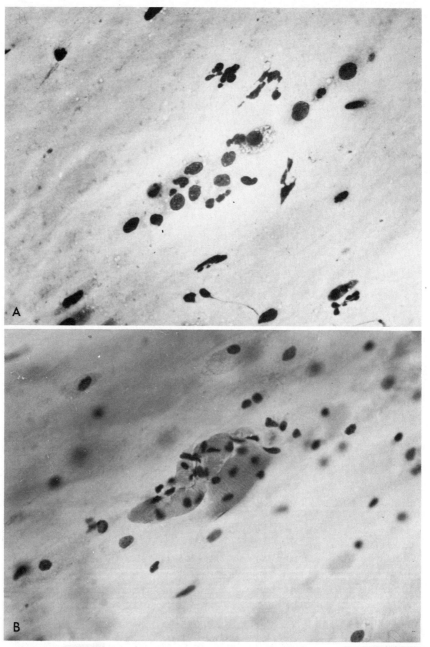

Figure 5–18   Mucocele of submaxillary gland. Abundant mucoid stroma contains a few epithelial cells with both finely vacuolated and dense cytoplasm. Note the resemblance of this pattern to that of low-grade mucoepidermoid carcinoma (Fig. 5–5), from which this lesion must be differentiated. If the mucocele cannot be completely evacuated or if it recurs after aspiration, it should be excised to avoid missing a low-grade carcinoma. A, Diff-Quik × 375. B, Papanicolaou × 375.

have been diagnosed as a pleomorphic adenoma if it were not clinically an obvious carcinoma. The metachromatic background failed to demonstrate any stromal cells (Fig. 5–5).

   With intermediate and high-grade mucoepidermoid carcinoma, the cytology is clearly that of a malignant tumor. The intermediate grade demonstrated in one case the clear cell appearance that has been described histologically (Figs. 5–19 and 5–20). The high-grade mucoepidermoid carcinomas (Fig. 5–21) are not distinguishable from poorly differentiated squamous cell malignant neoplasms, but they have larger cells than the typical undifferentiated anaplastic carcinomas (Figs. 5–22 and 5–23). Both

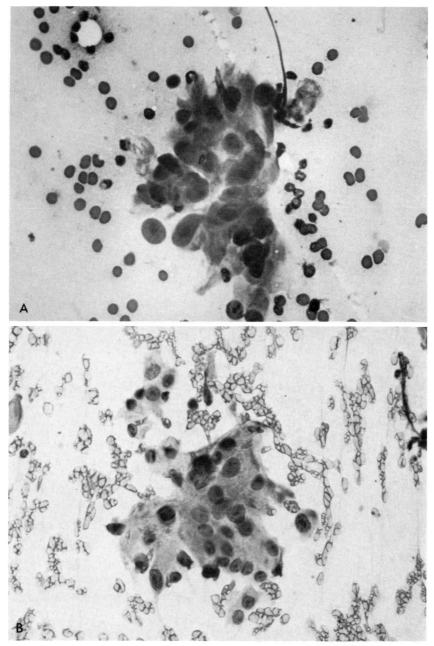

Figure 5–19 Mucoepidermoid carcinoma, intermediate grade. Tumor cells are more plentiful and pleomorphic than in low-grade mucoepidermoid carcinoma. The contrast between mucin-positive cells and squamous cells is not as obvious, but it can be identified by differences in density and vacuolization of the cytoplasm. These cytoplasmic variations are more apparent with Romanovsky stains. A, Diff-Quik × 375. B, Papanicolaou × 375.

cancers are usually clinically malignant. The aspiration biopsy merely confirms the undifferentiated nature of an aggressive salivary gland carcinoma. Distinction between these neoplasms and malignant mixed tumor is also arbitrary for the same reason.

Lymphoma. Malignant lymphoma involving the salivary glands has been a secondary lesion in two cases reported by this author. The monomorphic pattern of lymphocytes provides the best clue to the diagnosis. The cells also exhibit the pale nuclear centers described in Chapter 4 (Fig. 5–24). Only one other case of lymphoma was found in a reported series of salivary gland aspiration biopsies.[4] Details of that case are not provided.

Text continued on page 146

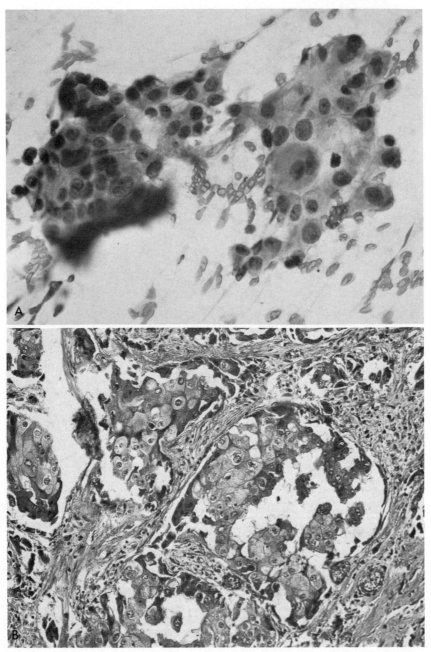

Figure 5–20 Mucoepidermoid carcinoma, intermediate grade. Another field of the smear from the case illustrated in Figure 5–19. Cell pleomorphism makes the diagnosis of malignancy relatively easy, but the exact classification of the tumor can not be determined unless the features of cells with sharp boundaries and the variable texture of the cytoplasm are appreciated. These characteristics of the intermediate grade of mucoepidermoid carcinoma are also apparent in the tissue pattern. A, Papanicolaou × 375. B, Hematoxylin and eosin × 150.

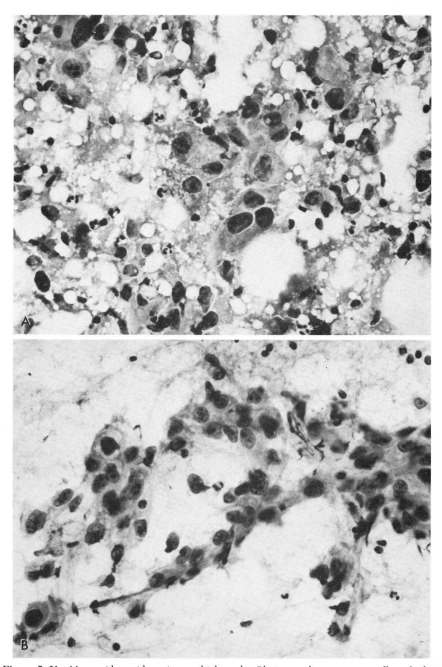

Figure 5–21 Mucoepidermoid carcinoma, high grade. Obvious malignant tumor cells with abnormal nuclear chromatin structure. Sheets of cells suggest a squamous cell carcinoma, but the lacy appearance of the cytoplasm favors the presence of some cells that might be positive for mucopolysaccharides. Tumors with this aggressive cytologic picture are usually clinically malignant, so an exact classification is not particularly important. *A*, Metachrome B × 375. *B*, Papanicolaou × 375.

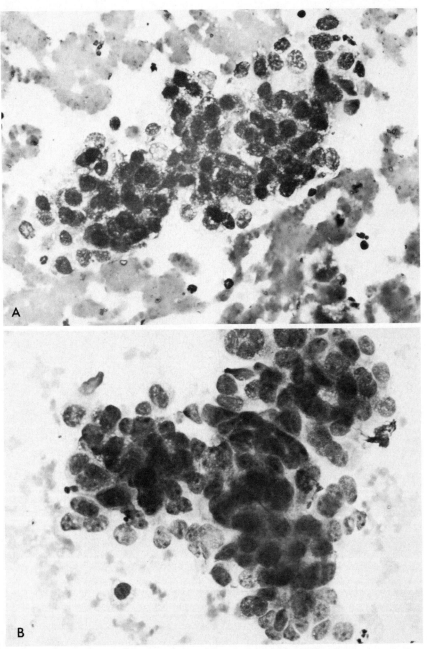

Figure 5–22   Anaplastic carcinoma. Undifferentiated malignant tumor cells with a very high nuclear-cytoplasmic ratio but with no other distinguishing features. This pattern appears in undifferentiated areas of malignant mixed tumors. A and B, Diff Quik × 375.

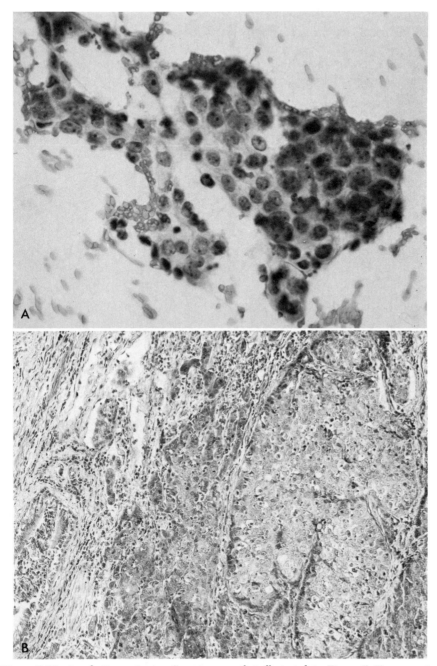

Figure 5–23 Anaplastic carcinoma. Same case as that illustrated in Figure 5–22, comparing the histologic section of an undifferentiated carcinoma with a Papanicolaou-stained smear. Sheets of malignant tumor cells have no definitive features that would identify this mass as anything other than anaplastic carcinoma. *A*, Papanicolaou × 375. *B*, Hematoxylin and eosin × 100.

OTHER CONDITIONS

Mesenchymal Tumors.   No mesenchymal tumors have been encountered by this author in the aspiration of salivary glands. Five mesenchymal tumors, four neurofibromas, and one lipoma were reported by Mavec and colleagues. Two of these demonstrated pleomorphism, suggesting sarcoma, but in each case the patient had received radiation prior to aspiration biopsy. The same two tumors were also considered neurofibromas; malignancy, suggested by the surgically removed specimen, was uncertain.[2] Whether these cases are actually tumors of the salivary gland is not known.

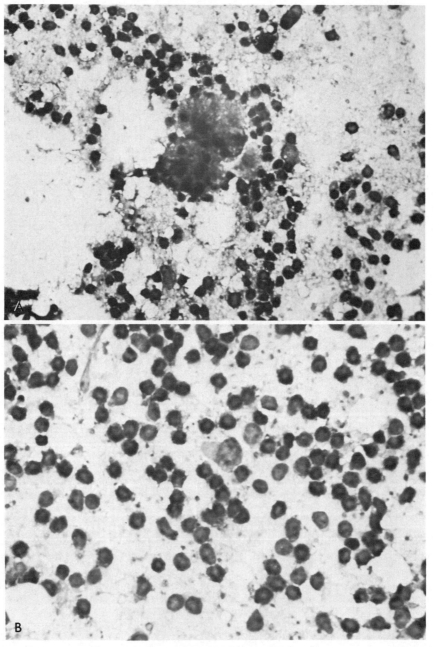

Figure 5–24   Non-Hodgkin's lymphoma, poorly differentiated lymphocytic, presenting as submaxillary swelling. Massive, bland lymphocytic infiltrate is visible in these smears. *A* depicts a small collection of salivary gland acinar cells showing some degeneration. The open, pale centers and immaturity of the lymphocytes are apparent in *B*. *A*, Diff-Quik × 375. *B*, Diff-Quik × 600.

Nontumerous Inflammation (Sialadenitis).   While a variety of processes may occur in salivary glands that are non-neoplastic, the only ones that can be broadly recognized, on the basis of aspiration biopsy, are inflammations. Many of these cases show nothing but normal salivary gland epithelium in small amounts (Fig. 5–25), while others reveal both salivary gland epithelium, some of it undergoing degeneration, and abundant inflammatory cells (Fig. 5–26). The basic objective, which is to rule out tumor, is accomplished by aspiration. Follow-up in this author's series has revealed no tumor, except in four cases in which the sialadenitis was concurrent with metastatic tumor to the parotid duct lymph node with duct obstruction. All the remaining patients

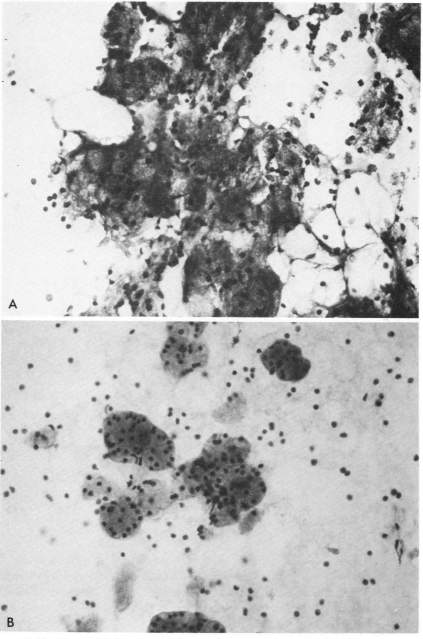

Figure 5–25   Chronic sialadenitis, mild. Aspirate from an enlarged parotid gland. Salivary gland acini with a surrounding infiltrate of lymphocytes are visible. Swelling of the salivary gland had occurred without clinically evident cause. A diagnosis of neoplasm was ruled out after aspiration was performed. *A*, Diff-Quik × 240. *B*, Papanicolaou × 240.

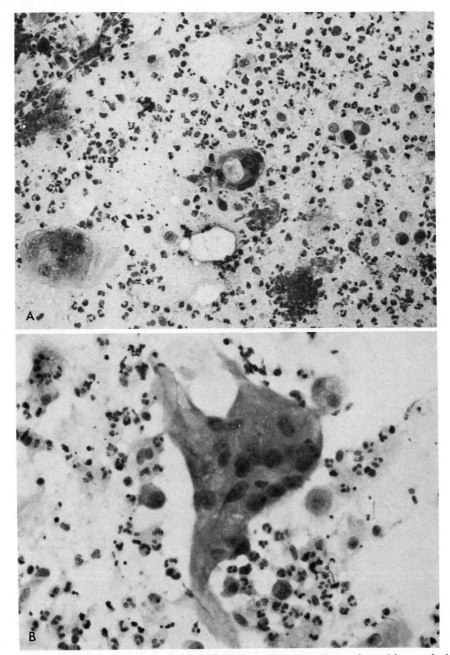

Figure 5–26 Acute and chronic sialadenitis. Aspirate from a swollen and painful parotid gland. Destruction of salivary gland cells and abundant exudate are evident. With strong clinical evidence of sialadenitis, aspiration biopsy of the salivary glands is not indicated. The pattern is easily distinguished from that of a neoplasm. *A,* Diff Quik × 240. *B,* Papanicolaou × 375.

had a benign course or surgical removal of the enlarged salivary gland demonstrated only sialadenitis.[17] The only other false-negative in the current series was a case of an ossified benign mixed tumor that had been present for more than 20 years and whose capsule could not be penetrated by the needle.

RESULTS OF SALIVARY GLAND ASPIRATIONS

This author's personal series is summarized in Table 5–1. Sensitivity for the presence of a neoplasm is 93 per cent; that is, tumor, either benign or malignant, was

TABLE 5–1.   THIN-NEEDLE ASPIRATION BIOPSY OF SALIVARY GLANDS

Aspirates	Parotid	Submaxillary	Sublingual	Accessory
Benign tumors	(34)	(12)	—	(3)
Mixed	30*	10	—	3
Warthin's	3	2	—	—
Other	2	—	—	—
Malignant tumors	(17)	(7)	—	(3)
Mixed	2	—	—	—
Squamous cell	3	—	—	1
Adenoid cystic	1	—	—	—
Mucoepidermoid	2	2	—	—
Anaplastic	2	3	—	1
Metastatic	7	—	—	1
Lymphoma	—	2	—	—
No tumor cells	27	11	1	—
Inflammation	35	32	2	1
Unsatisfactory	1	3	—	2
False-negative	(4)†	—	—	(1)
False-positive	(1)*	—	—	—
TOTALS	114	65	3	9

*Suspected mixed tumor that was sialadenitis.
†Small tumors causing obstruction of salivary gland duct with aspiration only of enlarged inflamed gland.

diagnosed in 75 of 81 cases. Specificity, the absence of a neoplasm, in this series is 99 per cent, accounting for 109 of 110 cases. Among the four cases of metastasis to the parotid lymph node with duct obstruction, persistence of clinical findings in the face of a benign aspiration diagnosis prompted exploration and discovery of the spread of tumor to the lymph node.

Upon review, the false-positive diagnosis of a benign mixed tumor was clearly erroneous: Only inflamed salivary gland epithelium was evident. This misinterpretation was based on observation of a degenerated stroma that revealed some confusing metachromasia without clearly identified chondroid cells. A second case, for a while considered a false-positive diagnosis, was a suspected anaplastic carcinoma. Sheets of degenerated small cells were obtained from a firm, nontender parotid mass that had been slowly enlarging for several months. None of the cells in the aspirate had the appearance of polymorphonuclear leukocytes, yet the diagnosis of the resected gland was abscess. Review of the histologic slides and multiple sections of the blocks revealed a central necrotic mass with a thick, fibrous outer wall. It was unclear, despite careful study, what this mass was. All the tissue showed only necrosis. The typical exudate of an abscess, however, was not present. Six months later, a mass appeared in the same area. Histologic diagnosis of that mass was poorly differentiated non-Hodgkin's lymphoma.

One other case, a potential false-positive, has been seen in consultation. The aspirate and subsequent surgical pathologic findings are depicted in Figure 5–27. The smears were obtained from aspiration of a soft, cystic, upper cervical mass present for some months in an elderly man. Head and neck examination was otherwise unremarkable. The smears contained many polymorphonuclear leukocytes as well as small sheets and single pleomorphic squamous cells. The cells appeared both dysplastic and degenerated. The necrotic background suggested a diagnosis of a cystic metastasis of squamous cell carcinoma. No definite malignant tumor cells could be seen. A biopsy was requested and carried out. The tumor was a papillary cystadenoma lymphomatosum with many areas of squamous metaplasia. Some of the metaplastic foci were atypical. Compare the cells of the aspirate with part of the metaplastic lining in this Warthin's tumor (Fig. 5–27). Also compare the cells in this aspirate with those from a true cystic metastasis of a squamous cell carcinoma to a cervical lymph node (see Chapter 4, Fig. 4–36).

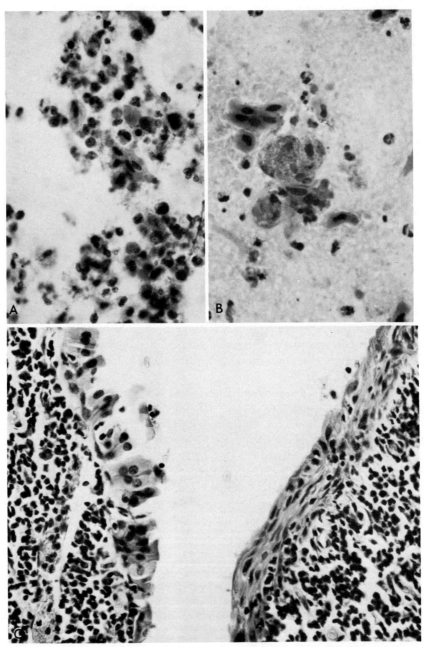

Figure 5–27 Papillary cystadenoma lymphomatosum with squamous metaplasia and focal atypia. Aspirate from an soft upper cervical mass in an elderly patient revealed much exudate and many small dysplastic squamous cells that appeared both singly and in sheets. No definitely malignant squamous cells were evident. A diagnosis of suspected metastatic squamous cell carcinoma with necrosis and cystic degeneration was made. Tissue removed at the requested biopsy revealed a Warthin's tumor with areas of squamous metaplasia and some atypia. Compare the cells in the aspiration smears with the metaplastic portion of this Warthin's tumor and also with a smear from proven cystic metastasis of squamous cell carcinoma (see Fig. 4–36). A, Diff-Quik × 375. B, Papanicolaou × 375. C, Hematoxylin and eosin × 375. (Courtesy of Dr. L. Mohanty.)

COMPLICATIONS OF SALIVARY GLAND ASPIRATIONS

Complications have not occurred in this series of aspiration biopsies of salivary gland tumors, even in those involving intraoral minor salivary gland masses. Mavec and colleagues noted an occasional small hematoma among a series of 652 aspirations that his group performed on salivary glands.[2]

Concern has been expressed with regard to aspiration biopsy of benign mixed tumors that tumor might be deposited in the needle track and so increase the risk of recurrences appearing after excision. Engzell and colleagues summarized their findings from 157 cases of benign mixed tumor treated surgically and followed for 10 years after fine-needle aspiration biopsy. There were three recurrences in this group of patients. Two of those were in patients considered to have had an original incomplete excision of their tumor. None of the recurrences involved the skin or the site of the aspiration.[18] In a personal communication from Eneroth, Mavec noted that in a study of seven cases of benign mixed tumor in which the needle track was excised with the tumor after aspiration, serial section of the track failed to reveal any tumor.[2] This author has yet to see any recurrence of benign mixed tumor in his own series.

REFERENCES

1. Zajicek, J., and Eneroth, C. M.: Cytological diagnosis of salivary-gland carcinomata from aspiration biopsy. Acta Otolaryngol. *263*:183–185, 1970.
2. Mavec, P., Eneroth, C. M., Franzen, S., et al.: Aspiration biopsy of salivary gland tumours. I. Correlation of cytologic reports from 652 aspiration biopsies with clinical and histologic findings. Acta Otolaryngol. *58*:472–484, 1964.
3. Eneroth, C. M., Franzen, S., and Zajicek, J.: Cytologic diagnosis on aspirates from 1000 salivary gland tumours. Acta Otolaryngol. (Suppl.) *224*:168–171, 1967.
4. Persson, P. S., and Zettergren, L.: Cytologic diagnosis of salivary gland tumors by aspiration biopsy. Acta Cytol. *17*:351–354, 1973.
5. Eneroth, C. M., and Zajicek, J.: Aspiration biopsy of salivary tumors. III. Morphological studies on smears and histologic sections from 368 mixed tumors. Acta Cytol. *10*:440–454, 1966.
6. Koivuniemi, A., Saksela, E., and Holopainen, E.: Cytological aspiration biopsy in otorhinolaryngological practice: A preliminary report with special reference to method. Acta Otolaryngol. *263*:189, 1970.
7. Droese, M., Tute, M., and Haubrich, J.: Aspiration biopsy cytology of salivary gland tumours. Laryngol. Rhinol. Otol. *56*:703–710, 1977.
8. Droese, M., Haubrich, J., and Tute, M.: The significance of aspiration cytology in the diagnosis of salivary gland tumors. Schwiez. Med. Wochenschr. *108*:933–935, 1978.
9. Zajicek, J., Eneroth, C. M., and Jakobsson, P.: Aspiration biopsy of salivary gland tumors. VI. Morphologic investigation on smears and histologic sections of 24 cases with mucoepidermoid carcinoma. Acta Cytol. *20*:35–41, 1976.
10. Eneroth, C. M., Jakobsson, P., and Zajicek, J.: Aspiration biopsy of salivary gland tumors. V. Morphologic investigation on smears and histologic sections of acinic cell carcinoma. Acta Radiol. (Suppl.)*310*:85–93, 1971.
11. Batsakis, J. G.: Basal cell adenoma of the parotid gland. Cancer *29*:226–230, 1972.
12. Eneroth, C. M., and Zajicek, J.: Aspiration biopsy of salivary gland tumors. II. Morphologic studies on smears and histologic sections from oncocytic tumors. Acta Cytol. *9*:355–361, 1965.
13. Woyke, S., Olszewski, W., Domagala, W., et al.: Cytodiagnosis of acinic cell carcinoma. Ultrastructural study of material obtained by fine needle aspiration biopsy. Acta Cytol. *19*:110–116, 1975.
14. Hagelqvist, E.: Light and electron microscopic studies on material obtained by fine needle biopsy. A methodological study on aspirates from tumours of the head and neck region with special emphasis 136
15. Frable, W. J., and Goplerud, D. R.: Adenoid cystic carcinoma of Bartholin's gland. Diagnosis by aspiration biopsy. Acta Cytol. *19*:152–153, 1975.
16. Eneroth, C. M., and Zajicek, J.: Aspiration biopsy of salivary gland tumors. IV. Morphologic studies on smears and histologic sections from 45 cases of adenoid cystic carcinoma. Acta Cytol. *13*:59–63, 1969.
17. Frable, W. J., and Frable, M. A. S.: Thin-needle aspiration biopsy. The diagnosis of head and neck tumors revisited. Cancer *43*:1541–1548, 1979.
18. Engzell, U., Esposti, P. L., Rubio, C., et al.: Investigation on tumor spread in connection with aspiration biopsy. Acta Radiol. *10*:385–398, 1971.

Chapter Six

Thyroid

ASPIRATION OF THYROID LESIONS

Needle biopsy of the thyroid gland has had a few proponents for some time. Vim-Silverman needle biopsy, however, has never become the general practice in the diagnosis of thyroid conditions.[1-6] Why tissue needle biopsy of this type has not been an accepted procedure is still unclear. Its proponents have reported few complications, and only one implant of a malignant tumor has been described.[1] Since the 1950's, Europeans have embraced wholeheartedly the fine-needle aspiration biopsy technique for thyroid lesions, particularly cold nodules. Some very large series have been reported.[7-18] The feasibility of this biopsy method is also recently attested to by American researchers. Some of these investigators employed both fine-needle aspiration biopsy and tissue needle biopsy in their series, basing their choice in each case on the clinical situation and the type of suspected disease..[19-24]

TECHNIQUE

The basic technique of fine-needle aspiration biopsy of the thyroid is similar to that performed on palpable lumps in other sites. There are a few additional technical considerations that include the availability of both scan imaging and ultrasonography for visualization of the thyroid as well as correct positioning of the patient to maximize both the prominence and exposure of an isolated nodule. This is the best accomplished by placing the patient in a supine position with a small pillow beneath the shoulders and upper back so that the neck is fully extended. Because this may prove to be uncomfortable for some patients, all preliminary examination of the thyroid is best completed prior to positioning. Slides as well as other equipment essential to performing the aspiration should also be in place.

A few thyroid nodules may actually be more prominent when the patient is sitting upright. Fine-needle aspiration can be performed with the patient in this position if there is an appropriate headrest on the back of the examining chair. This author has employed a small skin-marking pencil to outline the area of the mass in a manner that will allow the needle to traverse as little soft tissue as possible before entering the nodule. It is usually possible to avoid the sternocleidomastoid muscle with either lateral rotation of this muscle or extension of the neck so that the sternocleidomastoid does not have to be traversed during the aspiration.[20, 25]

Since the majority of thyroid masses, even single cold ones, are areas of goiter, the aspirate is likely to demonstrate blood in the hub of the syringe quite quickly. For this reason, a test needling has been advocated to determine the consistency of thyroid nodules.[26] The standard technique of aspiration described in Chapter 2 is usually quite rapid unless a very firm, fibrous process is encountered, as may be the case in Hashimoto's thyroiditis and in some tumors.[27]

After suitable smears are made, the remaining aspirate may be allowed to clot and a cell block prepared if a large amount of blood is obtained (see Chapter 2). Fluid aspirated from a cyst is processed using standard filter techniques or smears from the centrifuged specimen. When a cyst is encountered, every attempt is made to aspirate the lesion completely; afterwards, the patient should be carefully reexamined for any residual mass. As in breast aspirations, a repeat aspiration should be performed to sample any mass that remains.

This author's personal series includes 281 aspirations performed on 270 patients during the period ranging from 1973 through 1980. There were 21 unsatisfactory aspirations, six of which were satisfactorily repeated and yielded suitable material. The principal failure in these unsatisfactory aspirations is missing the lesion. In the clinical follow-up to date, no tumors have been overlooked in the remaining 15 patients who did not have repeat aspirations. The majority of the aspirations were performed on four common non-neoplastic conditions: nodular goiter, toxic hyperplasia, thyroiditis, and cysts.[28]

NONNEOPLASTIC LESIONS

Nodular Goiter. Whether they occur as multiple or single masses, nodular areas of colloid or adenomatous goiter are the most commonly encountered lesions in fine-needle aspiration biopsy. The aspiration smears may appear disappointing because they are relatively acellular, particularly if the goiter is predominantly composed of large colloid-filled follicles. Thyroid epithelium is found in sheets or small clusters. The individual thyroid cells are quite uniform (Fig. 6–1). There is much intervening blood and colloid. As Zajicek, Franzen, and others have emphasized, if colloid is seen on an aspiration smear of the thyroid, the presumption is that the mass is benign and not a true neoplasm. This rule proves extremely useful and practical although it is not absolute.[20, 25, 26] Colloid material will stain bluish-purple with Romanovsky stains and is variably stained orange, green, or yellow with the Papanicolaou stain. It lies in free masses, but, occasionally, whole thyroid acini containing a central mass of colloid will appear (Fig. 6–2).

Many histiocytes (Fig. 6–3), some with hemosiderin pigment, will be found in aspirates from goiter and reflect areas of hyperplasia with involution and old hemorrhage. Sheets of fibroblasts may also be found when there is cystic degeneration and areas of old hemorrhage. This mixed pattern of cellular elements with blood and colloid is the typical picture of nodules of goiter, regardless of whether they are multiple or single. When studying the several illustrations presented, one should remember that the cellular elements being emphasized occur in a wide background of blood and colloid. The overall pattern of aspirates from goiters is relatively acellular.

Toxic Hyperplasia. Because the clinical and biochemical findings are so classic, it is not usually necessary to aspirate toxic hyperplasia (Graves' disease). In the few cases that this author has encountered, the thyroid epithelium has been uniform, but nuclear size has been variable (Fig. 6–4). There may be some colloid, but it is rather thin and scanty. The cytoplasm of thyroid cells in Graves' disease has been described as finely vacuolated, and the vacuoles are small and nearly invisible.[25] With the absence of colloid, the differential diagnosis would involve follicular neoplasms.[29] The clinical picture of generalized thyroid enlargement should make the diagnosis of toxic goiter relatively easy. One investigator has described thyroid cells with nuclear segmentation. This finding is more frequently seen in toxic goiter than in nontoxic

Text continued on page 158

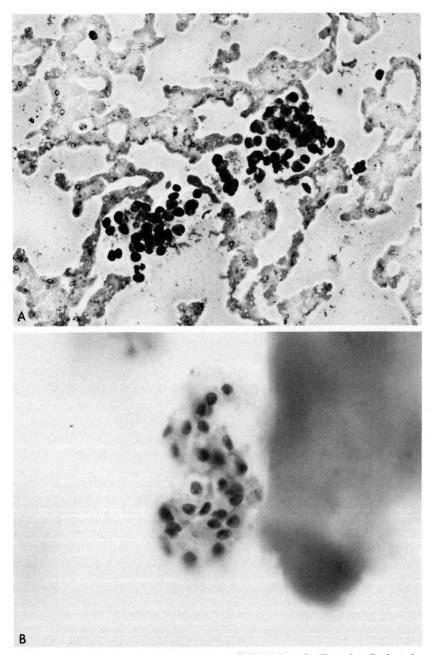

Figure 6–1 Colloid goiter. Sheets and clusters of uniform thyroid cells with colloid. *A* depicts the colloid as a diffuse background mixed with blood. In *B*, the colloid is a homogeneous gray mass adjacent to the epithelium. *A*, Diff-Quik ×375. *B*, Papanicolaou ×375.

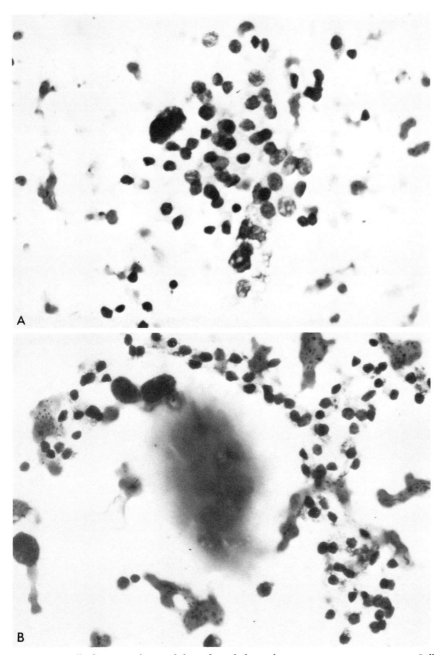

Figure 6–2 Colloid goiter. Sheets of thyroid epithelium showing some variation in size. Colloid is present in several foci, with the largest inspissated mass partly surrounded by thyroid epithelium in *B* (center). *A,* Diff-Quik × 375. *B,* Papanicolaou × 375.

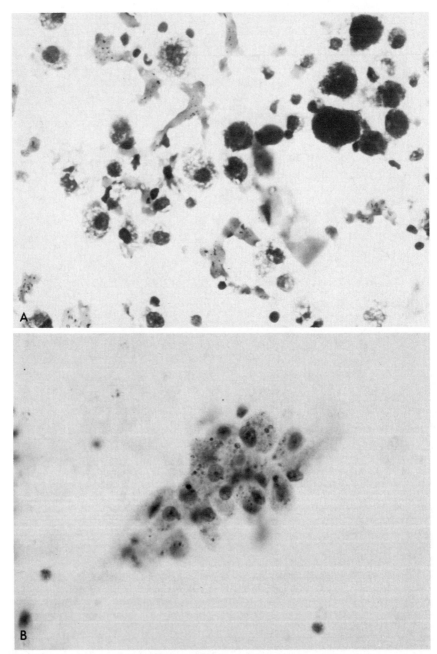

Figure 6–3   Colloid goiter. Histiocytes predominate in both *A* and *B*, with some masses of colloid present in the upper right of *A*. Hemosiderin pigment is visible in the histiocytes in *B*. *A*, Diff-Quik × 375. *B*, Papanicolaou × 375.

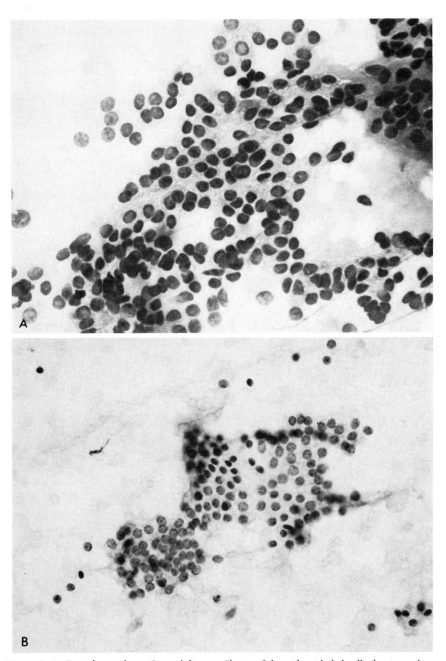

Figure 6–4   Toxic hyperplasia, Graves' disease. Sheets of thyroid epithelial cells dominate the smears without visible evidence of colloid. The cytoplasm has a finely vacuolated texture. This smear pattern cannot be differentiated from adenoma without clinical and laboratory data. *A*, Diff-Quik ×375. *B*, Papanicolaou ×375.

forms.[36] This author has not been able to find this differential feature in the few cases so far encountered.

Hashimoto's Thyroiditis.   If a patient presents with typical features of Hashimoto's thyroiditis, aspiration biopsy will easily confirm this diagnosis. The smear reveals abundant lymphocytes with focal collections of degenerating thyroid cells. In some areas, the lymphocytes will appear to be attached to the thyroid cells (Fig. 6–5). The cellular infiltrate is mixed: Not only lymphocytes but also plasma cells and large, pale,

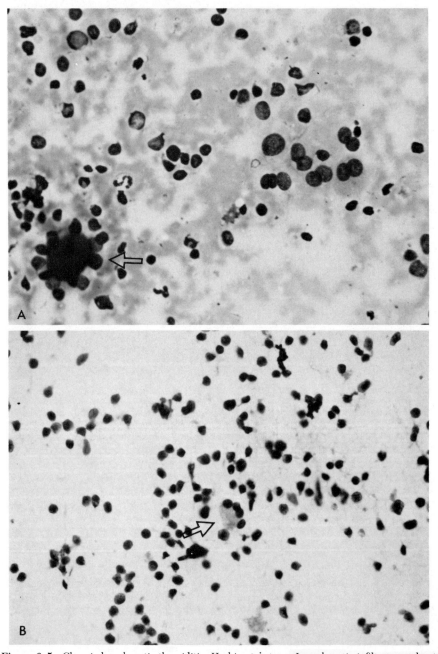

Figure 6–5   Chronic lymphocytic thyroiditis, Hashimoto's type. Lymphocytic infiltrate predominates in both smears, with degenerating thyroid follicle also present (arrows). *A*, Diff-Quik × 375. *B*, Papanicolaou × 375.

lightly metachromatic cells with lobulated nuclei and abundant cytoplasm are present (Fig. 6–6). These latter cells are the oncocytic, or Askanazy, cells that are found in histologic sections of Hashimoto's thyroiditis. Essentially no colloid is present on these smears. If both lobes are enlarged, the bilaterality of the disease can be confirmed by performing several aspiration biopsies. The pattern is usually quite uniform.

Some authors prefer tissue needle biopsy for cases of Hashimoto's thyroiditis, whereas others believe that needle biopsy is not a good idea because of the potential

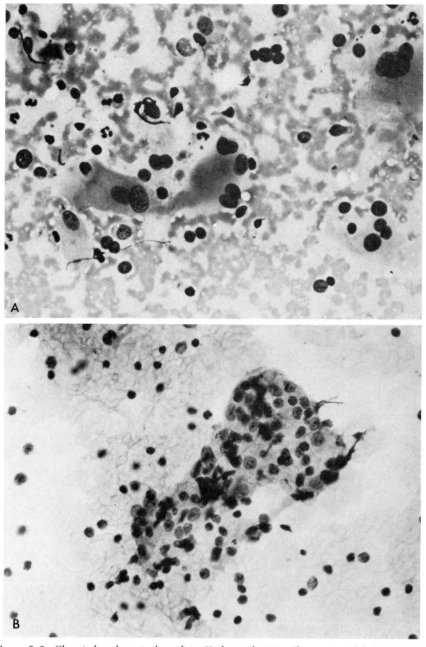

Figure 6–6 Chronic lymphocytic thyroiditis, Hashimoto's type. Characteristic lobulated or multinucleated oncocytic (Askanazy) cells or both are seen in the center and upper right of the illustrations. These cells are conspicuous in aspirates from typical cases of Hashimoto's thyroiditis. A, Diff-Quik ×375. B, Papanicolaou ×375.

of missing a carcinoma.[2, 31] In the series of Crile, the number of carcinomas ultimately detected in the Hashimoto's group was small, and they were all incidental findings.[2] Other authors think that fine-needle aspiration biopsy in cases of both Hashimoto's and nonspecific thyroiditis is very useful.[16, 32, 33] In this author's tabulated series, (Table 6–1), the aspiration biopsy picture is quite typical, with diffuse enlargement of the thyroid due to Hashimoto's disease. In a localized area of similar involvement, the pattern may or may not be diagnostic, but, usually, some lymphocytic and plasma cell infiltrate is noted on the aspiration. In the single nodules, the number of Askanazy cells may be low. Occasionally, atypical cells may also appear (Figs. 6–7 and 6–8). These regressive cell changes that occur in a variety of non-neoplastic thyroid diseases are well described in the monograph of Droese.[29]

Nonspecific Thyroiditis. Acute and chronic thyroiditis may present a rather nonspecific smear pattern. The diagnosis is based on both clinical features and cytopathologic consistency. This author has not had any experience with acute suppurative or subacute thyroiditis, but several investigators believe that these patterns are sufficiently specific for accurate cytologic diagnosis.[25, 33] In this author's personal reports of cases of localized chronic thyroiditis, scattered sheets or clusters of thyroid epithelial cells were mixed with a sprinkling of lymphocytes and plasma cells. Oxyphil cells were observed rarely or not at all. In nonsuppurative cases of acute thyroiditis, there were small numbers of thyroid epithelial cells in either a scant or relatively

TABLE 6–1.   THIN-NEEDLE ASPIRATION BIOPSY OF THE THYROID

	Correct Diagnosis	False-Positive	False-Negative
Neoplasms			
Benign	(19)	—	—
Follicular adenoma	17	(3)*	—
Hürthle cell adenoma	1	—	—
Schwannoma	1	—	—
Malignant	(24)	—	—
Follicular carcinoma vs. adenoma	4	—	—
Papillary carcinoma	7	(1)†	—
Hürthle cell carcinoma	1	—	—
Medullary carcinoma	1	—	—
Giant-cell and anaplastic carcinoma	8	—	—
Metastatic carcinoma	2	—	(1)‡
Lymphoma	1	—	(1)§
Non-neoplastic lesions			
Goiter	113	—	(3)‖
Hyperplasia	5	—	—
Normal thyroid	33	—	—
Cysts	23	—	—
Thyroiditis	(43)	—	—
Lymphocytic (Hashimoto's)	15	—	—
Acute	2	—	—
Chronic nonspecific	24	—	(1)**
Granulomatous	2	—	—
Unsatisfactory aspirations	21	—	—
Total aspirations	281	—	—

*Three cases of diagnosis of adenoma proved to be goiter.
†One case diagnosed as papillary carcinoma proved to be adenoma with intranuclear inclusions.
‡Unsatisfactory aspiration on first attempt. Correct diagnosis made on repeat aspiration.
§Aspiration diagnosis of Hashimoto's thyroiditis proved at open biopsy to be lymphosarcoma.
‖Two diagnoses of goiter proved to be adenoma. One goiter patient had occult thyroid cancer in the same lobe.
**Diagnosis of chronic thyroiditis in one patient in whom a small adenoma was found after thyroid lobectomy.

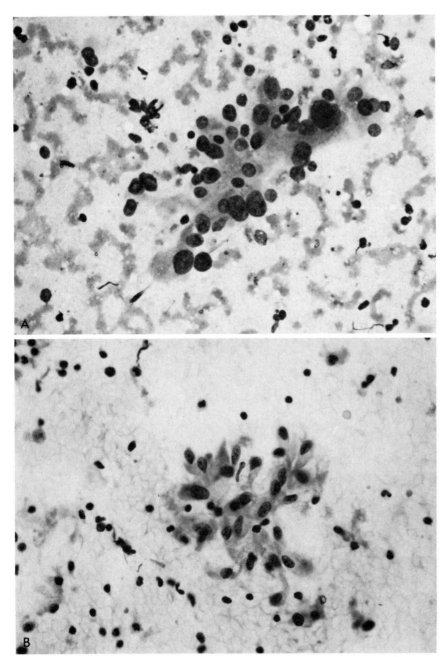

Figure 6–7 Chronic lymphocytic thyroiditis with regressive atypia. Atypical oncocytic cells with variation in size and shape in one field of an otherwise typical case of Hashimoto's thyroiditis (A). Spindle-shaped cells in another field from the same case (B). Cells in B suggest the general type of atypia seen in regeneration and repair. They could be either thyroid epithelial cells or fibroblasts. A, Diff-Quik × 375. B, Papanicolaou × 375.

abundant background of polymorphonuclear leukocytes. Aspirates from both chronic nonspecific and nonsuppurative acute thyroiditis tend to be mixed with a great deal of blood and also some colloid. The very clinically active thyroiditis in the present series demonstrated both inflammatory exudate and sheets of fibroblasts. In all cases of thyroiditis, the basic purpose of aspiration biopsy is to confirm the clinical diagnosis. Thus, an open biopsy or more extensive surgery is avoided, and the patient is reassured.

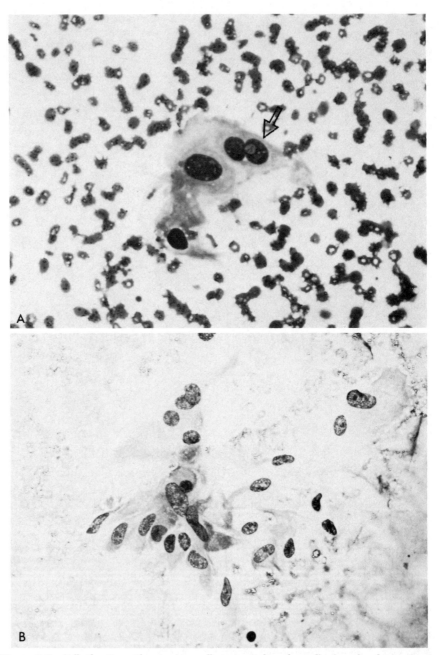

Figure 6–8   Colloid goiter with regressive cell atypia. Enlarged spindle-shaped and irregular thyroid epithelial cells from aspirate of a patient with nodular colloid goiter. Note that one cell has a glassy intranuclear inclusion (arrow). Such findings are not restricted to neoplasms or only cases of papillary thyroid carcinoma. A, Diff-Quik × 375. B, Papanicolaou × 375.

Cysts.   Morphologically, the least rewarding aspiration biopsy of a thyroid nodule is that of a cyst. However, this disadvantage is outweighed by the clinical usefulness of the procedure, which usually results in complete evacuation and elimination of the cyst. Hence, surgery is avoided. This author has aspirated 23 thyroid cysts followed from a period of six months to four years. Four cysts have recurred to date. Three incompletely evacuated cysts were later excised and proved to be cystic degeneration of colloid goiters.

The contents of cysts are usually produced by old hemorrhage and degeneration

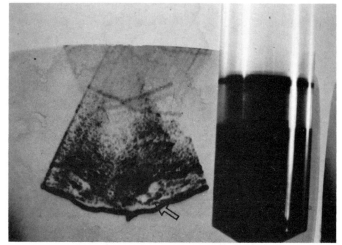

Figure 6–9   Thyroid cyst. Fluid removed from thyroid cyst detected with ultrasonography as two lucent areas in the left lobe (arrow). The cyst is greatly reduced in size on the ultrasonographic image. It contained about 15.0 ml of dark brown fluid.

within colloid and adenomatous goiter and appear as a turbid brown fluid or, occasionally, as a fluid that is clear, cloudy, or yellow. Most of the cells found in cyst fluid are histiocytic (macrophage) type and contain cytoplasmic deposits of hemosiderin. Rarely, thyroid epithelium may be found. It should be studied carefully for any indication of neoplastic alterations, specifically intranuclear inclusion bodies. Their presence might indicate papillary carcinoma of the thyroid, which may in part be cystic.[34-36] Crile prefers to inject sclerosing solution into cysts after aspiration, but the therapeutic value of this procedure is not established.[1, 3] Use of ultrasonography for evaluation of thyroid nodules in determining whether they are solid or cystic is quite helpful (Fig. 6–9).[36, 37]

NEOPLASTIC LESIONS

In most series of cold thyroid nodules, new growths account for about one fourth of the cases.[38] Therefore, there is great potential for a simple diagnostic technique such as fine-needle aspiration biopsy to detect those patients who truly require surgical excision of a nonfunctioning nodule. This has been the major thrust of needle biopsy of both tissue and aspiration type.[3, 5, 39]

Follicular Neoplasms. Were it not for the close resemblance between follicular adenomas and low-grade follicular carcinoma of the thyroid, thin-needle aspiration biopsy would probably be extremely accurate. This differential diagnosis is by far the most difficult with aspiration smears, but it is also difficult from a histologic point of view, depending almost exclusively on the demonstration of vascular invasion for the diagnosis of carcinoma. The majority of authors agree that it is not possible to differentiate between these two neoplasms on the basis of the aspiration biopsy smear alone.[8, 9, 22, 25, 39, 41, 42] There is, however, some disagreement on this point. Krisch, who used morphometric diameter of the nuclei as an indicator of malignancy in follicular neoplasms, and Lang and colleagues, who used very fine cytologic criteria, successfully made the differential diagnosis.[14, 43] Springer and colleagues measured nuclear DNA in aspiration biopsy smears from low-grade follicular carcinoma and follicular adenoma and found no difference in values or predominance of polyploidy in the carcinoma smears.[44] Because differentiating between these two tumors is difficult with even the most sophisticated cytologic methods, the preferred report in such cases is "follicular neoplasm, adenoma versus low-grade follicular carcinoma." Several examples of both these neoplasms are illustrated in Figures 6–10, 6–11, 6–12, and 6–13. Compare the adenoma aspiration smears with those of low-grade follicular carcinoma.

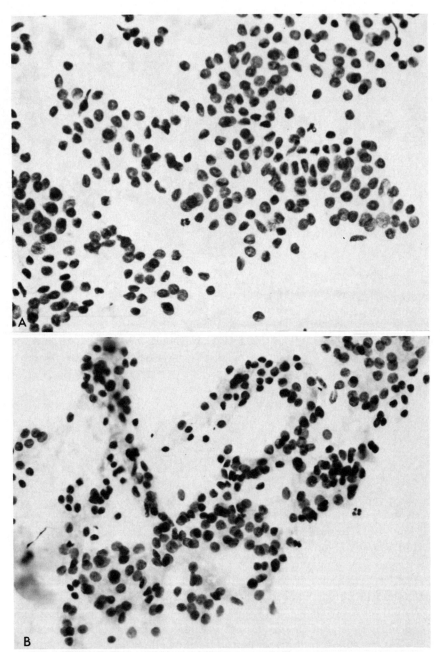

Figure 6–10 Follicular neoplasm, adenoma. Sheets of thyroid epithelium without evidence of colloid. A microfollicle pattern is present in the spindle-shaped cells in another field from the same case (*B*). Cells in *B* suggest the general type of atypia seen in regeneration and repair. *A*, Diff-Quik × 375. *B*, Papanicolaou × 375.

Thin-needle aspiration biopsies from adenomas, low-grade follicular carcinomas, or other definite thyroid cancers are usually <u>highly cellular</u> and <u>have no colloid</u>. With follicular adenoma, the nuclei appear slightly larger than those of normal thyroid epithelium. Uniform nucleoli are present but not in every cell. Chromatin structure tends to be finely granular and similar for follicular adenoma and low-grade follicular carcinoma. It is not surprising, therefore, that the measurements of the nuclear DNA have failed to reveal any significant differences between the two tumors.

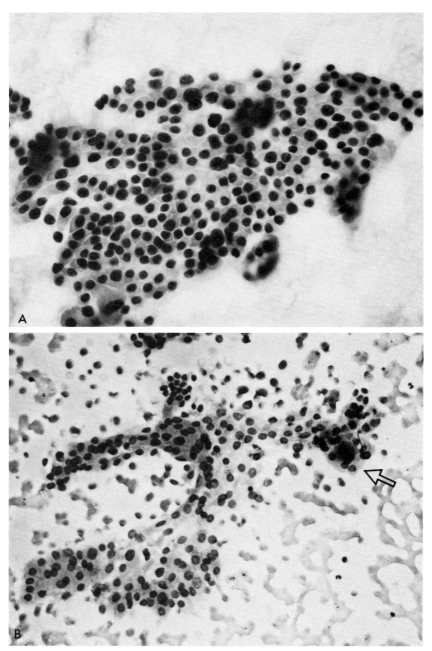

Figure 6–11 Follicular neoplasm, adenoma. Another example of an aspirate of follicular adenoma demonstrating more variation in cell size and shape. A microfollicle pattern is visible, and one follicle contains colloid (*B*, arrow). *A*, Diff-Quik ×375. *B*, Papanicolaou ×375.

This author has aspirated 17 nodules that were reported as follicular neoplasms strongly resembling adenomas. Of these diagnoses, 14 were correct and corroborated by histologic studies. There were three cases diagnosed as adenoma that proved to be only adenomatous goiter. In all these aspirations, the smears were cellular; however, there was scant but definite evidence of colloid. As has been pointed out, the presence of some colloid is a consistent finding among some aspirations of goitrous nodules, regardless of the cellularity. One of two Hürthle cell adenomas was recognized specifically. The aspiration from the second tumor did not have many of the cells with

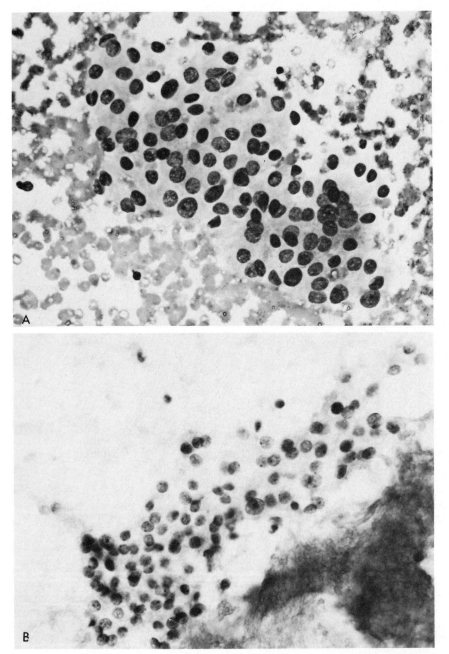

Figure 6–12   Follicular neoplasm, low-grade follicular carcinoma. Sheets of cells vary somewhat in size but do not differ from those seen in follicular adenoma aspirates. Slightly more distinct chromatin pattern and presence of nucleoli are evident, but these features do not reliably distinguish follicular adenomas from carcinomas. Red blood cells and fibrin, rather than colloid, are apparent in the lower right of *B. A,* Diff-Quik × 375. *B,* Papanicolaou × 375.

abundant granular cytoplasm that are typical of the Hürthle cell neoplasm. That case was reported as a follicular neoplasm.

There were four cases in this series reported as adenoma versus low-grade follicular carcinoma. All of them proved to be carcinoma, a result that has been consistent with the findings of other authors, even though this neoplasm is difficult to predict definitively. What is important in this series is that all these nodules were

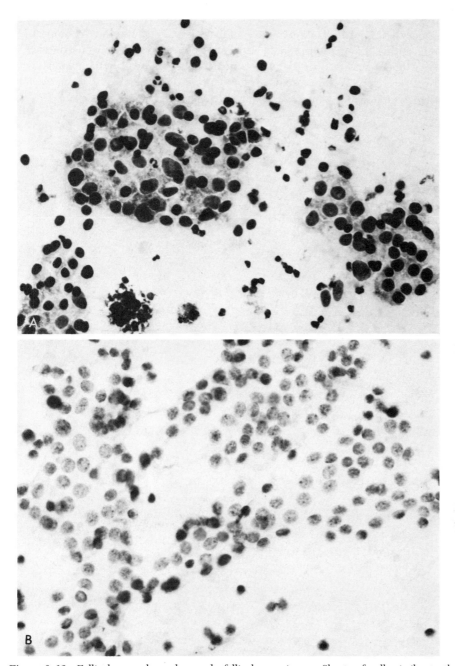

Figure 6–13 Follicular neoplasm, low-grade follicular carcinoma. Sheets of cells similar to those illustrated in Figure 6–12 but from a different case. Some variation in size and shape of the cells is evident. The fixed, Papanicolaou-stained smear demonstrates a distinct chromatin pattern throughout most of the nuclei *(B)*. A, Diff-Quik × 375. B, Papanicolaou × 375.

cold, single thyroid masses. The aspiration biopsy reinforced the decision to remove them surgically. It cannot be overemphasized that this is the principal function of aspiration biopsy in cold thyroid tumors.[10, 12, 21-23, 39, 45]

Non-Hodgkin's Lymphoma. The other malignant neoplasms of the thyroid are usually easily recognized. This author has experience with at least one case of each variety, including one non-Hodgkin's lymphoma. Unfortunately, this condition was the first thyroid case in this series of aspiration biopsies. It was incorrectly interpreted and reported as Hashimoto's thyroiditis. In retrospect, it is clear that with more experience with the aspiration biopsy of lymph nodes involved by non-Hodgkin's lymphoma, this neoplasm would have easily been recognized. Non-Hodgkin's lymphoma of the thyroid has been diagnosed correctly by other cytopathologists.[12, 25] The smear pattern in this case demonstrated a uniform population of small but very abnormal lymphocytes with no cellular cohesion (Fig. 6–14). This lack of cohesion

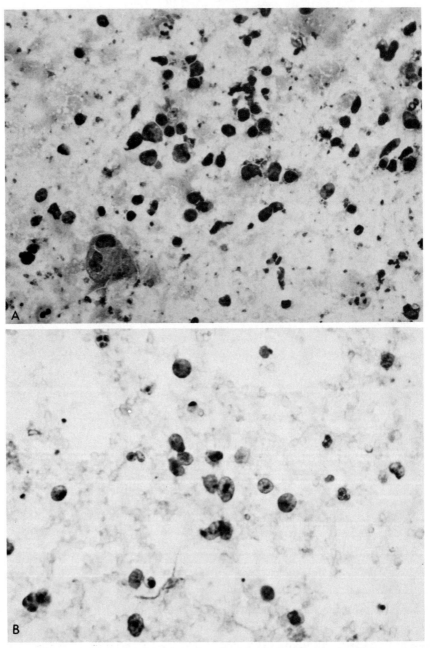

Figure 6–14 Lymphosarcoma of the thyroid. Scattered individual lymphoid cells varying in size and shape are visible. The pattern simulates that of Hashimoto's thyroiditis, with the cell in the lower left of *A* thought to be an Askanazy cell. Note the marked nuclear atypia and prominent angular nucleoli illustrated in some of the cells in *B*. These cells should have been the clue to the correct diagnosis of lymphosarcoma. *A*, Diff-Quik × 375. *B*, Papanicolaou × 600.

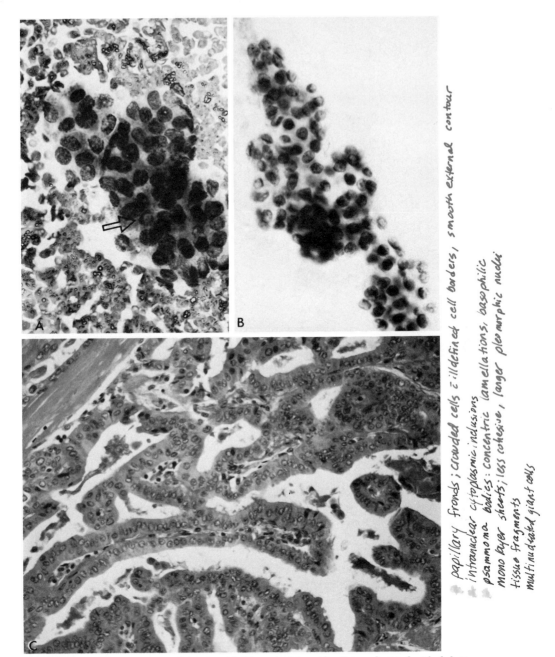

papillary fronds; crowded cells c̄ ill-defined cell borders, smooth external contour
intranuclear cytoplasmic inclusions
psammoma bodies: concentric lamellations, basophilic
mono layer sheets; less cohesive, larger pleomorphic nuclei
tissue fragments
multi nucleated giant cells

Figure 6–15 Papillary carcinoma of the thyroid. Clusters of thyroid cells are depicted with definite depth of focus present in the fixed smear (*B*). <u>Intranuclear inclusion</u> is apparent in *A* (arrow). *A*, Diff-Quik × 375. *B*, Papanicolaou × 375. *C*, Hematoxylin and eosin × 240.

would rule against a diagnosis of anaplastic small-cell carcinoma. Almost every cell in the smear had a prominent nucleolus. No oxyphil cells or plasma cells were detected. Many of the lymphoid cells in the Romanovsky-stained smear demonstrated pale centers, a consistent finding in lymph node aspirates from non-Hodgkin's lymphoma. The usefulness of this artefact has been discussed previously (see Chapter 4). Because the clinical course in this patient continued to be severe dyspnea, an open biopsy was promptly performed and revealed the correct diagnosis. The bilateral swelling of the thyroid and the symptoms of tracheal compression responded quickly to radiation therapy.

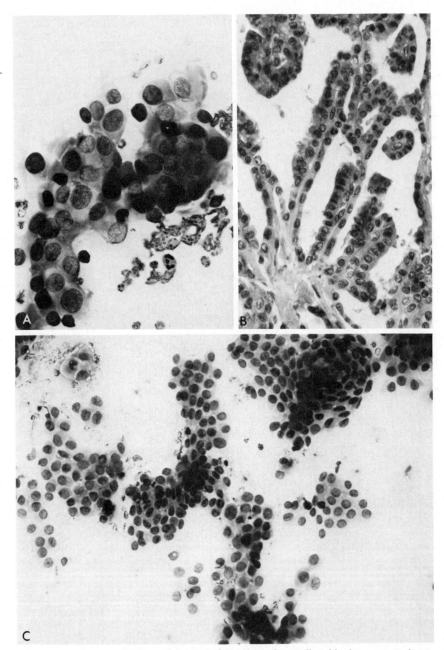

Figure 6–16   Papillary carcinoma of the thyroid. Compare the papillary-like fragments in the aspiration smears with the tissue pattern. Intranuclear inclusions were few in these aspirates but significant ones are seen in a few cells in *B*. *A*, Diff-Quik × 375. *B*, Hematoxylin and eosin × 375. *C*, Papanicolaou × 240.

Papillary Carcinoma.   Papillary carcinoma is probably one of the easiest tumors to diagnose by aspiration biopsy because its smear may contain two important identifying features: (1) three-dimensional papillary fragments, and (2) some cells with characteristic intranuclear inclusions ("Orphan Annie" nuclei).[46] Kini and colleagues analysed 87 surgically confirmed cases of papillary thyroid cancer and found four features of aspiration biopsy smears important to the correct cytologic diagnosis: (1) monolayered sheets, (2) tissue fragments, (3) psammoma bodies, and (4) multinucleated giant cells.[47]

The general pattern of the smears reveals a total <u>absence of colloid</u> and many sheets as well as true clusters of thyroid cells. The cells may not always appear in papillary formation. One therefore cannot rely exclusively on this particular feature. Hence, the consistent appearance of some cells with <u>glassy intranuclear inclusions</u> is extremely important. This author has found them in all his cases of papillary thyroid carcinoma, while Christ and Haja found them in 16 of 18 cases.[48] Several examples, with variations in smear pattern of papillary carcinoma of the thyroid, are illustrated in Figures 6–15 to 6–18.

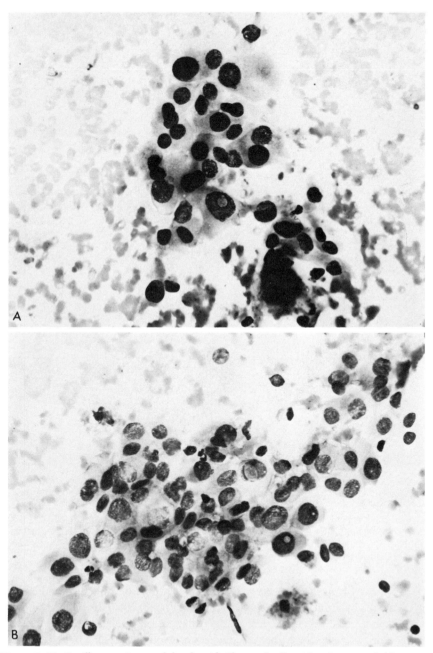

Figure 6–17 Papillary carcinoma of the thyroid. <u>Sheets of cells with rather remarkable variation in size and shape.</u> Several cells in both *A* and *B* have excellent examples of <u>glassy intranuclear inclusions.</u> The dark mass of material at the bottom of *A* is not colloid but a homogeneous fragment of metachromatic stroma. Both *A* and *B* Diff-Quik × 375.

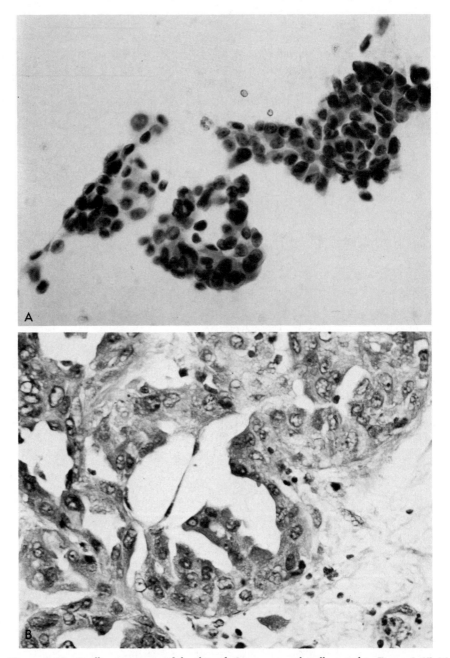

Figure 6–18   Papillary carcinoma of the thyroid. Same case as that illustrated in Figure 6–17. More papillary-like configuration is visible in the Papanicolaou-stained smear. Glassy nuclei are not evident in this cell cluster. Compare with the tissue pattern of the papillary carcinoma in *B*. *A*, Papanicolaou × 375. *B*, Hematoxylin and eosin × 375.

Hürthle Cell Carcinoma.   One Hürthle cell carcinoma was biopsied and did not differ cytologically from Hürthle cell adenoma (Fig. 6–19). Clinically, this neoplasm was malignant and was therefore readily diagnosed. Hürthle cell tumors are as unpredictable cytologically as they are histologically. This has also been true in several reported series of thyroid aspirations.[10, 14, 22, 25, 36]

Medullary Carcinoma.   This author has seen and aspirated only <u>one case</u> of medullary carcinoma, which was a <u>bilateral irregular</u> mass in a 12-year-old male with

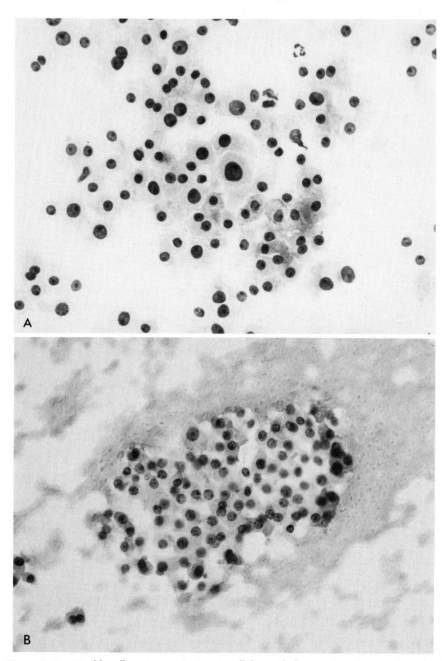

Figure 6–19 Hürthle cell carcinoma. Aspirate is cellular, with the cytoplasm having a fine granularity that is best seen with Romanovsky stains. There is some variation in nuclear size, not an unexpected feature of Hürthle cell neoplasms. Predicting from the aspiration smear alone that this tumor is malignant is not possible. A, Diff-Quik × 375. B, Papanicolaou × 375.

Sipple's syndrome. Romanovsky staining revealed a spindle cell pattern with irregular clumps of acellular metachromatic material. Characteristic red granularity of the cytoplasm was seen in many of the tumor cells. Unlike colloid, the acellular stroma did not stain very well with the Papanicolaou technique, which gave it a pale, glassy appearance. Also noted were dense bluish-black structures that later were determined to be calcification of the stroma. These features are illustrated in Figures 6–20 and 6–21. Several authors have identified this neoplasm correctly with aspiration biopsy,

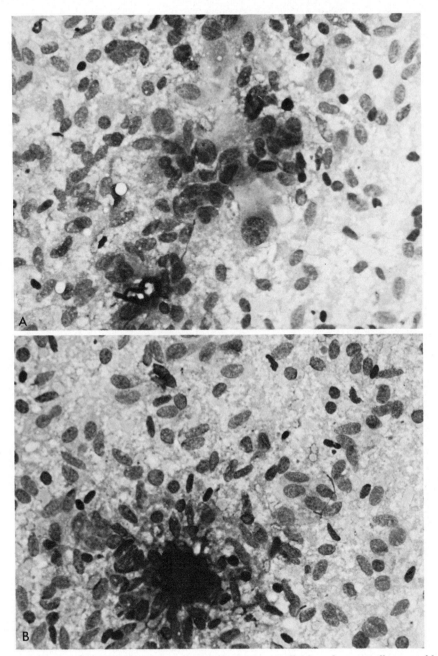

Figure 6–20 Medullary carcinoma with amyloid stroma. Spindle-shaped tumor cells are visible in a background of amorphous stroma, or the amyloid. The tumor cells will also exhibit fine red granules in the cytoplasm with Romanovsky stains. The stroma in *B* has become partially calcified, appearing as a dark homogeneous mass near the bottom of the figure. Both *A* and *B*, Diff-Quik × 375.

basing their diagnoses on observations of the characteristic cell pattern and identification of the amyloid material.[22, 42, 49-52]

Anaplastic Carcinoma. The giant-cell, anaplastic thyroid carcinomas are easily recognized by aspiration biopsy, just as they are readily suspected clinically. Aspiration biopsy is important because it is probably the simplest and most convenient way to confirm the diagnosis.[53] The disease of our patients followed the usual course of undifferentiated thyroid cancers, except for one woman who survived for two years

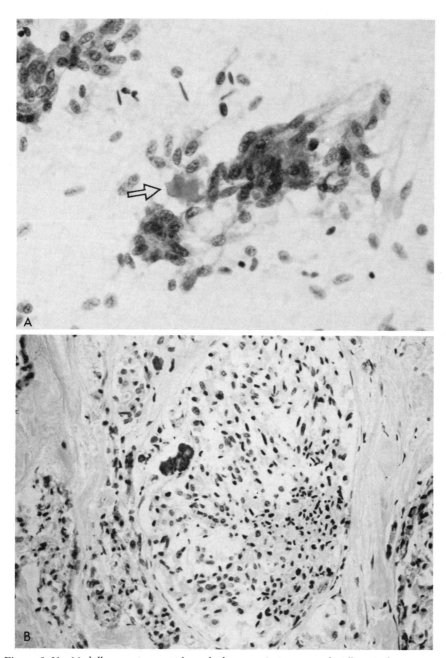

Figure 6–21   Medullary carcinoma with amyloid stroma. Same case as that illustrated in Figure 6–20, but in this figure a Papanicolaou-stained smear is compared with a tissue section. A small fragment of the amyloid stroma is apparent in the center of *A* (arrow). *A*, Papanicolaou × 375. *B*, Hematoxylin and eosin × 240.

after surgery and postoperative radiation therapy. Her thyroid mass, while clinically suspect for giant-cell carcinoma, was smaller than the others and proved operable. This patient never developed a recurrence in the neck, but she expired eventually from pulmonary metastases, the diagnosis of which was confirmed by transthoracic needle aspiration biopsy. Figures 6–22 and 6–23 depict this lethal carcinoma. The smears reveal both the marked cellularity and the pleomorphism that characterize giant-cell thyroid cancer. Anaplastic carcinomas of the small-cell type may be mistaken

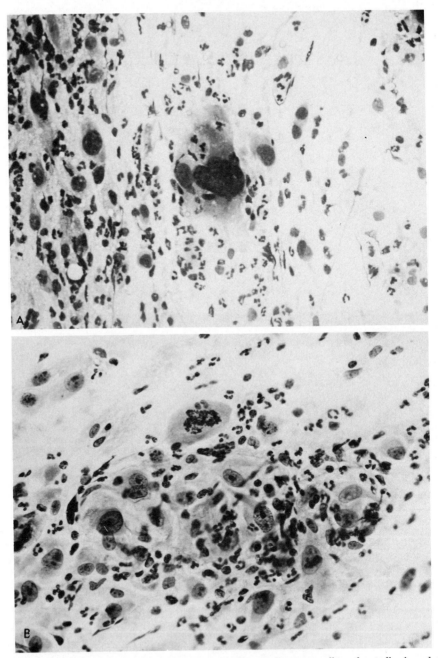

Figure 6–22   Spindle and giant cell carcinoma. Pleomorphic giant cells and spindle-shaped tumor cells as well as an irregular mitotic form are evident. The giant cells in this tumor have also engulfed polymorphonuclear leukocytes *(A)*. *A*, Diff-Quik × 240. *B*, Papanicolaou × 375.

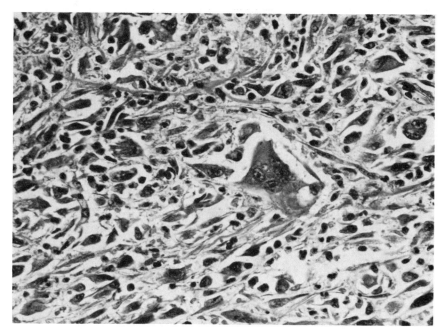

Figure 6–23   Spindle and giant carcinoma of the thyroid. Tissue section from the case illustrated in Figure 6–22. Hematoxylin and eosin × 375.

for lymphomas, and one must be careful to look for cellular cohesion.[8, 42, 49] So far, this series does not contain an example. Droese illustrates some typical cases in his monograph.[29]

RESULTS OF THYROID ASPIRATIONS

In this author's personal series, the false-positive rate is 1.5 per cent (Table 6–1). Of the four incorrect diagnoses, three were lesions reported as benign neoplasms. One was reported as suspected papillary carcinoma. No incorrect aspiration biopsy report was followed by radical surgery. Since all these patients had cold nodules, exploration was sufficiently justified. The problem was judging the significance of even a small amount of colloid in a relatively cellular smear with respect to a diagnosis of goiter versus one of adenoma.

There were six cases either missed or incorrectly classified, and the most potentially serious mistake involved the rather rare form of non-Hodgkin's lymphoma (PDLL). Experience would indicate that this tumor should be recognizable and easily differentiated from thyroiditis. Three adenomas were reported as goiters because of the confusing smear pattern that resulted from areas of hemorrhage within the adenomatous nodule and the presence of a small amount of colloid (Fig. 6–24). This produced a pattern simulating that demonstrated in aspiration biopsy smears from goiters. This error is probably unavoidable, but it should be infrequent.

One incidental occult carcinoma occurred in the same lobe in which a nodular goiter had been successfully aspirated. This carcinoma was not clinically detected either. Because this patient was a child but with no prior history of radiation therapy, surgery was undertaken. Based on previous experience with occult lesions, it is uncertain whether this carcinoma would have ever been clinically manifest. One incidental adenoma was found in a resected lobe showing chronic thyroiditis. Aspiration

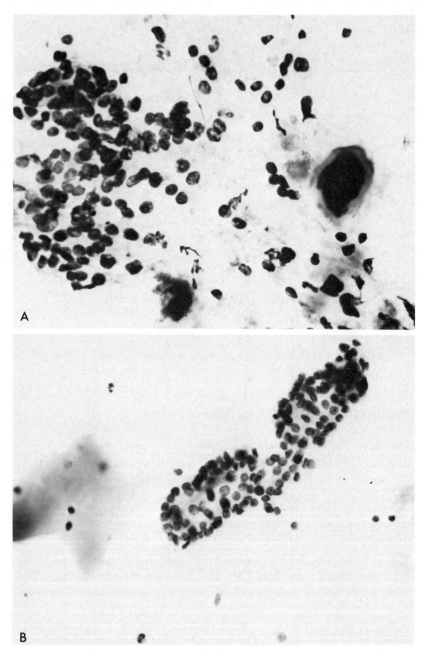

Figure 6–24 Follicular adenoma with colloid. Aspiration smear with a cellular pattern but easily discernible colloid. Several homogeneous masses of colloid are evident in *A* and at the left edge of *B*. Histiocytes with hemosiderin pigment were present in other fields. Excision of the thyroid nodule revealed a follicular adenoma with central hemorrhage. *A*, Diff-Quik ×375. *B*, Papanicolaou ×375.

biopsy had correctly diagnosed the thyroiditis. Neither the smear nor palpation revealed the adenoma.

In a previous publication, this author has summarized the results of several series of thin-needle aspiration biopsies of the thyroid. False-negative and false-positive rates were compared, as were the percentages of unsatisfactory smears. The rate of false-negatives ranged from 0.3 per cent to 6.0 per cent; the rate of false-positives ranged from 0.0 per cent to 2.5 per cent. It should be emphasized that these percentages are derived from a total series.[28] When it is remembered that cold thyroid nodules that are actually neoplasms occur no more commonly than in about 20 per cent of the cases, calculating the figures in this manner seems reasonable, since obtaining histologic confirmation for every cold nodule would lead to a great deal of unnecessary and potentially hazardous surgery. If, however, one wishes to be a purist and calculate the number of false-negatives using the number of malignant tumors actually determined, then the rate of missed neoplasms is much higher. These reported rates range from 2 per cent to 37 per cent.[20, 54]

It is difficult to evaluate other series because of what appear to be incomplete data. Some have shown very high false-negative rates for carcinoma. For example, Kolendorf diagnosed only 15 of 20 thyroid neoplasms correctly, missing two and overdiagnosing three.[32] In the 4555 cases reported by Galvan, one fourth of the patients had subsequent surgery. There were 129 cytologic reports of malignancy based on aspiration biopsy, and only 40 per cent of these were confirmed histologically. The very high false-positive rates in this series were attributable to adenomas and Hürthle cell neoplasms that were diagnosed unequivocally as carcinomas. Eight malignancies were actually missed. Five were well-differentiated follicular carcinomas. In three cases, the aspiration biopsy failed to produce a sample from the nodule.[10, 34]

Walfish has used a somewhat larger needle (18-gauge) instead of the 21- or 22-gauge needle. He reported an overall accuracy of 95 per cent for 150 aspirations. His diagnostic accuracy for cysts was 88 per cent. Of note, however, was that ultrasonography alone was only 71 per cent accurate in his series.[36, 37] A very large series of 9230 aspirations of cold nodules of the thyroid has been reported by Lang. Of these, 1097 were followed by surgical excision and histologic study. Included in those histologically examined were 311 simple adenomas, 42 atypical adenomas, and 69 carcinomas, including both well-differentiated and anaplastic types. There were only two false-positives for carcinoma reported, but there was a 27 per cent false-negative rate for the diagnosis of malignant neoplasms. This, however, is similar to other series in which the number of false-negatives are calculated against the number of malignant tumors actually found.[14]

Einhorn and Frazen observed no false-positives in a series of 84 malignant thyroid tumors. There were, however, five false-negative reports. While these authors perform their own aspiration biopsies, they do not interpret their own histopathologic findings. The series is, therefore, probably not biased. They believe very strongly that the clinical examination of the patient by whomever actually performs the aspiration is vitally important.[9] This author's personal experience confirms that contention.

At least in terms of total number of cases diagnosed, fine-needle aspiration biopsy has now surpassed the Vim-Silverman tissue needle biopsy preferred by Crile and Hawk as well as by Wang. The accuracy seems to be essentially similar. The results of tissue needle biopsy series *also* suffers to some extent from lack of histologic study, but complete follow-up would involve a significant amount of unnecessary surgery.[4, 5] In fact, Crile states that needle biopsy can eliminate 90 per cent of thyroid nodule surgery. His recent articles summarize the use of both tissue needle biopsy and fine-needle aspiration biopsy in the following situations:

1. Enlargement thought to be struma lymphomatosa (Vim-Silverman needle preferred).

2. A nodule thought to be benign (requires a 15-gauge needle for aspiration but a cell block for preparation).

3. Cyst or hemorrhage within an adenoma (requires a 20-gauge needle for aspiration followed by injection of sclerosing solution when a cyst is encountered).[1-3]

Miller and colleagues reported a very large and complete series of 455 thyroid nodules that were evaluated by either aspiration biopsy or tissue needle biopsy, compared with 1094 nodules evaluated by clinical methods. In their report, these authors emphasized that both biopsy procedures substantially reduced the number of patients with suspected cancer and doubled the number of patients to be observed in follow-up. They also emphasized that the number of patients at high or intermediate risk for thyroid cancer was increased by 75 per cent, while the number of operations for benign disease was decreased by 70 per cent. Reductions in morbidity and cost are obvious advantages of this approach.[23]

The many series of thin-needle aspiration biopsies taken together indicate that the test is best viewed as a simple screening method for cold thyroid nodules. To substantiate this conclusion, this author has calculated predictive value, sensitivity, and specificity from the data of several reports using the methodology of Galen and Gambino.[28, 55] Predictive value of a positive aspiration for the presence of a neoplasm was better than 90 per cent in all the series except one. Results of predictive value for a negative aspirate ruling out a neoplasm were somewhat better in the same series.[28] Sensitivity for the presence of a neoplasm in this author's expanded series is 91 per cent, after deleting two cases in which an incidental neoplasm was detected by a thyroid lobectomy performed after aspiration biopsy. Sensitivity for all the collected series is also better than 90 per cent. Specificity for the absence of tumor is 98 per cent in this series.

The calculated results as well as those of the present series support the concept that thin-needle aspiration biopsy is an excellent screening method despite its limitations in differentiating follicular adenoma from low-grade follicular carcinoma. Hence, performing thin-needle aspiration biopsy of the thyroid when a cold nodule is discovered confirms the need for surgery. When a non-neoplastic condition is discovered by aspiration biopsy, the risk in delaying surgery is very minimal.

COMPLICATIONS OF THYROID ASPIRATIONS

As in other sites, aspiration biopsy of the thyroid has been virtually free of complications. This author has observed one case of hematoma that developed several hours after aspiration and delayed surgery for two weeks until it resolved. The patient demonstrated a cold nodule lying on the medial border of the left lobe of the thyroid that was correctly diagnosed as papillary carcinoma by aspiration biopsy. While performing the aspiration, the operator thought that the nodule was penetrated completely and that the needle impinged upon thyroid cartilage. A small vein overlying the thyroid cartilage probably bled slowly in the hours following the biopsy. The patient suffered no ill effects as a result of the hematoma. Two other patients experienced transient lightheadedness, probably a vagus reflex, immediately after aspiration biopsy of the thyroid.

Complications following Vim-Silverman needle biopsy of the thyroid have been documented in the literature. One case of hematoma, one of suspected needle tract implantation of a malignant tumor, and one of transient paralysis of a vocal cord have been reported by Crile and collaborators.[2, 40] Wang and colleagues noted in a series of

1200 biopsies three cases of ecchymosis that occurred after use of the short 14-gauge tissue needle.[5] No needle tract implantations developed in their series, and none were recorded in the other series reviewed here.

REFERENCES

1. Crile, G., Jr.: Management of thyroid disease: With particular reference to thyroid nodules. Postgrad. Med. *60*:105–108, 1976.
2. Crile, G., Jr.: Struma lymphomatosa and carcinoma of the thyroid. Surg. Gynecol. Obstet. *147*:350–352, 1978.
3. Crile, G., Jr., and Hawk, W. A., Jr.: Aspiration biopsy of thyroid nodules. Surg. Gynecol. Obstet. *136*:241–245, 1973.
4. Hawk, W. A., Jr., Crile, G., Jr., Hazard, J. B., et al.: Needle biopsy of the thyroid gland. Surg. Gynecol. Obstet. *122*:1053–1065, 1966.
5. Wang, C., Vickery, A. L., Jr., and Maloof, F.: Needle biopsy of the thyroid. Surg. Gynecol. Obstet. *143*:365–368, 1976.
6. Yao, Y.: Thyroid nodules — benign or malignant? 1. Diagnosis. Postgrad. Med. *61*:65–70, 1977.
7. Bolis Ferranti, M. G., and Monico, S.: Cytological diagnosis of carcinoma of the thyroid. Lav. Ist. Anat. Istol. Patol. Univ. Studi Perugia. *38*:25–40, 1978.
8. Cornillot, M., Granier, A. M., and Houcke, M.: Cyto-puncture of thyroid lesions: Anatomo-clinical comparisons. I. Malignant lesions (300 cases). Arch. Anat. Cytol. Pathol. *25*:325–333, 1977.
9. Einhorn, J., and Franzen, S.: Thin-needle biopsy in the diagnosis of thyroid disease. Acta Radiol. *58*:321–328, 1962.
10. Galvan, G., Pohl, G. B., and Skerblisch, I.: Fine needle biopsy of "cold" struma nodules in 4555 patients of an endemic goiter area. Results and clinical significance. Schweiz. Med. Wochenschr. *106*:1247–1251, 1976.
11. Galvan, G.: Fine needle biopsy of cold goiter nodules (author's translation). Muench. Med. Wochenschr. *119*:229–232, 1977.
12. Heikkinen, J., Lehtinen, M., and Poyhonen, L.: Gamma imaging and thin needle biopsy in diagnosis of thyroid cancer. Duodecim. *95*:192–197, 1979.
13. Kempken, K., Droese, M., Bayer-Pietsch, E., et al.: Scintigraphy and fine needle biopsy in nodular goiter. Results in 548 patients. Fortschr. Med. *96*:1369–1372, 1978.
14. Lang, W., Atay, Z., and Georgii, A.: The cytological classification of follicular tumours in the thyroid gland (author's translation). Virchows Arch. Pathol. Anat. *378*:199–211, 1978.
15. Pedio, G., Nadig, J., Hedinger, C.: Significance of fine-needle puncture in the diagnosis of thyroid malignancies. Comparative cytological and histological examinations. Schweiz. Med. Wochenschr. *107*:1928–1931, 1977.
16. Schnurer, L. B., and Widstrom, A.: Fine-needle biopsy of the thyroid gland: A cytohistological comparison in cases of goiter. Ann. Otol. Rhinol. Laryngol. *87*:224–227, 1978.
17. Wildmeister, W.: Early diagnosis of malignant thyroid neoplasms. Fortschr. Med. *95*:923–930, 1977.
18. Stavric, G. D., Karanfilski, B. T., Kalamaras, A. K., et al.: Early diagnosis and detection of clinically non-suspected thyroid neoplasia by the cytologic method. Cancer *45*:340–344, 1980.
19. Chu, E. W., Hanson, T. A., Gershengorn, M. C., et al.: Studies of cells in fine needle aspiration of thyroid gland. Acta Cytol. *23*:309–314, 1979.
20. Friedman, M., Shimaoka, K., and Getaz, P.: Needle aspiration of 310 thyroid lesions. Acta Cytol. *23*:194–203, 1979.
21. Gershengorn, M. C., McClung, M. R., Chu, E. W., et al.: Fine-needle aspiration cytology in the preoperative diagnosis of thyroid nodules. Ann. Intern. Med. *87*:265–269, 1977.
22. Kini, W., Miller, J. M., and Hamburger, J. I.: The cytopathology of the thyroid nodule by fine needle aspiration. Acta Cytol. *22*:605–606, 1978.
23. Miller, J. M., Hamburger, J. I., and Kini, S.: Diagnosis of thyroid nodules. Use of fine needle aspiration and needle biopsy. JAMA *24*:481–484, 1979.
24. Hamburger, J. I., Miller, J. M., and Kini, S.: *Preoperative Clinical-Pathological Diagnosis of Thyroid Nodules. Handbook and Atlas.* Associated Endocrinologists — Northland Thyroid Laboratory, Southfield, MI, 1979.
25. Zajicek, J.: *Aspiration Biopsy Cytology. Part I. Cytology of Supradiaphragmatic Organs.* New York, S. Karger, 1974, pp. 67–89.
26. Zajicek, J.: Personal communication.
27. Frable, W. J.: Thin-needle aspiration biopsy. A personal experience with 469 cases. Am. J. Clin. Pathol. *65*:168–182, 1976.
28. Frable, W. J., and Frable, M. A. S.: Fine-needle aspiration biopsy of the thyroid. Histopathologic and clinical correlations; *in* Fenoglio, C. M. and Wolff, M. (Eds.): *Progress in Surgical Pathology,* Vol. 1. New York, Masson, 1980, pp. 105–118.
29. Droese, M.: *Cytological Aspiration Biopsy of Thyroid Gland.* Stuttgart, F. K. Schattauer Verlag, 1980.
30. Nilsson, G.: Nuclear segmentation in goitre aspirates. Acta Pathol. Microbiol. Scand. Sect. A. *87*:11–13, 1979.

31. Holmes, H. B., Jr., Kreutner, A., and O'Brien, P. H.: Hashimoto's thyroiditis and its relationship to other thyroid diseases. Surg. Gynecol. Obstet. *144*:887–890, 1977.
32. Kolendorf, K., Hansen, J. B., Engberg, L., et al.: Fine needle and open biopsy in thyroid disorders. Acta Chir. Scand. *141*:20–23, 1975.
33. Persson, P. S.: Cytodiagnosis of thyroiditis. A comparative study of cytological, histological, immunological and clinical findings in thyroiditis, particularly in diffuse lymphoid thyroiditis. Acta Med. Scand. (Suppl.)*483*:7–100, 1968.
34. Galvan, G., and Maurer, H.: Emptying of goitre cysts by small-needle aspiration (author's translation). Dtsch. Med. Wochenschr. *102*:829–830, 1977.
35. Jensen, F., and Rasmussen, S. N.: The treatment of thyroid cysts by ultrasonically guided fine needle aspiration. Acta Chir. Scand. *142*:209–211, 1976.
36. Walfish, P. G., Hazani, E., Strawbridge, H. T., et al.: A prospective study of combined ultrasonography and needle aspiration biopsy in the assessment of the hypofunctioning thyroid nodule. Surgery *82*:474–482, 1977.
37. Walfish, P. G., Hazani, E., Strawbridge, H. T., et al.: Combined ultrasound and needle aspiration cytology in the assessment and management of hypofunctioning thyroid nodule. Ann. Intern. Med. *87*:270–274, 1977.
38. Ackerman, L. V., and Rosai, J.: *Surgical Pathology.* 5th Ed. St. Louis, C. V. Mosby Co., 1974.
39. Bain, J., and Walfish, P.: The assessment of thyroid function and structure. Otolaryngol. Clin. N. Am. *11*:419–443, 1978.
40. Crile, G., Jr., Esselstyn, C. B., Jr., and Hawk, W. A.: Needle biopsy in the diagnosis of thyroid nodules appearing after radiation. N. Engl. J. Med. *301*:997–998, 1979.
41. Droese, M.: Cytologic identification of follicular carcinoma of the thyroid by fine needle aspiration biopsy (author's translation). Med. Klin. *71*:908–911, 1976.
42. Löwhagen, T., and Sprenger, E.: Cytologic presentation of thyroid tumors in aspiration smear. Acta Cytol. *18*:192–197, 1974.
43. Krisch, K., Jakesz, R., Erd, W., et al.: Punctate cytology of benign and malignant changes in the thyroid gland (author's translation). Muench. Med. Wochenschr. *118*:1383–1386, 1976.
44. Sprenger, E., Löwhagen, T., Vogt-Schaden, M.: Differential diagnosis between follicular adenoma and follicular carcinoma of the thyroid by nuclear DNA determination. Acta Cytol. *21*:528–530, 1977.
45. Hasselstrom, K., and Henriques, U. V.: Fine needle aspiration of the thyroid gland. Dan. Med. Bull. *22*:259–263, 1975.
46. Hapke, M. R., and Dehner, L. P.: The optically clear nucleus. A reliable sign of papillary carcinoma of the thyroid? Am. J. Surg. Pathol. *3*:31–38, 1979.
47. Kini, S., Miller, J. M., Hamburger, J. I., et al.: Cytopathology of papillary carcinoma of the thyroid by fine needle aspiration. Acta Cytol. *24*:511–521, 1980.
48. Christ, M. L., and Haja, J.: The frequency and significance of intranuclear cytoplasmic inclusions in fine needle aspirations of the thyroid gland. Acta Cytol. *23*:327–331, 1979.
49. Atay, Z., Lang, W., and Georgii, A.: Classification of thyroid carcinoma by cytology. Zentralbl. Allg. Pathol. *122*:160–161, 1978.
50. DeLellis, R. A., Rule, A. H., Spiler, I., et al.: Calcitonin and carcino-embryonic antigen as tumor markers in medullary thyroid carcinoma. Am. J. Clin. Pathol. *70*:587–594, 1978.
51. Ljungberg, O.: Cytologic diagnosis of medullary carcinoma of the thyroid gland. Acta Cytol. *16*:253–255, 1972.
52. Soderstrom, N., Telenius-Berg, M., and Akerman, M.: Diagnosis of medullary carcinoma of the thyroid by fine needle aspiration biopsy. Acta Med. Scand. *197*:71–76, 1975.
53. Schneider, V., and Frable, W. J.: Spindle and giant cell carcinoma of the thyroid. Cytologic diagnosis by fine needle aspiration. Acta Cytol. *24*:184–189, 1980.
54. Russ, J. E., Scanlon, E. F., and Christ, M. A.: Aspiration cytology of head and neck masses. Am. J. Surg. *136*:342–347, 1978.
55. Galen, R. S., and Gambino, S. R.: *Beyond Normality: The Predictive Value and Efficiency of Medical Diagnosis.* New York, John Wiley and Sons, 1975.

Chapter Seven

Lung and Mediastinum

ASPIRATION OF LUNG AND MEDIASTINAL LESIONS

HISTORY AND TECHNIQUE

In 1883, Leyden reported the first aspiration biopsy, a puncture of the lung performed for the diagnosis of pneumonia.[1] Only three years later, Menetrier made the first diagnosis of a lung carcinoma by transthoracic aspiration. That aspiration confirmed a previous diagnosis formed by conventional cytologic studies of sputum.[2] No other significant reports appeared until Craver and Benkley published their studies in 1938.[1] They used an 18-gauge needle along with x-ray guidance and a set of calipers for localization of tumors with diameters less than 4 cm. Films were even placed against the patient's chest, and the clavicle and the sternum served as specific landmarks when the patient was in the sitting position.[1] With the assistance of a knowledgeable thoracic surgeon, this author has used these same methods of localization and placement of the needle for both central and peripheral lung tumors. The overall results of Craver and Benkley indicated a diagnostic accuracy of about 60 per cent, with an emphasis on diagnosis of malignant tumors. There were seven false-positive results in a series of 92 different pulmonary conditions.[1]

Only two reports on aspiration biopsy of the lung were published during the 1940s: one by Rosemond and colleagues and another by Gledhill and coworkers.[3, 4] Both groups employed an 18-gauge needle. The degree of accuracy was 61 per cent in Rosemond's series, and 78 per cent in Gledhill's series. The latter report demonstrated that the diagnostic value of aspiration biopsy is considerably superior to that of bronchoscopy. Both groups of authors noted that the procedure had been criticized by Ochsner and De Bakey, based on the documented complication of implantation occurring in a case reported by Dolley and Jones after aspiration of pleural fluid containing carcinoma cells. It is appreciated today that although this is not an unusual complication, it is not related to the technique of transthoracic thin-needle aspiration biopsy of solid malignant pulmonary tumors.[5-7] An early report in the English literature actually advocated using a large bore needle for aspiration as well as pulling the needle out of the chest wall with the vacuum fully applied.[8] The publication of Reincke as cited in a review by Grunze was believed to have been the first report of tumor implantation. It was also a study of the same type of case previously described in which fluid was aspirated from a patient with carcinomatosis.[9, 10]

Despite its relatively favorable early reception by a few authors, aspiration biopsy of the lung failed to gain general acceptance. A single series was reported in 1954 by Woolf, but this nearly exclusively involved the use of aspiration biopsy for the diagnosis of infectious disease of the lung. While this biopsy method was diagnostically valuable in this series, an unusual number of complications developed. Thirty-four per cent of the patients experienced hemoptysis, and one patient died, probably from air embolism.[11] Interest in the Vim-Silverman tissue needle biopsy of lung developed at about this time. A report by Aronovitch describes a small series of peripheral localized tumors sampled in this manner. Most of these were malignant. A diagnosis was obtained in 60 per cent of the cases. Although the report mentions one case of needle track spread of tumor, there is no further documentation of this complication.[12]

Largely because of the interest of radiologists, the development of thin-needle aspiration biopsy paralleled that of tissue needle (Vim-Silverman) biopsy during the 1960s. Various marking techniques, as well as fluoroscopy, either single plane or biplane, were employed in many of the series. Some reports emphasized the study of cytologic smears, whereas others relied on the observation of tiny tissue fragments that were fixed, embedded, and sectioned as a cell block. A few investigators prepared a filter from a rinse of the needle, but most prepared the aspirate using a combination of methods to obtain optimal results.[13-18]

Increasing acceptance of this diagnostic biopsy method is evident in the summary of Stevens and colleagues, who found references to 2700 transthoracic aspirations.[14] The best data from this literature seemed to be that of King and Russell, who reported a diagnostic rate of 87.5 per cent for malignant tumors. Cancerous lesions in that series ranged from 1.5 cm to 15 cm in diameter.[15] The rate of false-negative results for all the series was approximately 10 per cent, whereas the rate of false-positive diagnoses ranged from less than 1 per cent to 2 per cent.[13, 18]

During this period, Dahlgren and Nordenström published their monograph *Transthoracic Needle Biopsy*. This is, to date, the most comprehensive report of fine-needle aspiration biopsy of the lung.[19] Nordenström, in particular, pioneered many of the techniques of aspiration of the lung and mediastinum, including some innovative therapeutic approaches to lung cancer.[20, 21]

Simultaneously, a comparable but smaller series of transthoracic biopsies of the lung performed with the Vim-Silverman needle were being reported.[22-28] Tissue needle biopsy seemed to be preferred by some authors, specifically for masses near the periphery of the lung or for pleural-based tumors. Thus, Janower recommended that a tissue needle be used when the diameter of the mass exceeded 2 cm and when thoracotomy was contraindicated.[23] Core biopsy was also preferred when there was diffuse parenchymal disease. Youmans and colleagues reported that specimens were obtained from 90 per cent of 61 patients with diffuse parenchymal disease and that a diagnosis was possible in 85 per cent of the cases. However, a chest tube was left indwelling in all patients because a substantial number of complications developed. For example, 19 of the patients had an air leak, and in 11 of these patients the condition persisted for more than 24 hours.[25]

The number of complications has probably inhibited the universal acceptance of the Vim-Silverman method of tissue needle biopsy for lung disease. Adamson and Bates reported significant complications in 23 per cent of patients.[26] Krumholz and colleagues noted hemoptysis in 30 per cent of patients in their series, and 16 per cent of these patients developed a pneumothorax that required some type of therapy.[27] In a collected series, Zavala and Bedell reported four deaths among 792 patients undergoing transthoracic tissue needle biopsy.[22]

Recent Trends. The remarkable increase in incidence of lung cancer and the development of new imaging techniques perhaps account for the recent general acceptance of fine-needle aspiration biopsy of lung lesions. A cursory review revealed 27 references from the American and the European literature that specifically detail series of cases, methods, and results reported during the past 10 years. Most of this data has been compiled by either radiologists working independently or radiologists, pathologists, and thoracic surgeons working together.[29-56] Results of the larger series from this review, including rates of complications, are summarized in Table 7–1. It can be seen that accuracy depends to some extent on evaluation of individual malignant tumors or specific sites versus overall results.

Some authors prefer the screw needle for transthoracic biopsy, an outer sheath needle with an internal stylus having protrusions on the end. This internal needle extends 1.5 cm beyond the external needle.[36, 45] The screw needle was designed by Nordenström, who also described a number of unique approaches to needle aspiration biopsy of lung and mediastinal neoplasms.[57-60] The screw needle has been especially useful for transthoracic biopsy of hamartomas, although Ramzy has successfully used a conventional long-beveled, 19- or 20 gauge fine-needle in the diagnosis of these nodules.[61-63] Ultrasonography has also been advocated for diagnosis of tumors lying against the chest wall.[38]

Only a few authors have compared fine-needle aspiration biopsy for the diagnosis of lung tumors with conventional cytologic methods of studying sputum, bronchial washings, and bronchial brushings. Nasiell reported such a comparison in a series of 83 cases. Aspiration biopsy provided a positive diagnosis in 72 per cent of the total cases and in 59 per cent of the 49 cases in which cytologic studies of sputum had also been performed. He felt that an adequate comparison could be made in only 42 cases, in which there were both an aspiration and an adequate examination involving the usual methods of pulmonary cytology. In 19 of these cases, results of both techniques were positive. In 13 additional cases, aspiration biopsy provided a positive diagnosis, and exfoliative cytologic studies resulted in a negative diagnosis. In seven cases, aspiration biopsy yielded a negative diagnosis, and exfoliative cytologic studies provided a positive diagnosis. Results of both methods were negative in three patients. The superiority of aspiration biopsy was clearly demonstrated in the cases in which the conventional cytologic specimens, in terms of quality or quantity or both, were unacceptable.[48]

Dahlgren also reported a similar series with suitable comparison in 101 cases. Ninety four specimens were diagnosed by aspiration biopsy, while only 42 were diagnosed by cytologic studies of sputum. In the latter group, only 27 were clearly positive, while the remaining 15 were suspicious. Cytologic examination of sputum did prove more valuable for diagnosis of central neoplasms, providing positive results in 56 per cent of the cases, while aspiration biopsy provided a positive diagnosis in only 17 per cent. More than half the tumors in this series had a diameter less than 5.0 cm. No complications were reported by Dahlgren in this total group of over 3000 aspiration biopsies.[49]

As documented by Landsman and colleagues, the rate of diagnostic accuracy of cytologic studies of brushings compared favorably with that of needle aspiration (89 per cent versus 72 per cent) in a series composed only of bronchogenic cancers situated both centrally and peripherally. No other types of malignant lung tumors in this series were diagnosed by brushing, but 88 per cent were diagnosed by needle aspiration.[52] Borgeskov and Francis also noted the superiority of fine-needle aspiration biopsy to brushings obtained through the flexible bronchoscope. Their series included only tumors that were not diagnosed by sputum studies and bronchial washings and that were not visualized directly by bronchoscopy with the flexible scope. Blind brushing and biopsy yielded a diagnostic accuracy of 30 per cent, whereas fine-needle aspiration biopsy provided positive results in 62 per cent of cases.[42]

Localization Method. Figure 7–1 illustrates one useful marking technique for localization of a lung tumor in the lower lobe. Paper clips or other suitable metallic markers are attached to a piece of adhesive tape at uniform intervals, and this is then

TABLE 7–1.   SUMMARY OF RESULTS OF SELECTED SERIES OF TRANSTHORACIC FINE-NEEDLE ASPIRATION BIOPSIES

Reference	Positive Diagnosis	Complications	False-Positive	False-Negative
Polak and Helbich[29]	80% of 150 cases	25% of cases	NR	NR
Sinner[30]	90.7% of 2726 cases	27% (rare to require treatment)	2.4%	3.0%
Tao et al.[31]	88.8% of 712 cases	NR*	NR	NR
Heal[33]	92.0% of 80 cases	NR	NR	8.0%
Zornoza et al.[34]	87.0% of 100 cases discrete nodules	14.0% pneumothorax, 1.0% required chest tube	NR	NR
Atay and Brandt[35]	84.0% of 1841 cases	NR	NR	NR
House and Thomson[36]	95.0% of 57 cancer cases using screw needle	6.8% pneumothorax requiring chest tube	4.0%	3.0%
Jereb amd Us-Krasovec[37]	75% of 50 cases	16.0% symptomatic	NR	2.0%
Walls et al.[39]	95.0% of 27 Pancoast tumors	8.0% symptomatic	0	0
Dick et al.[40]	73.0% of 223 cases	5.0% pneumothorax requiring treatment	NR	NR
Pavy et al.[41]	80.0% of 59 cancer cases	7.0% pneumothorax requiring treatment	NR	NR
Sinner[43]	95.0% of small peripheral lesions 4.0 mm to 2.0 cm; 302 cases.	1.1% pneumothorax requiring treatment	1.3%	1.3%
Sargent et al.[44]	83.0% of 230 lung cancers	NR	NR	17.0%
Hayata et al.[45]	84.4% of 225 lung cancers	7.6% total complications	NR	15.6%
Yam and Levine[46]	90.0% of 24 lung cancers	NR	NR	15.0%
Sassy-Dobray et al.[47]	84.0% of all lesions of lung intraoperative	NR	4.7%	11.3%
Nordenström[54]	87.0% all lesions of lung	NR	NR	NR

*NR = Not reported.

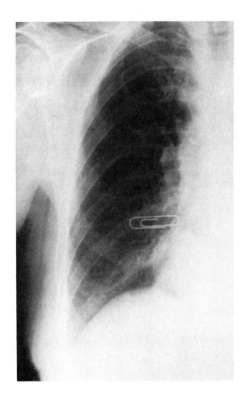

Figure 7–1 Marking technique for mass in the right lower lobe. Paper clip taped to the patient's back is evident on the film at the upper border of the mass. A second marker is just barely visible in the roentgenogram at the lower margin of the tumor.

taped to the patient's back in the approximate area of the tumor. Films are taken with the patient in the position that he or she will occupy during the subsequent aspiration. The patient and the films are then taken to the operating room. Removing the tape reveals that the metallic markers leave a small skin impression. Comparing the location of these marks with the radiographs quite accurately determines the precise site for the puncture. Figures 7–2 and 7–3 illustrate the cytomorphologic appearance of an aspirate from this case, demonstrating syncytial masses of tumor cells with fairly large nuclei and prominent nucleoli. The actual gland-like spaces reflect the adenocarcinoma pattern of this cancer seen in the subsequent lobectomy specimen (Fig. 7–4).

MALIGNANT TUMORS

Carcinoma. As suggested by this author's own experience with approximately 140 cases, the aspiration biopsy method is most suitable for the diagnosis of malignant tumors. In fact, the cytomorphologic evidence of malignancy is usually quite a bit more convincing in aspirates than in sputum or bronchial washings, simply because of the large number of tumor cells visible on the smears. A typical example is illustrated in Figures 7–5 and 7–6: The first figure depicts a radiograph of a superior sulcus tumor with destruction of the posterior third rib; the second represents an aspiration demonstrating multiple pleomorphic and keratinized squamous cancer cells. Figures 7–7 and 7–8 depict a midlung mass just beneath the pleura in a patient with severe emphysema. The aspirate demonstrates undifferentiated small malignant cells in a hemorrhagic and necrotic background. The obvious linear arrangement of the cells is typical of oat cell carcinoma. As in bronchial brushings, the cells of oat cell carcinoma in aspiration smears appear about 2 to 2½ times as large as those seen in exfoliative cytologic studies of sputum or bronchial washings.

Text continued on page 192

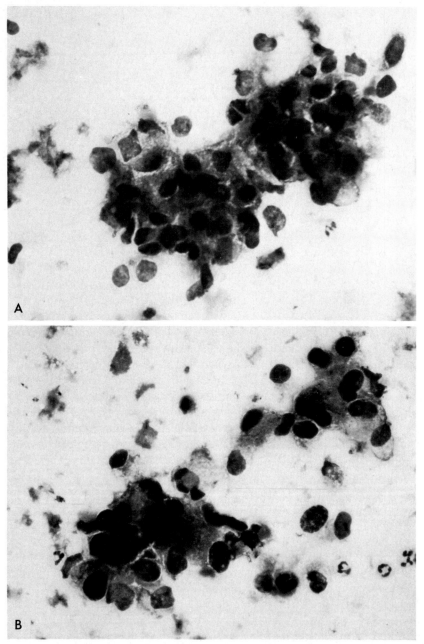

Figure 7–2   Adenocarcinoma, poorly differentiated. Clusters and sheets of the tumor cells have a finely vacuolated cytoplasm. High nuclear-cytoplasmic ratio and irregular nuclear configuration are evident. A and B, Diff-Quik × 375.

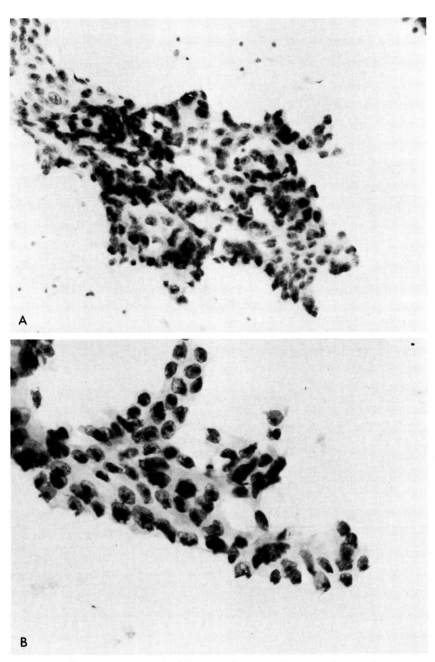

Figure 7–3 Adenocarcinoma, poorly differentiated. Papanicolaou-stained smear from same case as that illustrated in Figure 7–6. Actual glandular spaces are seen within the sheets of cells. A squamous component cannot be completely excluded on the basis of the aspirate, but no cells have well-defined boundaries. *A*, Papanicolaou × 240. *B*, Papanicolaou × 375

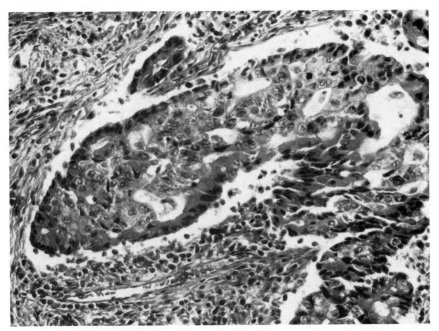

Figure 7–4 Adenocarcinoma, poorly differentiated. Histology of the tumor illustrated in preceding two figures. Hematoxylin and eosin × 240.

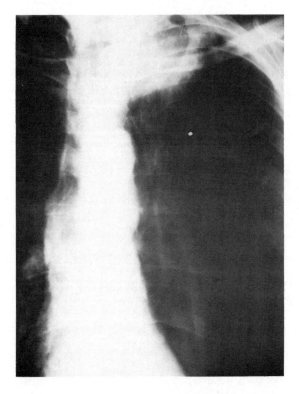

Figure 7–5 Superior sulcus tumor with probable destruction of the fourth rib. Aspiration was performed through the supraclavicular space.

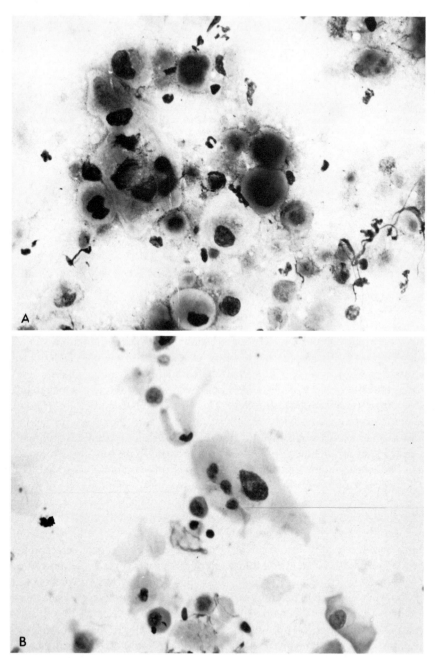

Figure 7–6   Keratinizing squamous cell carcinoma. Pleomorphic cells with irregular nuclei are evident in both smears. *A*, Diff-Quik × 375. *B*, Papanicolaou × 375.

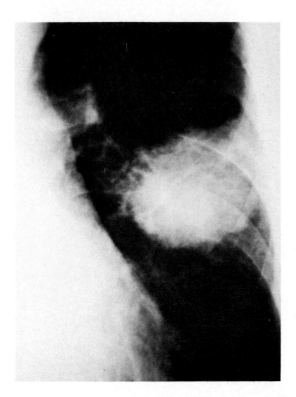

Figure 7–7 Mid-lung mass with evidence of extension to the pleura. Patient inoperable because of severe emphysema.

Other examples of poorly differentiated squamous cell carcinomas are represented in Figures 7–9 and 7–10, and another example of a poorly differentiated adenocarcinoma is illustrated in Figure 7–11. The poorly differentiated squamous tumors are distinguished by the sheet-like arrangement of cells with some definite cytoplasmic borders and intercellular cytoplasmic attachments. The nuclear abnormalities are quite evident, and the cytomorphologic features are almost identical with those seen in the bronchial brushing specimens. In contrast, the poorly differentiated adenocarcinoma demonstrates a syncytial arrangement of cells. Differentiating between the cytomorphologic features of adenocarcinoma and those of squamous cell carcinoma is probably not that important, since it seems from recent work that the most common type of lung cancer is the mixed adenosquamous variety.[64] This might explain much of the diagnostic variability that is associated with aspiration smears and even with conventional cytologic studies of sputum and bronchial washings.

There has been only one case of terminal bronchioalveolar carcinoma in this author's personal experience. The radiograph of this tumor (Fig. 7–12) showed multiple areas of infiltration of the left lung with some similar but focal densities on the right. There was a left pleural effusion. The aspirate demonstrated very large clusters of tumor cells with considerably varied morphologic features (Fig. 7–13). Although the cell groups demonstrated a three-dimensional configuration, they seemed to have a smooth outer border and a remarkable cohesiveness. Some cells even appeared to be ciliated; however, no terminal plate was identified. Vacuolization of the cells was rather prominent. These criteria for differential diagnosis of primary and metastatic adenocarcinoma of the lung have been referred to in other studies.[65] Some of the tumor cells even appeared in a squamous arrangement, further confusing the picture (Fig. 7–14). Examination of pleural fluid obtained at the same time as the aspiration revealed papillary clusters of malignant cells. This finding confirmed the diagnosis of a lung carcinoma and strongly suggested that the tumor was a terminal bronchiolar

Text continued on page 197

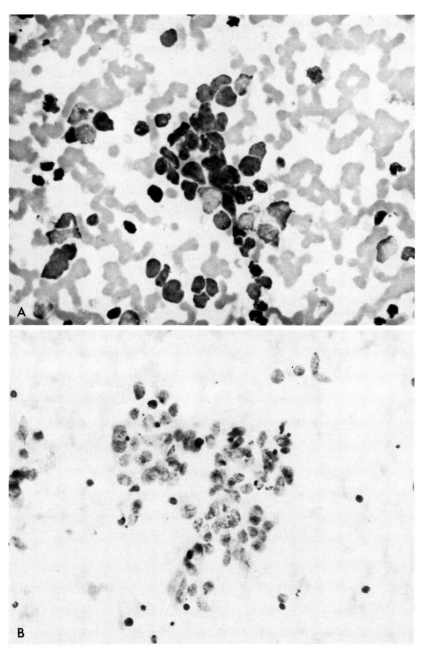

Figure 7–8   Small-cell undifferentiated carcinoma. Both *A* and *B* depict sheets of small undifferentiated cells. Good nuclear molding is evident in the air-dried smear *(A)*. A coarsely granular chromatin pattern and small nucleoli are found in the neoplastic cells in *B*. *A*, Diff-Quik × 375. *B*, Papanicolaou × 375.

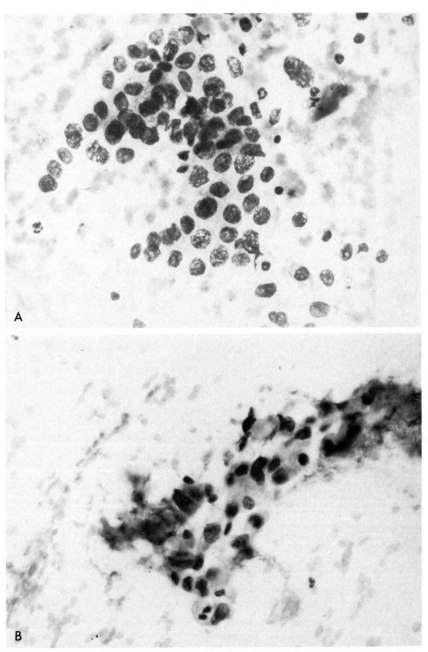

Figure 7–9   Squamous cell carcinoma, poorly differentiated. In *A*, the tumor cells are undifferentiated in morphology and poorly preserved. The fixed aspirate in *B* demonstrates some spindle-shaped cells and other cells that have eosinophilic and dense cytoplasm. *A*, Diff-Quik × 375. *B*, Papanicolaou × 375.

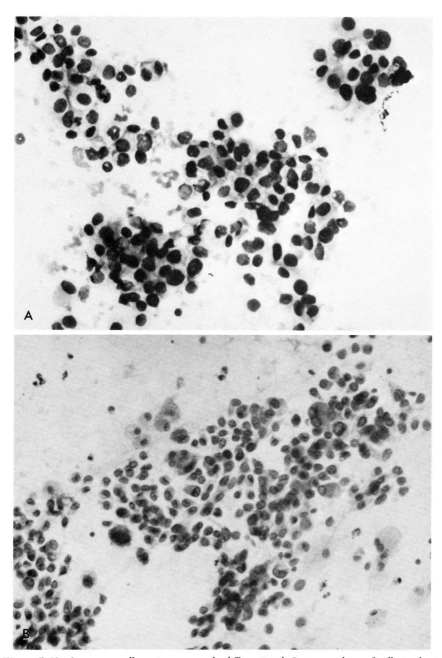

Figure 7–10 Squamous cell carcinoma, poorly differentiated. Large numbers of cells in sheets are present. Cytoplasmic borders are somewhat better defined than in the case illustrated in Figure 7–9. The consistently eccentric nuclear position in many cells might suggest an adenocarcinoma. No true glandular features were seen. *A,* Diff-Quik × 240. *B,* Papanicolaou × 240.

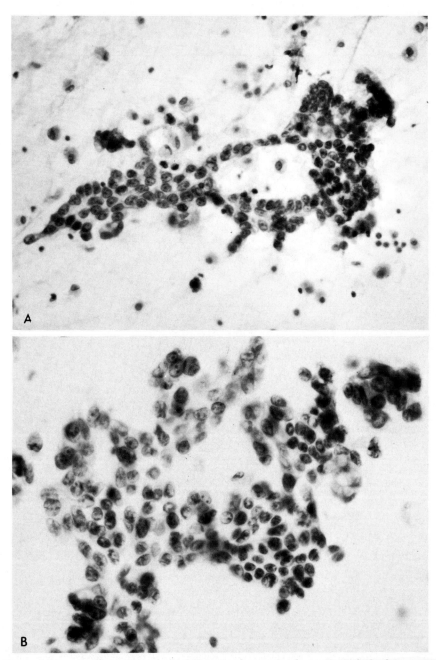

Figure 7–11 Adenocarcinoma, poorly differentiated. Aspirate depicts several glandular spaces that may be present in monolayers of cells from cases of adenocarcinoma. Clustering of the cells with some depth of focus is evident at higher-power magnification (B). Resection of the tumor confirmed the aspiration diagnosis of adenocarcinoma. A, Papanicolaou × 240. B, Papanicolaou × 375. (Courtesy of Dr. R. L. Smith.)

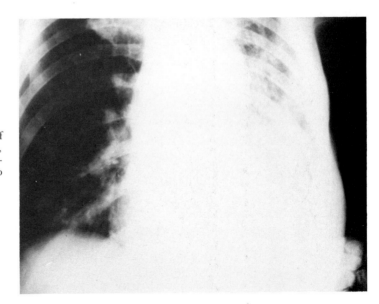

Figure 7–12 Multiple areas of nodular infiltrate in the left lung, with some pleural fluid. Some involvement of the right lung is also evident.

type (Fig. 7–15). This patient was inoperable, so it was not possible to obtain histologic confirmation.

Carcinoid Tumor. As a participant in a diagnostic seminar concerned with pulmonary cytopathology, this author had the opportunity to review two cases of carcinoid tumors of the lung. The first was an asymptomatic mass in a 67-year-old female that was discovered on routine chest film after admission and treatment for a stroke. Radiographically, the tumor measured 9.0 cm in diameter. The aspirate, even at low-power magnification (Fig. 7–16*A*), suggests an organoid tumor composed of small cells. The ribbons and cords of cells are not well defined, and they might even be mistaken for lymphocytes. A close examination of the illustration reveals the proximity of these small cells to a curving capillary. One can then appreciate the endocrine-like structure of the aspiration smear, which immediately suggests a carcinoid tumor. Figure 7–16*B* shows the uniform, distinct nuclear structure of these tumor cells with a small but definite nucleolus. The cells are arranged in a circular pattern with a fibril of cytoplasm pointing toward the central lumen. Figure 7–17 shows the tissue pattern of the mass, which confirms the diagnosis of carcinoid tumor.

The aspirate of the second tumor had a very different pattern. This was also an asymptomatic 2.5 cm nodule discovered on routine chest film in an elderly male admitted for cataract surgery. Figure 7–18 illustrates the small, spindle-shaped tumor cells. In the larger group of cells *(A)*, there are definite glandular lumens. In both *A* and *B*, the individual cells have glassy intranuclear inclusions, as in papillary carcinoma of the thyroid. That feature is confusing, particularly in view of the fact that there was neither a history of thyroid problems nor physical findings indicating a thyroid mass. The tissue from the tumor (Fig. 7–19) does show a typical spindle carcinoid of the lung.

Mesothelioma. Two cases of malignant mesothelioma have been diagnosed by this author with transthoracic aspiration. A radiograph of the first tumor (Fig. 7–20) revealed obviously thickened pleura surrounding the entire lung and extending into the mediastinum, a fairly typical feature of a pleural mesothelioma. The aspirate (Fig. 7–21) showed sheets of undifferentiated malignant cells that interdigitated in the manner of a squamous cell carcinoma. Some pleomorphism was present. This inoperable patient was treated with radiation therapy. It was unexpectedly discovered at

Text continued on page 206

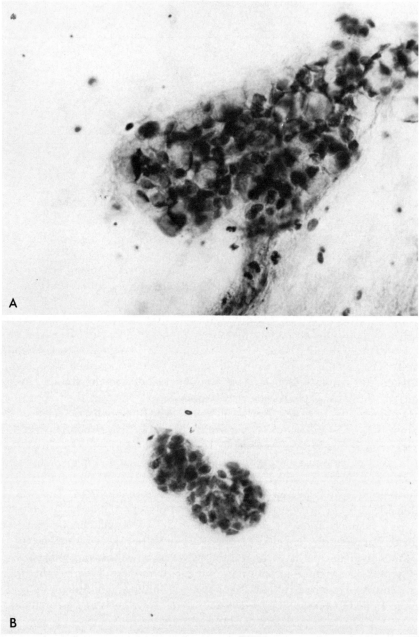

Figure 7–13   Aspirate of the left lung shows multiple clusters of cells, some with coarsely vacuolated cytoplasm. Nuclear atypia is not very striking, but the pattern of the cells suggests alveolar cell carcinoma. *A* and *B*, Papanicolaou × 375.

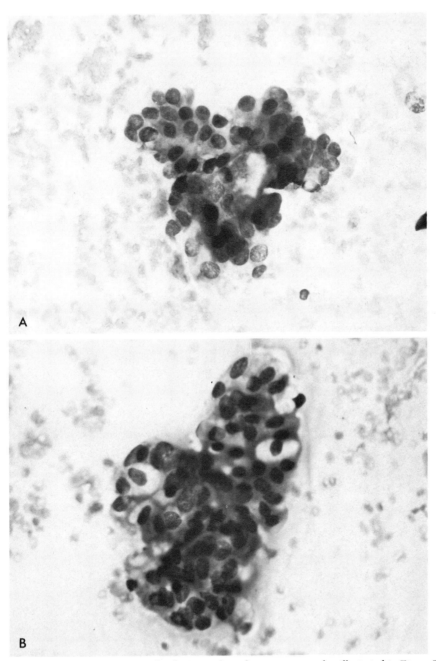

Figure 7–14 Cell features in air-dried aspirate from the same case as that illustrated in Figure 7–13. Three-dimensional, glandular-papillary configuration is evident in both cell groups. Cytoplasmic density and some cells with well-defined borders suggest squamous cell carcinoma *(B)*. This latter feature confused the diagnosis in this case. Both *A* and *B*, Diff-Quik × 375.

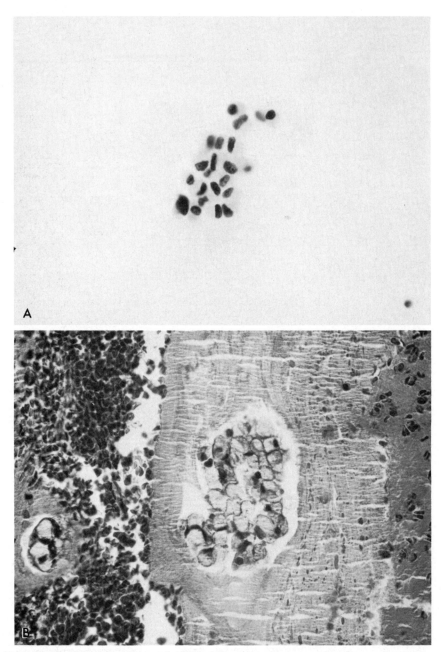

Figure 7–15 Pleural fluid filter and cell block from the same case as that illustrated in Figures 7–13 and 7–14. Papillary clusters of malignant cells are visible and diagnosed in conjunction with the aspiration biopsy as alveolar cell carcinoma. *A*, Papanicolaou × 375. *B*,-Hematoxylin and eosin × 375.

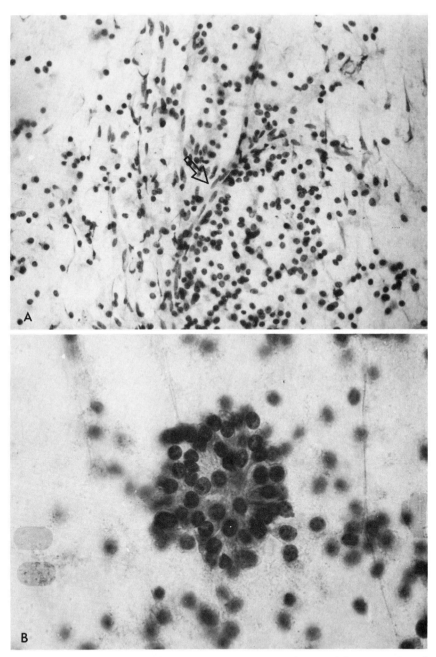

Figure 7–16 Carcinoid tumor of the lung. Lower-power magnification of this aspirate reveals small round tumor cells in a suggestive acinar pattern bounded by a thin capillary blood vessel (arrow) in A. Details of the tumor cells and the rosette-like pattern are apparent in B. A, Papanicolaou × 240. B, Papanicolaou × 600. (Courtesy of Dr. R. Vauclair.)

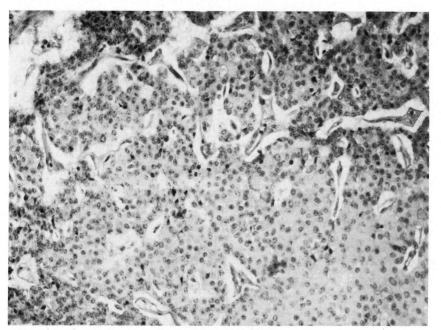

Figure 7–17   Carcinoid tumor. Histology of the tumor diagnosed from the aspiration illustrated in Figure 7–16. Hematoxylin and eosin × 240. (Courtesy of Dr. R. Vauclair.)

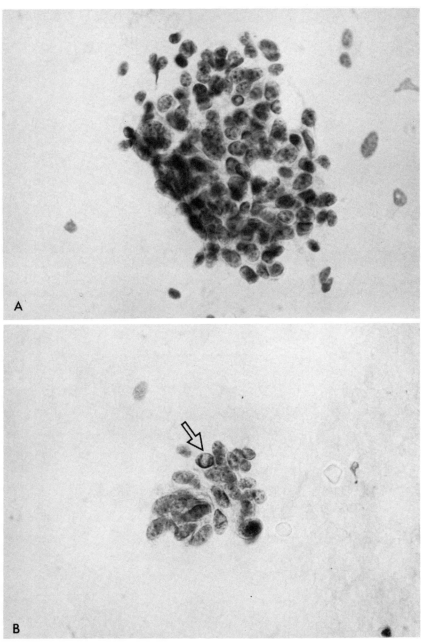

Figure 7-18 Spindle carcinoid tumor. Aspirate from a spherical lung mass, with clusters of small uniform cells. Note the slight spindle shape of the cells and the occasional intranuclear inclusion (arrow). Both *A* and *B*, Papanicolaou × 375. (Courtesy of Dr. J. Chenard.)

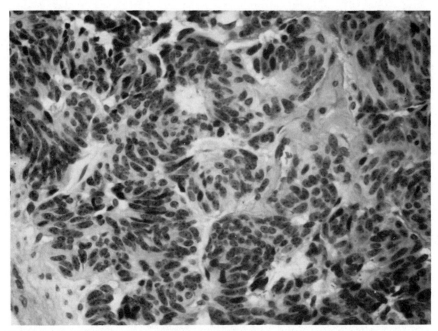

Figure 7–19 Spindle carcinoid tumor. Histology of the tumor seen on aspiration in Figure 7–18. Typical spindle cell carcinoid pattern. Hematoxylin and eosin × 240. (Courtesy of Dr. J. Chenard.)

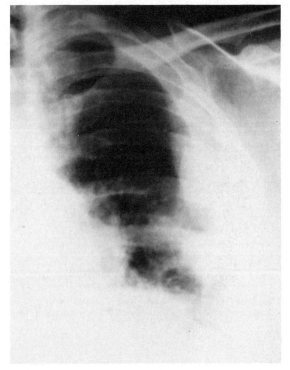

Figure 7–20 Mesothelioma. Film of the tumor involving the pleura, diaphragm, and mediastinum.

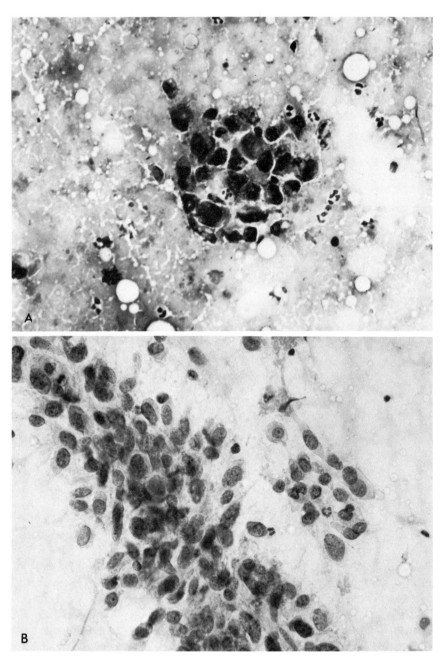

Figure 7–21 Malignant mesothelioma. Sheets of undifferentiated tumor cells, interdigitating in the manner of squamous cell carcinoma. Note the spindle-cell pattern in *B*. *A*, Diff-Quik × 375. *B*, Papanicolaou × 375.

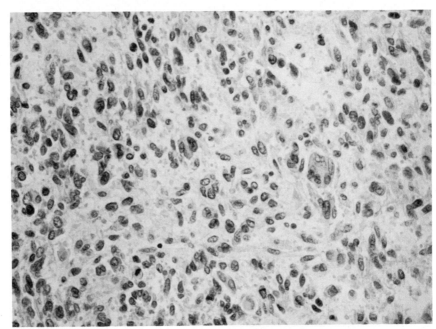

Figure 7–22 Fibrosarcomatous mesothelioma. In view of the aspiration smears, which appeared epithelial, the finding of a fibrosarcomatous pattern was surprising. Hematoxylin and eosin × 375.

subsequent autopsy that this tumor was a fibrosarcomatous mesothelioma rather than an epithelial variety (Fig. 7–22).

The other patient with mesothelioma presented with a very precisely localized acute pain in the back between the shoulder blades. A radiograph showed a small mass adjacent to the vertebral column and destruction of the adjacent rib. Because of the tenderness of the affected area, it was easy to localize the site for biopsy. The aspirate contained undifferentiated, relatively small malignant cells (Fig. 7–23). The results of the original aspiration suggested an anaplastic, poorly differentiated carcinoma in a peripheral location. This patient responded very well to radiation therapy and continued to do well until approximately four years later, when she returned with pain in the same area and an obvious recurrent tumor. Repeat aspiration demonstrated the same tumor. Exploration was undertaken to determine resectability. Tissue biopsy and clinical features at that time revealed mesothelioma (Fig. 7–24). This patient had worked in the shipyards for some years. During this time she was exposed to asbestos, and mesothelioma subsequently developed, presumably from that exposure.

Leukemia.   Several examples of metastatic tumors, lymphomatous infiltrates, or leukemia involving the lungs have also been seen in aspiration biopsies by this author. The most interesting case involved a 12-year-old boy who, with chemotherapy, was in remission for acute lymphatic leukemia. He developed cough and dyspnea and was found to have a reticulated perihilar lung infiltrate (Fig. 7–25). Transthoracic aspiration biopsy revealed only reactive alveolar pneumocytes, but these cells demonstrated prominent nucleoli and abundant cytoplasm (Fig. 7–26). Previous experience suggested that this condition was probably caused by a drug reaction. Steroid therapy resulted in prompt and dramatic improvement. The child was not seen again until a year and a half later, when he returned to the hospital with identical symptoms and radiographic findings. This time, however, aspiration revealed lymphoblastic cells, which indicated relapse of leukemia in the lung. The patient was totally unresponsive to chemotherapy and died within three weeks of the second aspiration (Fig. 7–27).

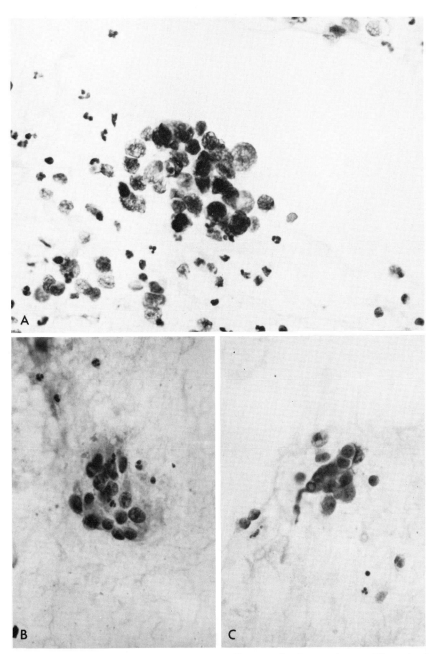

Figure 7–23 Undifferentiated malignant tumor cells originally diagnosed as undifferentiated carcinoma, not further classified. No specific pattern is evident in this aspirate. A, Diff-Quik × 375. B and C, Papanicolaou × 375.

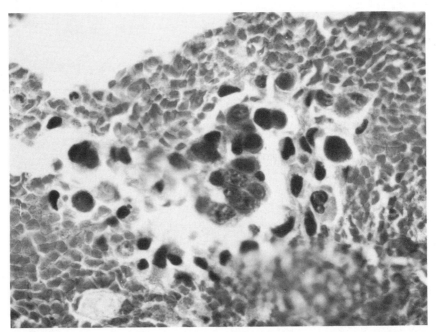

Figure 7–24   Needle biopsy of the pleura taken at the same time as the aspirate reveals small sheets of undifferentiated tumor cells. This biopsy was taken four years after an original aspiration biopsy and diagnosis of carcinoma and a course of radiation therapy. Exploration revealed that the patient was inoperable and that the tumor had the clinical features of a mesothelioma. Biopsy is too limited for more than a diagnosis of malignant tumor.

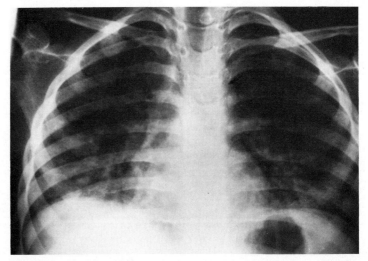

Figure 7–25   Hazy radiating infiltrate of the lung in a 12-year-old male in clinical remission under treatment for acute lymphoblastic leukemia. (From Johnston, W. W., and Frable, W. J.: Diagnostic Respiratory Cytopathology: 290–309, 1979. Copyright © by Masson Publishing U.S.A., Inc., New York.)

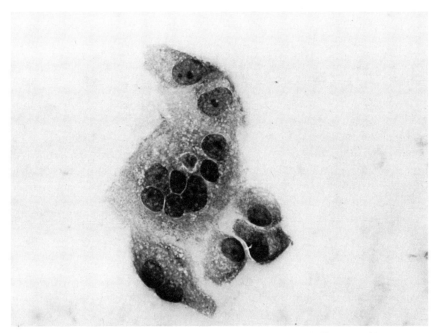

Figure 7–26   Reactive alveolar cells. Aspirate from the right lung infiltrate visible in Figure 7–25. Cells have prominent nucleoli and abundant cytoplasm. Without clinical correlation, such cells might be regarded as malignant. Diff-Quik × 375. (From Johnston, W. W., and Frable, W. J.: Diagnostic Respiratory Cytopathology: 290–309, 1979. Copyright © by Masson Publishing U.S.A., Inc., New York.)

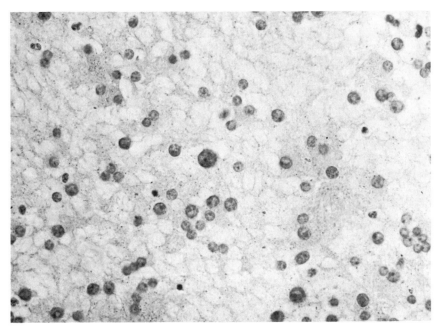

Figure 7–27   Acute lymphoblastic leukemia involving the lung. Same patient as that illustrated in Figures 7–25 and 7–26, one and one-half year later. As previously, clinical presentation and roentgenographic findings were identical. Aspiration this time revealed that recurrence of the leukemia in the lung accounted for the infiltrate. Papanicolaou × 375.

Typing of Lung Tumors

References to studies on typing of lung tumors from aspiration biopsy alone are relatively few. Pavy and colleagues cite Dahlgren and Nordenström's experience, noting 87 per cent accuracy in the diagnosis of malignant tumors and 77 per cent accuracy in classification. This study was based on histologic follow-up.[41] Francis and Hojgaard studied 100 transthoracic aspiration biopsies examined by two pathologists. One was familiar with the technique, but the other was given only a short introduction to this type of preparation. Comparison of results showed that there was excellent reproducibility. The basic difference between the results of the two pathologists was in the diagnosis of malignant tumor cells.[66] Sinner reported the diagnosis of oat cell carcinoma by aspiration biopsy, since confirmation of that tumor type has a signficant impact on subsequent therapy. In 54 cases, 31 of which provided histologic material, 28 were correctly reported as oat cell carcinoma. There was one carcinoid tumor, one adenocarcinoma, and one non-Hodgkin's lymphoma. In the 23 remaining cases, clinical follow-up and mode of death strongly supported the diagnosis of oat cell carcinoma.[51]

BENIGN TUMORS

Hamartoma.   This author has not aspirated any hamartomas, benign lung tumors that are important in differential diagnosis among coin lesions of the lung. One case, seen in consultation (Fig. 7–28), was correctly diagnosed. The air-dried smears stained with Diff-Quik primarily demonstrated sheets of epithelial cells, reactive histiocytes, and alveolar pneumocytes with only one tiny fragment of metachromatic material that resembled cartilage. This stroma is illustrated in Figure 7–28A. A larger fragment, more typical of the cartilaginous matrix of a hamartoma, is depicted in the Papanicolaou-stained, fixed aspirate *(B)*. The small area of hematoma in the center of the tumor indicates where the tumor was aspirated (Fig. 7–29B). Several reports stress that it is important to diagnose this condition successfully so that an open thoracotomy can be avoided. Dahlgren favors the screw needle for this tumor. More of the stromal material is entrapped on the burrs of this needle than can be aspirated with the fine needle.[59, 62]

Other Tumors.   A few of the collected series mention isolated cases of other benign lung tumors diagnosed by aspiration biopsy, such as "bronchial adenomas." None specifically discusses tumors metastatic to the lung. A very rare case of a meningioma metastatic to the lung diagnosed by a percutaneous needle aspiration biopsy is reported by Peck and colleagues.[67]

ASPIRATION FOR DIAGNOSIS OF INFECTIOUS DISEASE

Pneumocystosis.   While fine-needle aspiration biopsy of the lung has been most frequently used in the diagnosis of malignant tumors, the technique is occasionally useful in the diagnosis of infiltrative or inflammatory disease. This is particularly true if a specific organism can be detected. One of the more frequent uses of aspiration is in the identification of *Pneumocystis carinii.*[68, 69, 71] A continuing debate occurs in the literature, however, over the accuracy of the fine-needle aspiration method versus that of open lung biopsy with touch preparations.[70] Figure 7–30 depicts a fine-needle aspirate that demonstrates typical features of pneumocystis. This patient was a 26-year-old male who had been under treatment for Hodgkin's disease when he developed shortness of breath and the typical infiltrative pattern radiographically consistent with pneumocystis. Aspiration biopsy and immediate staining of the smears by May-Grunwald-Giemsa revealed a flocculent, slightly metachromatic background and a few reactive alveolar pneumocytes. Figure 7–30B illustrates the definitive trophozoites arranged around the periphery of the cyst as seen with the Giemsa stain. The cyst

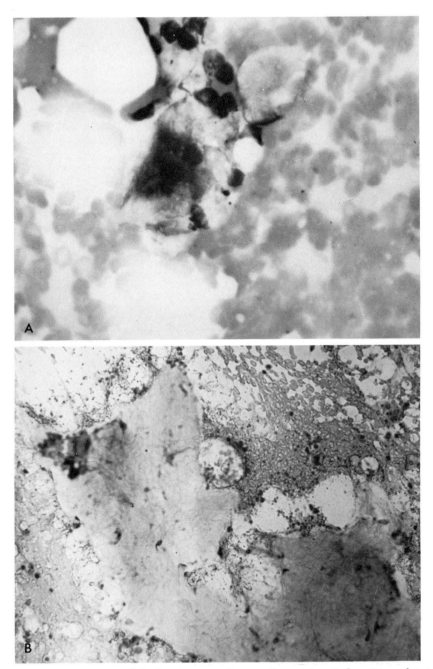

Figure 7–28 Hamartoma of the lung. Aspirate from small asymptomatic lung tumor detected on routine chest film. Irregular mass in center of *A* was the only metachromatic stroma seen on the air-dried smear. Masses of uniform cartilage marix are present in the Papanicolaou-stained preparation *(B)*. A, Diff-Quik × 375. *B*, Papanicolaou × 240. (Courtesy of Dr. F. Gutierrez.)

wall does not actually stain, but the number and morphologic appearance of the trophozoites are thought to be specific for pneumocystis. A confirmatory Gomori methenamine silver stain was also performed.

Gaucher's Disease. A similar problem involving differentiation of infiltrative disease from pneumocystis has occurred in the interpretation of a lung aspirate from a two-year-old child with known Gaucher's disease. This case has been described previously.[65] The smears demonstrated large cells that resembled histocytes with linear

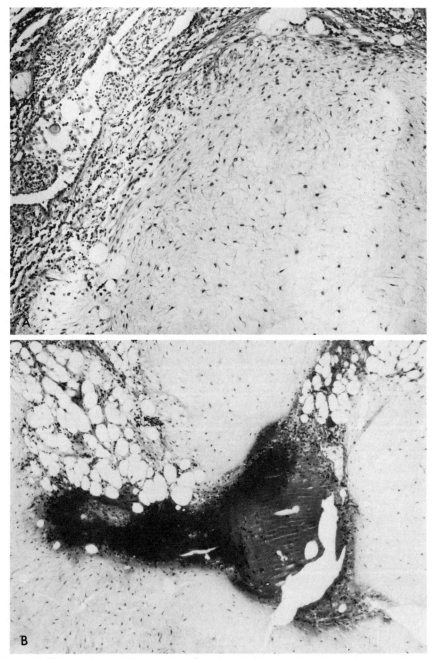

Figure 7–29 Hamartoma. Two sections demonstrate the typical histology of this lung hamartoma. Area of hemorrhage in *B* outlines the needle puncture site. *A*, Hematoxylin and eosin × 100. *B*, hematoxylin and eosin × 60. (Courtesy of Dr. F. Gutierrez.)

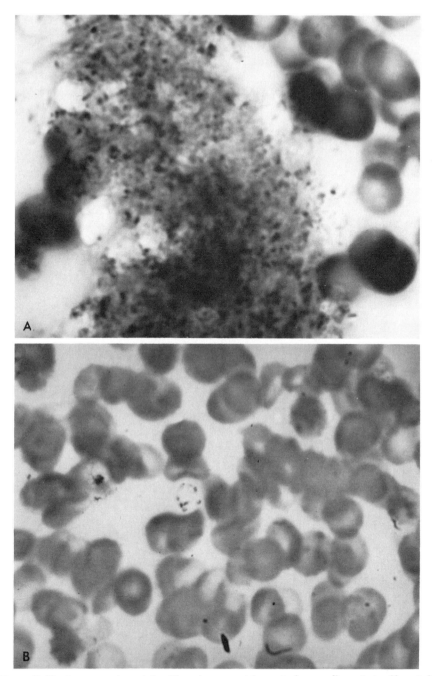

Figure 7–30 *Pneumocystis carinii.*   Flocculent material seen in fine-needle aspirate of lung infiltrate in patient with Hodgkin's disease. Trophozoites within the cyst are seen in the air-dried smear, stained with Diff-Quik. Note the single cyst with the trophozoites arranged about the periphery, a definitive diagnostic feature of *Pneumocystis carinii.* Both *A* and *B*, Diff-Quik × 1000.

striated cytoplasm, which are typical of Gaucher's cellular infiltrate. The child had the rapidly progressive infantile form of Gaucher's disease. Later at autopsy, massive infiltration of Gaucher's cells into the lungs and tracheobronchial tree was documented.

Pulmonary Tuberculosis.   Dahlgren and Ekstrom have reported a series of patients in whom aspiration cytology of the lung was performed for the diagnosis of pulmonary tuberculosis. These authors used the Ziehl-Nielsen stain when there was adequate material or destained slides after initial review when there was a suspected or firmly positive diagnosis of tuberculosis. There were 186 cases in which this diagnosis was made positively. In 57 of these cases, bacteriologic or histologic evaluation was performed, and the diagnosis was confirmed in 42 cases. Nine were considered to be false-positive for tuberculosis. In 136 cases, neither histologic nor bacteriologic studies were performed; in 129 of these cases, clinical and radiographic follow-up of not less than five years revealed findings consistent with tuberculosis. The cytologic diagnosis was based on observation of a finely granular background, necrosis, an increased number of lymphocytes, Langhans type giant cells, epithelioid cells, and occasional small calcium fragments in the aspiration smear.[72]

Mycotic Infections.   Transthoracic aspiration biopsy has also been useful in the definitive diagnosis of mycotic infections. Whitaker and Sterrett used aspiration to diagnose a case of cryptococcosis.[73] Bhatt and colleagues employed transthoracic aspiration biopsy to diagnose opportunistic infections caused by the organisms *Mucor* and *Aspergillus.*[74]

Wegener's Granulomatosis.   Another unique case seen by this author during a diagnostic seminar involved Wegener's granulomatosis. The patient was 53 years old and presented with cough and bloody sputum that developed and increased over a two-month period. A 5.0 cm mass was found on chest film and was believed to be a neoplasm. The aspirate revealed a variety of cells, but none of them looked malignant. Figure 7–31 illustrates inflammatory cells in a granular background that stained eosinophilic, probably representing fibrin. Some of these cells are histiocytes. Figure 7–32 reveals cells in a more cohesive structure with finely granular cytoplasm and eccentrically placed nuclei. These cells also lack malignant features. No giant cells were seen. Trying to account for all the various cells presented a problem in interpreting these smears, especially because the mass was presumed to be a malignant neoplasm. The histologic specimen demonstrates inflammatory and granulomatous features (Fig. 7–33) with a prominent vasculitis. The sheets of cells with the granular cytoplasm that are visible in the smear seem to correspond to swollen endothelial cells present in the inflamed vessels or macrophages or both. Kidney lesions were later observed.

SUMMARY

COMPLICATIONS OF LUNG AND MEDIASTINAL ASPIRATIONS

Table 7–2 summarizes the current experience that this author has had at the Medical College of Virginia with transthoracic needle aspiration biopsy. The cases have been divided according to diagnosis and complications. There is no specific type of disease process related to particular complications, which in this series have been those traditionally reported, principally pneumothorax.

Pneumothorax.   Radiographically, pneumothorax can be demonstrated in about 30 per cent to 40 per cent of patients after thin-needle aspiration biopsy. In experienced hands, less than 10 per cent of these should require chest tube and drainage treatment. In some patients who experience mild symptoms, the air can be aspirated.[75] Among our own patients, those with a rapid respiratory rate, those under ventilatory assistance, and those who were bagged vigorously by the anesthesiologist during the procedure accounted for the majority of pneumothoraces requiring treatment. It can be anticipated that pneumothorax will occur in 100 per cent of patients on respirators. This does not preclude the performance of the aspiration biopsy, but the clinician should be aware that pneumothorax will ensue and require chest tube placement.

Hemoptysis.   One transient case of hemoptysis occurred in this series. The patient was a child being treated for acute lymphatic leukemia. Pneumocystis was suspected in this patient.

Air Embolism.   There was one fatality, which was probably due to air embolism. Several other examples of this complication have been reported. It can best be avoided

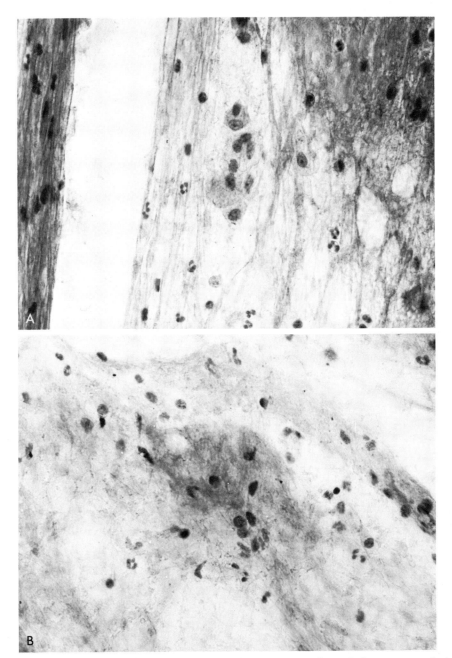

Figure 7–31 Wegener's granulomatosis. Aspirate from a patient with cough, hemoptysis, and a lung mass. Fibrin, inflammatory cells, and large pale histiocytic-appearing cells make up the illustrated fields. No specific diagnostic pattern is present. Both *A* and *B*, Papanicolaou × 375. (Courtesy of Dr. Y. Boivin.)

by not performing aspiration biopsy on those patients with severe emphysema or on patients in a sitting position and by not changing the position of the patient after aspiration biopsy, as occurred in this author's case.[11, 75, 76] This complication has also been reported with Vim-Silverman needle biopsy of the lung.[26]

   Hemorrhage.   Complications of serious pulmonary hemorrhage have occurred more frequently with the large Vim-Silverman needle than with the thin needle.[40, 77]

   Needle Tract Seeding and Tumor Implantation.   Thin-needle aspiration biopsy, especially for lung cancers, has been challenged as an unsafe method because it is believed to cause needle tract seeding and tumor implantation. The reported cases

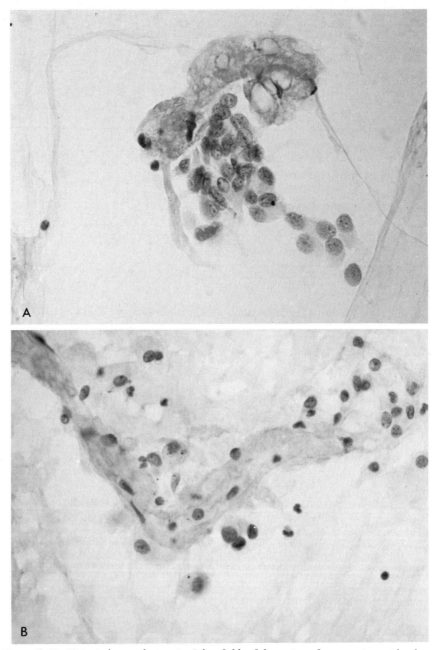

Figure 7–32 Wegener's granulomatosis. Other fields of the aspirate from a patient with a lung mass that was later diagnosed as Wegener's granulomatosis. In *A*, note the granular material bounded at one border by round uniform cells, possibly of bronchiolar type, without cilia. Cells with granular cytoplasm and small uniform nuclei extend into an almost tubular shape. One diagnostic consideration was granular cell myoblastoma, but the aspiration pattern was too inconsistent for any diagnosis. Both *A* and *B*, Papanicolaou × 375. (Courtesy of Dr. Y. Boivin.)

involving this complication are summarized in Table 7–3. It is obvious that the case against the Vim-Silverman needle is well established for this complication. The early studies report the complications of aspirating fluid with tumor cells already in it. Needles with a bore larger than thin needles were probably used in these patients. Sinner and Zajicek report the only documented case in which this complication occurred with the thin-needle method. This tumor was a very large carcinoma that in all probability had already invaded the chest wall at the time of aspiration.[80]

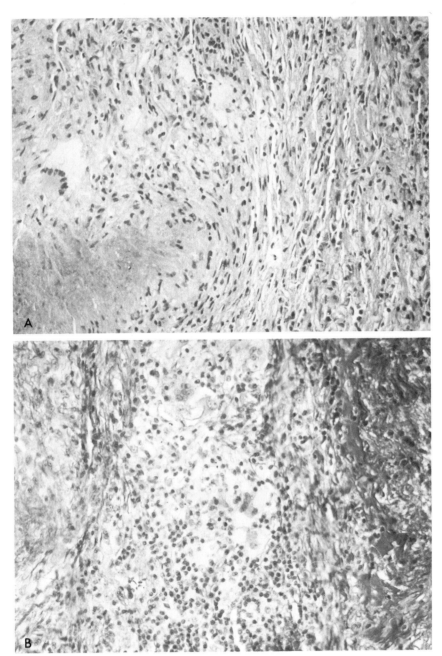

Figure 7–33 Resected lung mass demonstrating granulomas with giant cells, necrosis, and vasculitis. Some of the large round granular cells are found in both *A* and *B*. This lesion was diagnosed as Wegener's granulomatosis. Renal lesions were subsequently documented. Both *A* and *B*, hematoxylin and eosin × 240. (Courtesy of Dr. Y. Boivin.)

INDICATIONS AND CONTRAINDICATIONS FOR ASPIRATION OF LUNG AND MEDIASTINAL LESIONS

Dick and colleagues have summarized the indications for transthoracic thin-needle aspiration biopsy as follows:

1. To confirm suspected malignancy when the lesion is inoperable owing to evident metastasis to mediastinal structures or chest wall or because of poor respiratory function.

2. To differentiate between benign and malignant conditions.

TABLE 7–2. RESULTS AND COMPLICATIONS OF THIN-NEEDLE ASPIRATION BIOPSIES OF THE LUNG

Primary Malignant Tumors	Metastatic Tumors	Benign Tumor, Inflammation, or Other	False-Positive	False-Negative	Complications by Diagnosis
62	25	35	(2)*	(7)†	0
6	2	6	—	—	Pneumothorax‡
—	—	1	—	—	Vagal reflex
—	—	1	—	—	Air embolism
1	—	—	—	—	? Bleeding
—	—	1	—	—	Hemoptysis
1	—	1	—	—	Subcutaneous emphysema

142 Aspirations in 128 patients

Unsatisfactory aspirations	7
Sensitivity for tumor	93%
Specificity for *no* tumor	95%
Overall complication rate	14%

*One case of carcinoma suspected; correct diagnosis was organizing pneumonia. One case of suspected malignant fibrous mesothelioma; correct diagnosis was benign fibrous mesothelioma.

†One case of mesothelioma proved at thoracotomy. Two cases proved tumors metastatic to distant sites; lung was the most likely primary. Four cases of primary lung cancer missed on first aspirate; three of these diagnosed on second attempt.

‡Pneumothorax rate requiring treatment: 9%.

TABLE 7–3.   CASE REPORTS OF NEEDLE TRACT SEEDING IN TRANSTHORACIC ASPIRATION BIOPSIES

Reference and Date	Type of Case	Notes
Reincke[10] 1870	Aspiration from peritoneal carcinomatosis	Probably used large bore needle
Dolley and Jones[7] 1939	Aspiration of pleural fluid with cancer cells	Probably used large bore needle
Ochsner and DeBakey[5,6] 1941 to 1942	Citation of Dolley's case	No documented personal cases
Aronovitch et al.[12] 1953	Lists one case of spread; no documentation as to type of cancer.	Used Vim-Silverman needle for 111 biopsies
Dutra[78] 1954	One case of carcinoma	Used Vim-Silverman needle
Wolansky and Lischner[79] 1969	One case of carcinoma	Used Franklin modification of Vim-Silverman needle
Sinner and Zajicek[80] 1976	One case in 5300 biopsies for malignant tumors	Large, inoperable squamous cell carcinoma originally invading the pleura; thin needle used.

3. To distinguish metastatic tumor from known primaries or a second primary malignancy of the lung.

4. To diagnose multiple tumors in the lung.

5. To identify infectious organisms.

6. To obtain material for tissue culture and bacteriologic studies.[40]

Contraindications are also important and should be carefully observed in performing this procedure, particularly in elderly patients. They have been summarized by Sanders and colleagues as follows:[81]

1. When there is evidence of a hemorrhagic diathesis.

2. When the patient is receiving anticoagulant therapy.

3. When severe pulmonary hypertension is present.

4. When there is a suspected or definite pulmonary hydatid cyst.

5. When uncontrollable cough is present.

6. When advanced pulmonary emphysema is evident.

7. When there is evidence or suspicion of pulmonary arteriovenous malformation.

REFERENCES

1. Craver, L. F., and Binkley, J. S.: Aspiration biopsy of tumors of the lung. J. Thorac. Surg. 8:436–463, 1939.
2. Menetrier, P.: Cancer primitif du poumon. Bull. Soc. Anat. (Paris) 11:643, 1886.
3. Rosemond, G., Burnell, W. E., and Hall, J.: Value and limitations of aspiration biopsy for lung lesions. Radiology 52:506–510, 1949.
4. Gledhill, E. Y., Spriggs, J. B., and Binford, C. H.: Needle aspiration in diagnosis of lung carcinoma. Am. J. Clin. Pathol. 19:235–242, 1949.
5. Ochsner, A., and DeBakey, M.: Carcinoma of the lung. Arch. Surg. 42:209–258, 1941.
6. Ochsner, A., and DeBakey, M.: Significance of metastasis in primary carcinoma of the lung. J. Thorac. Surg. 11:357–387, 1942.
7. Dolley, F. S., and Jones, J. D.: Lobectomy and pneumonectomy for lung suppuration and malignancy. Lancet 59:162–168, 1939.
8. Horder, T. J.: Lung puncture: A new application of clinical pathology. Lancet 2:1345–1350, 1909.
9. Grunze, H.: A critical review and evaluation of cytodiagnosis in chest diseases. Acta Cytol. 4:175–198, 1960.
10. Reincke, J.: Zwei Falle von Krebsimpfung in Punctionskanalen bei carcinomatoeser Peritonitis. Virchows Arch. 51:391, 1870.
11. Woolf, C. R.: Application of aspiration lung biopsy with review of the literature. Dis. Chest 25:286–301, 1954.
12. Aronovitch, M., Chartier, J., Kahana, L. M., et al.: Needle biopsy as an aid to the precise diagnosis of intrathoracic disease. Can. Med. Assoc. J. 88:120–127, 1953.

13. Jamplis, R. W., Stevens, G. M., and Lillington, G. A.: Percutaneous needle aspiration of the lung. Am. J. Surg. *116*:243–250, 1968.

14. Stevens, G. M., Weigen, J. F., and Lillington, G. A.: Needle aspiration biopsy of localized pulmonary lesions with amplified flouroscopic guidance. Am. J. Roentgenol. *103*:561–571, 1968.

15. King, E. B., and Russell, W. M.: Needle aspiration biopsy of the lung. Technique and cytologic morphology. Acta Cytol. *11*:319–324, 1967.

16. Dahlgren, S. E.: Aspiration biopsy of intrathoracic tumors. Technic and results. Acta Path. Microbiol. Scand. *70*:566–576, 1967.

17. Rabinov, K., Goldman, H., Rosbach, H., et al.: The role of aspiration biopsy of focal lesions in lung and bone by simple needle and fluoroscopy. Am. J. Roentgenol. *101*:932–938, 1967.

18. Lauby, V. W., Burnett, E., Rosemond, G. P., et al.: Value and risk of biopsy of pulmonary lesions by needle aspiration. J. Thorac. Cardiovasc. Surg. *49*:159–172, 1965.

19. Dahlgren, S., and Nordenström, B.: *Transthoracic Needle Biopsy.* Chicago, Year Book Medical Publishers, 1966.

20. Nordenström, B. E. W.: Electrocoagulation of small lung tumors; *in* Potchen, E. J. (Ed.): *Current Concepts in Radiology.* Vol. III. St. Louis, C. V. Mosby Co., 1977, pp. 331–347.

21. Nordenström, B. E. W.: Preliminary clinical trials of electrophoretic ionization in the treatment of malignant tumors. IRCS Med. Sc.–Libr. Compend. 6:537, 1978.

22. Zavala, D. C., and Bedell, G. N.: Percutaneous lung biopsy with a cutting needle. An analysis of 40 cases and comparison with other biopsy techniques. Am. Rev. Respir. Dis. *106*:186–193, 1972.

23. Janower, M. L., and Land, R. E.: Lung biopsy. Bronchial brushing and percutaneous puncture. Radiol. Clin. N. Am. 9:73–83, 1971.

24. Turner, A. F., and Sargent, E. N.: Percutaneous pulmonary needle biopsy. An improved needle for a simple direct method of diagnosis. Am. J. Roentgenol. *104*:846–850, 1968.

25. Youmans, C. R., Middleton, J. M., Derrick, J. R., et al.: Percutaneous needle biopsy of the lung for diffuse parenchymal disease. Dis. Chest *54*:105–111, 1968.

26. Adamson, J. W., and Bates, J. H.: Percutaneous needle biopsy of the lung. Arch. Intern. Med. *119*:164–169, 1967.

27. Krumholz, R. A., Manfredi, F., Weg, J. G., et al.: Needle biopsy of the lung. Ann. Intern. Med. 65:293–307, 1966.

28. Sabour, M. S., Osman, L. N., Legolvan, P. C., et al.: Needle biopsy of the lung. Lancet 2:182–184, 1960.

29. Polák, J., and Helbich, P.: The technique and methodology of percutaneous aspiration biopsy of the lungs. Cesk. Radiol. 33:130–134, 1979.

30. Sinner, W. N.: Pulmonary neoplasms diagnosed with transthoracic needle biopsy. Cancer *43*:1533–1540, 1979.

31. Tao, L. C., Pearson, F. G., Delarue, N. C., et al.: Percutaneous fine-needle aspiration biopsy: I. Its value to clinical practice. Cancer *45*:1480–1485, 1980.

32. Snyder, R. N., Willie, S., Cove, J. K., et al.: Extended results of transthoracic fine needle aspiration cytology of lung lesions. Abstr. Acta Cytol. 22:597, 1978.

33. Heaf, R.: Aspiration cytology of lung lesions (meeting abstract). Acta Cytol. *21*:714–715, 1977.

34. Zornoza, J., Snow, J., Jr., Lukeman, J. M., et al.: Aspiration biopsy of discrete pulmonary lesions using a new thin needle. Results in the first 100 cases. Radiology *123*:519–520, 1977.

35. Atay, Z., and Brandt, H. J.: The importance of cytodiagnosis of peribronchial fine needle aspiration of mediastinal or hilar tumours. Dtsch. Med. Wochenschr. *102*:345–348, 1977.

36. House, A. J., and Thomson, K. R.: Evaluation of a new transthoracic needle for biopsy of benign and malignant lung lesions. A.J.R. *129*:215–220, 1977.

37. Jereb, M., and Us-Krasovec, M.: Transthoracic needle biopsy of mediastinal and hilar lesions. Cancer *40*:1354–1357, 1977.

38. Chandrasckhar, A. J., Reynes, C. J., and Churchill, R. J.: Ultrasonically guided percutaneous biopsy of peripheral pulmonary masses. Chest *70*:625–630, 1976.

39. Walls, W. J., Thornbury, J. R., and Naylor, B.: Pulmonary needle aspiration biopsy in the diagnosis of Pancoast tumors. Radiology *111*:99–102, 1974.

40. Dick, R., Heard, B. E., Hinson, K. F. W., et al.: Aspiration needle biopsy of thoracic lesions. An assessment of 227 biopsies. Br. J. Dis. Chest *68*:86–94, 1974.

41. Pavy, R. D., Antic, R., and Begley, M.: Percutaneous aspiration biopsy of discrete lung lesions. Cancer *34*:2109–2117, 1974.

42. Borgeskov, S., and Francis, D.: A comparison between fine-needle biopsy and fiberoptic bronchoscopy in patients with lung lesions. Thorax *29*:352–354, 1974.

43. Sinner, W.: Transthoracic needle biopsy of small peripheral malignant lung lesions. Invest. Radiol. 8:305–314, 1973.

44. Sargent, E. N., Turner, A. F., Bordonson, J., et al.: Percutaneous pulmonary needle biopsy. Report of 350 patients. Am. J. Roentgenol. *122*:758–768, 1974.

45. Hayata, Y., Oo, K., Ichiba, M., et al.: Percutaneous pulmonary puncture for cytologic diagnosis. Its diagnostic value for small peripheral pulmonary carcinoma. Acta Cytol. *17*:469–475, 1973.

46. Yam, L. T., and Levine, H.: Rapid cytologic diagnosis of percutaneous needle aspirates of peripheral pulmonary lesions. Am. J. Clin. Pathol. *59*:648–652, 1973.

47. Sassy-Dobray, G., Keszler, P., and Kompolthy, K.: Experience with respect to intraoperative cytodiagnosis. Acta Cytol. 16:478–482, 1972.
48. Nasiell, M.: Diagnosis of lung cancer by aspiration biopsy and a comparison between this method and exfoliative cytology. Acta Cytol. 11:114–119, 1967.
49. Dahlgren, S., and Lind, B.: Comparison between diagnostic results obtained by transthoracic needle biopsy and by sputum cytology. Acta Cytol. 16:53–58, 1972.
50. Steinmann, G., and Greul, W.: Effect of methods of sample taking on the cytologic diagnosis of lung tumors. Acta Cytol. 22:425–430, 1978.
51. Sinner, W. N., and Sandstedt, B.: Small-cell carcinoma of the lung. Cytological, roentgenologic, and clinical findings in a consecutive series diagnosed by fine-needle aspiration biopsy. Radiology 121:269–274, 1976.
52. Landsman, S., Burgener, F. A., and Lim, G. H. K.: Comparison of bronchial brushing and percutaneous needle aspiration biopsy in the diagnosis of malignant lung lesions. Radiology 115:275–278, 1975.
53. Dahlgren, S. E., and Lind, B.: Transthoracic needle biopsy or bronchoscopic biopsy? Scand. J. Respir. Dis. 50:265–272, 1969.
54. Nordenström, B.: Current concepts. Transthoracic needle biopsy. N. Engl. J. Med. 276:1081–1082, 1967.
55. Jensen, V., Enge, J., and Lexow, P.: The value of percutaneous lung puncture cytology in clinical work. Scand. J. Respir. Dis. 51:233–241, 1970.
56. McCarthy, W. J., Christ, M. L., and Fry, W. A.: Intraoperative fine needle aspiration biopsy of thoracic lesions. Ann. Thorac. Surg. 30:24–29, 1980.
57. Nordenström, B.: Paravertebral approach to the posterior mediastinum for mediastinography and needle biopsy. Acta Radiol. 12:298–304, 1972.
58. Nordenström, B.: Transjugular approach to the mediastinum for mediastinal needle biopsy. A preliminary report. Invest. Radiol. 2:134–140, 1967.
59. Nordenström, B.: A new technique for transthoracic biopsy of lung changes. Br. J. Radiol. 38:550–553, 1965.
60. Nordenström, B.: Paraxiphoid approach to the mediastinum for mediastinography and mediastinal needle biopsy. A preliminary report. Invest. Radiol. 2:141–146, 1967.
61. Nordenström, B.: New instruments of biopsy. Radiol. 117:474–475, 1975.
62. Dahlgren, S. E.: Needle biopsy of intrapulmonary hemartoma. Scand. J. Respir. Dis. 47:187–194, 1966.
63. Ramzy, I.: Pulmonary hamartomas: Cytologic appearances of fine needle aspiration biopsy. Acta Cytol. 20:15–19, 1976.
64. Hess, F. G., Jr., McDowell, E. M., and Trump, B. F.: The respiratory epithelium: VIII. Interpretation of cytologic criteria for human and hamster respiratory tract tumors. Acta Cytol. 25:111–134, 1981.
65. Johnston, W. W., and Frable, W. J.: Diagnostic Respiratory Cytopathology. New York, Masson Publishing, 1979, pp. 209–246.
66. Francis, D., and Hojgaard, K.: Transthoracic aspiration biopsy. A study on diagnostic reproducibility. Acta Pathol. Microbiol. Scand. 85:889–896, 1977.
67. Peck, A. G., Dedrick, C. G., and Taft, P. D.: Pulmonary metastases from intracerebral meningioma. Diagnosis by percutaneous needle aspiration biopsy. Am. J. Roentgenol. 126:419–422, 1976.
68. Kim, H., and Hughes, W. T.: Comparison of methods for identification of Pneumocystis carinii in pulmonary aspirates. Am. J. Clin. Pathol. 60:462–466, 1973.
69. Dutz, W., and Burke, B. A.: Cytologic diagnosis of Pneumocystis carinii. Natl. Cancer Inst. Monogr. 43:157–161, 1976.
70. Rosen, P. P.: Frozen section management of a lung biopsy for suspected Pneumocystis pneumonia. Am. J. Surg. Path. 1:79–84, 1977.
71. Jacobs, J. B., Vogel, C., Powell, R. D., et al.: Needle biopsy in Pneumocystis carinii pneumonia. Radiology 93:525–530, 1969.
72. Dahlgren, S. E., and Ekstrom, P.: Aspiration cytology in the diagnosis of pulmonary tuberculosis. Scand. J. Respir. Dis. 53:196–201, 1972.
73. Whitaker, D., and Sterrett, G. F.: Letter: Cryptococcus neoformans diagnosed by fine needle aspiration cytology of the lung. Acta Cytol. 20:95–107, 1976.
74. Bhatt, O. N., Miller, R., Le Riche, J., et al.: Aspiration biopsy in pulmonary opportunistic infections. Acta Cytol. 21:206–209, 1977.
75. Nordenström, B., and Sinner, W. N.: Needle biopsies of pulmonary lesions. Fortschr. Rontgenstr. 129:414–418, 1978.
76. Westcott, J. L.: Air embolism complicating percutaneous needle biopsy of the lung. Chest 63:108–110, 1973.
77. Smith, W. G.: Needle biopsy of the lung. Lancet 2:318, 1964.
78. Dutra, F. R., and Geraci, C. L.: Needle biopsy of the lung. J.A.M.A. 155:21–32, 1954.
79. Wolansky, H., and Lischner, M. W.: Needle track implantation of tumor after percutaneous lung biopsy. Ann. Intern. Med. 71:359–362, 1969.
80. Sinner, W. N., and Zajicek, J.: Implantation metastasis after percutaneous needle aspiration biopsy. Acta Radiol. Diagn. 17:473–480, 1976.
81. Sanders, D. E., Thompson, D. W., and Pudden, B. J. E.: Percutaneous aspiration lung biopsy. Can. Med. Assoc. J. 104:139–142, 1971.

Chapter Eight

Gastrointestinal System

ASPIRATION OF THE ORGANS OF THE GASTROINTESTINAL SYSTEM

TECHNIQUE

This chapter and the next describe fine-needle aspiration biopsy of intra-abdominal organs, including those in the retroperitoneal area. For convenience, aspiration of gastrointestinal and urogenital organs is discussed in two chapters, but this division is obviously arbitrary, as the technical considerations of the biopsy are quite similar for both.

Increased use of this type of biopsy is reflected in the remarkable advances made in recent years in imaging, specifically ultrasonography and computerized axial tomography (CAT scan).[1, 2, 3] Other methods that have been used, particularly in the diagnosis of masses in the pancreas, are selective angiography, either alone or combined with endoscopic retrograde cholangiopancreatography and fluoroscopy;[4, 19] angiography alone combined with fluoroscopy;[5, 6] and intraoperative aspiration biopsy.[7-10]

Regardless of the type of imaging, the aspiration itself is performed in a similar fashion using a 22- or 23-gauge needle 0.6 mm in external diameter and from 12 cm to 20 cm in length. Most authors have used local anesthesia for the skin and for subcutaneous tissue down to the peritoneum. A larger bore needle, such as an 18-gauge, is placed through the skin and subcutaneous tissue to avoid plugging up the aspiration biopsy needle or having it deflected by the heavy musculature of the abdominal wall found in some patients. If an intra-abdominal mass is palpable, imaging is not necessarily required. The aspiration biopsy may be performed directly after administration of local anesthesia to the skin, subcutaneous tissue, and peritoneum. This author has performed most of his aspiration biopsies in this manner.

THE PANCREAS

Tumors in the pancreas have been a favorite site for fine-needle aspiration biopsy because of both their gross inaccessibility and the complications associated with surgical and Vim-Silverman needle biopsy. Ultrasonography has been the preferred imaging method.[11-17] Excellent results, however, have been obtained using angiography and fluoroscopic control,[5, 6] cholangiography and fluoroscopic localization,[18, 19] or a combination of cholangiography and angiography with fluoroscopic control.[4] Some authors have preferred intraoperative aspiration biopsy of the pancreas and quick staining of the smears to obtain a diagnosis or at least to confirm that an adequate sample for diagnosis is present.[7, 9, 10, 20, 21]

One advantage of ultrasonography is that it allows the mass to be delineated while one is using a biopsy transducer with the needle passed through it directly into the mass. The ultrasonic equipment accurately calculates the depth of the tumor.[11, 12] An 18-gauge needle is often introduced through the biopsy transducer and the abdominal wall, since the 0.6 mm 23-gauge fine needles are quite flexible and may be deviated from the target, as previously described. Multiple attempts may be made to biopsy the mass through the short needle introduced via the transducer. The details of the technique have been described by Bartrum and Crow in their monograph on ultrasonography.[22]

This author would suggest as a modification of their biopsy method use of the syringe holder and the 20 ml syringe. This allows the application of more vacuum and better control of the depth of the needle as well as the performance of the biopsy itself, that is, moving the needle back and forth in the mass with the vacuum applied.

This author's experience with fine-needle aspiration biopsy of the pancreas is limited to only eight cases of a total of 74 aspiration biopsies of intra-abdominal organs. All except three of these aspirations were intraoperative. Recent biopsies were performed using ultrasonography.

Pancreatitis. An example of sheets of reactive pancreatic duct and acinar cells from an intraoperative aspiration biopsy of chronic pancreatitis is illustrated in Figure 8–1. The cells have a cohesive, well-organized structure, and the duct cells usually have a predominantly columnar shape or a honeycomb appearance resembling that of endocervical cells when viewed en face. The acinar cells occur in small clusters. They have abundant cytoplasm with a fine granularity, as described by Stormby.[15] The background exudate is variable, depending upon the activity of the inflammation.

In acute pancreatitis, there are polymorphonuclear leukocytes and debris with evidence of precipitation of necrotic fat and deposition of calcium (Fig. 8–2). In the more chronic stages, lymphocytes and plasma cells predominate but may be scanty if there is considerable fibrosis. The atypical epithelial cell changes seen with regeneration and repair have been described as potentially easy to confuse with carcinoma. Kline disputes this, indicating that the carcinomas are very obviously malignant.[10] Islet tissue is usually not identifiable in aspiration biopsy smears from normal pancreas, pancreatitis, or pancreatic neoplasms.[15]

Pancreatic Carcinoma. Pancreatic carcinoma is illustrated in Figures 8–3 to 8–7. The anaplastic nature of the cells, demonstrated by their very hyperchromatic, irregular nuclei and by the granular chromatin pattern, is evident in Figure 8–3. This neoplasm is very undifferentiated, as it shows conspicuous nuclear molding. It would be impossible to differentiate this aspirate from that of an oat cell carcinoma metastatic to the pancreas or retroperitoneal area because the cytomorphologic appearance of both is identical. That differential diagnosis would have to be made on the basis of clinical or other morphologic evidence. The original clinical presentation and follow-up information in this case would indicate that it was a primary carcinoma of the pancreas.

A better differentiated pancreatic carcinoma with the large papillary clusters of duct cells is depicted in Figure 8–4. Many of these cells are vacuolated with eccentric nuclei. There are prominent nucleoli evident in most of these tumor cells. This intraoperative aspirate was from a mass in the head of the pancreas producing painless jaundice. A comparison of the morphologic appearance and size of the tumor cells with the features of normal pancreatic cells from the pancreatitis smear should be made (Fig. 8–1).

Text continued on page 228

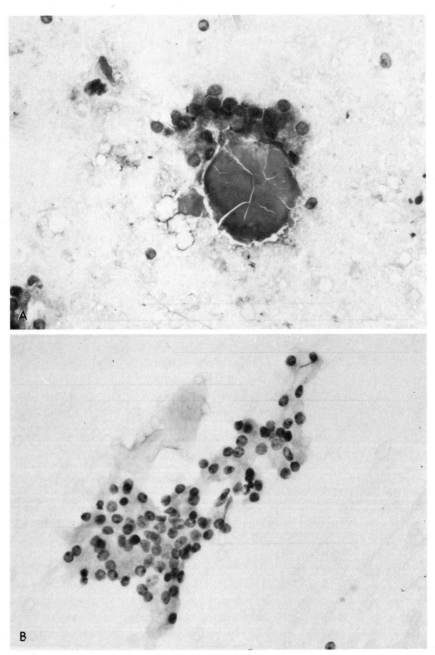

Figure 8–1   Chronic pancreatitis. Intraoperative aspiration composed of sheets of uniform epithelial cells, a few inflammatory cells, and some debris. Note the inspissated secretion from a small duct and the attached epithelial cells (upper panel). *A*, Diff-Quik × 375. *B*, Papanicolaou × 375.

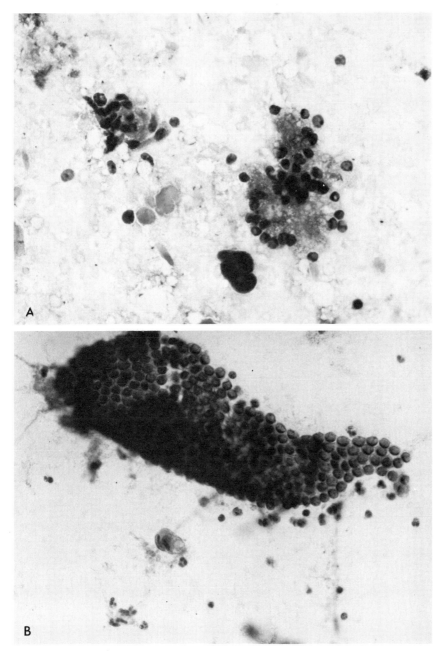

Figure 8–2 Acute and chronic pancreatitis. Intraoperative aspiration with more active-appearing epithelium, increased inflammatory cells, debris, and precipitated calcium (left center of *A*). The epithelial cells are of uniform size with minimal atypia. *A*, Diff-Quik × 375. *B*, Papanicolaou × 375.

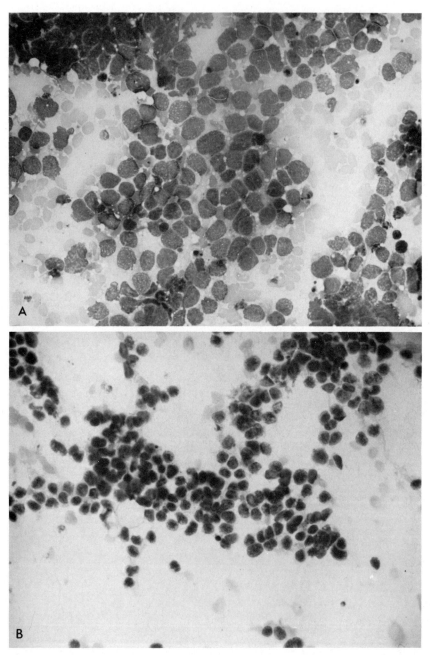

Figure 8–3   Anaplastic carcinoma of the pancreas. Aspiration of a mass in the head of the pancreas performed with ultrasound imaging. Note the undifferentiated nature of the cells with a pattern not unlike that of oat cell carcinoma. *A*, Diff-Quik × 375. *B*, Papanicolaou × 375.

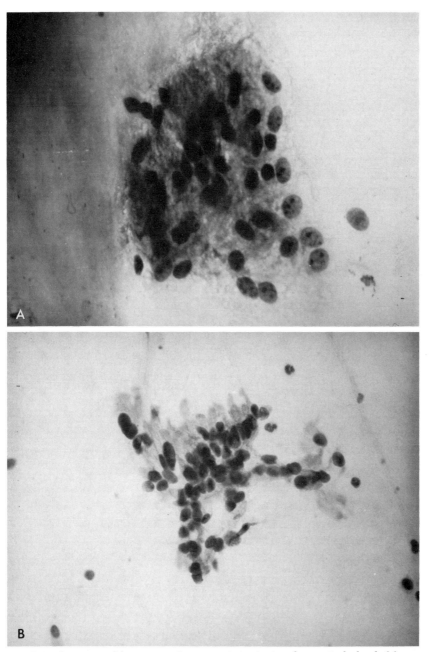

Figure 8–4   Carcinoma of the pancreas. Intraoperative aspiration of a mass in the head of the pancreas. Note the larger cell size with the somewhat granular nuclear chromatin and the prominent nucleoli. A definite acinar arrangement is also apparent in *B*. *A*, Diff-Quik × 375. *B*, Papanicolaou × 375.

Figures 8–5 and 8–6 depict an intraoperative aspirate from a less differentiated carcinoma of the body of the pancreas. With this cancer, there is substantial cellular atypia. The irregular clusters of cells should also be compared with normal pancreatic elements. Although clinically resectable, a mesenteric node revealed metastatic carcinoma on frozen section (Fig. 8–6B). Figure 8–7 demonstrates the use of ultrasonic imaging for placement of the needle and the resulting aspirate, diagnosed as pleomorphic carcinoma of the pancreas.

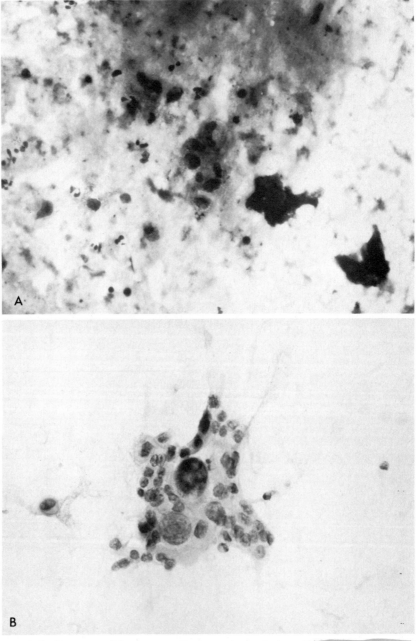

Figure 8–5   Carcinoma of the pancreas. Intraoperative aspiration with irregular sheets of cells and pleomorphic nuclei. A, Diff-Quik × 240. B, Papanicolaou × 375.

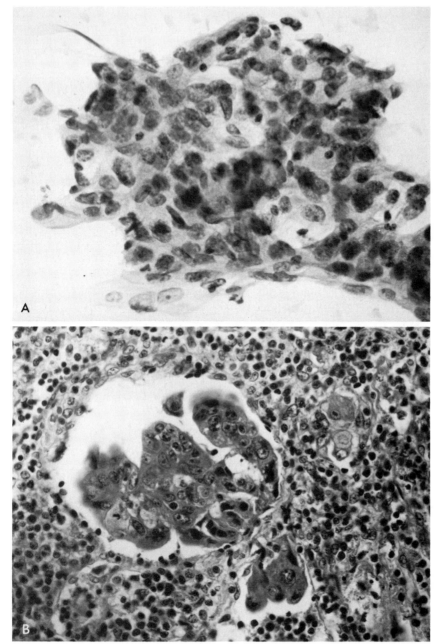

Figure 8–6 Carcinoma of the pancreas. Intraoperative aspiration showing another sheet of malignant cells (A) and microscopic metastasis to mesenteric lymph node (B). A, Papanicolaou × 375. B, Hematoxylin and eosin × 375.

Results of Pancreas Aspirations

Table 8–1 summarizes the results of several fine-needle biopsy series with calculations of both sensitivity for a malignant tumor and specificity for the absence of a pancreatic neoplasm. While many of the series are small, results appear to be quite good. Specificity for the absence of tumor is 100 per cent in nearly all reports because there is usually a strong clinical suspicion of pancreatic carcinoma before the aspiration biopsy is attempted. Hence, very few pancreatic masses that are diagnosed negative are actually examined.

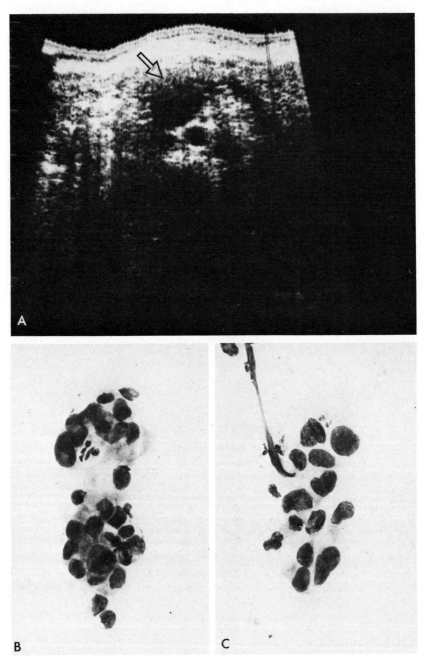

Figure 8–7 Pleomorphic carcinoma of the pancreas. Aspiration biopsy performed with ultrasonic imaging. A mass in the head of the pancreas is represented by the large dark area in *A* (arrow). In *B* and *C*, pleomorphic epithelial cells with hyperchromatic nuclei are illustrated. *B* and *C*, Diff-Quik × 375.

TABLE 8–1.   RESULTS FROM SELECTED SERIES OF FINE NEEDLE ASPIRATION BIOPSIES OF THE PANCREAS

Reference	True-Positive	False-Positive	True-Negative	False-Negative	Sensitivity (%)	Specificity (%)	Unsatisfactory
Holm et al.[1]	15	0	0	2	88	‡	0
Tao et al.[4]	24	0	8	2	92	100	0
Tyler et al.[5]	18	0	0	0	100	‡	0
Stormby et al.[8]	42(2)*	0	36	2	95	100	4
Koivuniemi et al.[9]	21(2)*	0	36	7	75	100	2
Kline et al.[10]	35(1)*	0	20	1	97	100	0
Hancke[11]	15	0	27	2	88	100	0
Zornoza[17]	32	0	12	20	61	100	0
McLoughlin et al.[18]	19†	0	5	4	82	100	0
Frederiksen et al.[20]	27(6)	1	33	3	90	97	0
Shorey[21]	18	0	3	0	100	100	0
Kirstaedter and Meyer-Burg[23]	15	0	27	4	79	100	0
Bodner et al.[24]	77(12)*	0	26	5	93	100	8
Dekker and Lloyd[25]	12(1)*	0	0	1	92	‡	0

*Cases reported as suspicious included in ( ) as part of the total true positives for carcinoma.
†Includes tumors near the biliary tree and pancreas.
‡No true-negative results in these series.

$$\frac{TP}{TP+FN} \quad \text{measure of true } (+)$$

$$\frac{TN}{TN+FP}$$

Data from other case studies could not be accurately evaluated in this tabular form. For example, the results of Evander and colleagues are less impressive. They performed 108 aspiration biopsies, using selective angiography and transhepatic cholangiography. This series included tumors both within the pancreas and around the biliary tree. The rate of accuracy for pancreatic carcinoma was 60 per cent in 52 tumors, while it was only 53 per cent in 19 patients with extrahepatic biliary tract carcinoma. There were no false-positive results, and in 17 patients the authors accurately ruled out a clinical suspicion of neoplasm after a negative aspiration biopsy.[26]

Commenting on these results, Stormby noted that 14 different radiologists performed the examinations and many of the tumors were quite small.[15] A recent series reported in the American literature by researchers at M.D. Anderson Hospital revealed an overall diagnostic accuracy rate of 85 per cent in 18 patients with pancreatic masses and in 19 others with abdominal tumors. Biopsy was performed under fluoroscopic guidance, and ultrasonography was used to determine the depth of the mass prior to biopsy.[27]

Complications of Pancreas Aspirations

Complications following either percutaneous or intraoperative pancreatic fine-needle aspiration biopsy have been extremely rare. Stormby noted that in 350 such aspirations there were no complications, while during the same period a summary of Vim-Silverman needle biopsies of the pancreas revealed a complication rate of 2 per cent to 20 per cent.

Of 15 reports concerning fine-needle biopsy of the pancreas, only two cited complications.[15] In the series by Holm and colleagues, there was one small intra-abdominal hematoma in 1200 ultrasonically-guided aspirations.[1] Koivuniemi and colleagues mentioned an occasional slight increase in amylase in pancreatitis patients after aspiration.[9] Obviously, one can conclude that the procedure is extremely safe.

Ferrucci and colleagues have reported the single well-documented case of needle tract implantation that occurred after fine-needle aspiration biopsy of pancreatic carcinoma guided by CAT scan. Ten aspirations of this mass were made on two successive days. The first five, which were obtained from the necrotic center of the tumor, yielded nondiagnostic material. The second five all yielded malignant cells reported as pancreatic carcinoma. Since the patient was inoperable, no harm was done. He developed progressive symptoms of pancreatic cancer, including jaundice. Two subcutaneous tumor nodules appeared along the course of the needle tract three months after the biopsies.

Some criticism can be leveled at the procedure in this case. First, the number of biopsies is excessive, particularly when five of them yielded tumor cells. Use of rapid stains and a quick diagnostic report could have prevented the unnecessary aspirations. Second, after obtaining only necrotic material from the center of the mass that was considered necrotic on the basis of the scan, the biopsy should have been made of the peripheral and solid part of the tumor at the first session. Nevertheless, this author believes that this single case of implantation does not detract from the utility of the thin-needle aspiration biopsy method.[28]

THE LIVER

In reports of several large series of fine-needle aspiration biopsies of the liver, authors advocate this technique because of its usefulness in diagnosing both malignant and benign disease.[29-33] Methodology is similar to that of other aspirations. A needle

0.6 mm to 0.8 mm in outer diameter and 8 cm to 15 cm in length is used. The approach is usually through the ninth or tenth intercostal space in the anterior axillary line, and the liver is punctured during deep expiration. Patients should be instructed to hold their breath during the puncture and aspiration. Hemorrhagic diatheses are considered an absolute contraindication, and the patient is made to rest for two hours after the procedure. Both air-dried smears stained with May-Grunwald-Giemsa and alcohol-fixed hematoxylin and eosin- or Papanicolaou-stained aspirates are prepared. Stormby and Akerman prefer wet fixation by alcohol with subsequent hematoxylin and eosin staining, particularly when a neoplasm is suspected.[29]

Lundquist estimates that fine-needle aspiration biopsy provides about one tenth the number of cells obtained with the traditional tissue needle biopsy. This yield is adequate for quantitative chemical analysis and special staining with dyes such as oil red O for fat; aminoacid naphthylamidase for bile canaliculi; alkaline phosphatase for enzymatic activity in canaliculi; and Prussian blue for hemosiderin.[31, 32] Puncture of the gallbaldder should be avoided.[31] This author has no personal experience with this type of biopsy for benign conditions. Lundquist, Soderstrom, Stormby, Akerman, and Wasastjerna provide excellent descriptions of the normal cellular composition of aspirates obtained with fine-needle biopsy of the liver and changes related to increases in fat, siderosis, bile stasis, hepatitis, myeloid metaplasia, and granulomatous disease.[29-32] This author believes, after reviewing their reports, that the findings are not that specific, particularly in cases of hepatitis and cirrhosis, and concludes that one must rely on traditional tissue needle biopsy for those diagnoses.

Carcinoma.   Fine-needle aspiration biopsy of the liver appears to be most effective with malignant disease, either a specific mass identified by an imaging technique or a palpable tumor.[17, 34-37] Figure 8–8 illustrates an aspirate from an adenocarcinoma of the duodenum metastatic to the liver.

An alternative and popular procedure that has been employed in this laboratory is to obtain the tissue by conventional needle biopsy and then prepare touch preparations on filters from saline washing of the biopsy needle. This was originally described by Sherlock and colleagues as an additional aid in the diagnosis of metastatic carcinoma to the liver. In that original paper, two additional cases of metastatic carcinoma were diagnosed exclusively by the cytologic preparation in a series of 62 patients. The authors also felt that even in benign cases, additional information was obtained from the touch preparations.[38]

Results of Liver Aspirations

This author's experience with the touch-preparation method and needle wash-out technique preferred for this type of liver aspiration is summarized in Table 8–2. The results indicate a false-negative group of diagnoses for both methods: 10 for touch preparation wash-out and five for core biopsy. Six cases identified by core biopsy were not seen with the cytologic smears, while four cases diagnosed cytologically were not present in multiple sections of the core biopsy, two more cases than Sherlock found in his reported series. In seven recent cases, CAT scan or ultrasonographically directed biopsy or both were used in the diagnosis of metastatic neoplasms. All were positive for carcinoma.

No correlation was established for benign disease (64 cases). A few cytologic studies did show reactive-inflammatory changes of hepatocytes or actual inflammatory cells. In those patients, tissue needle biopsy usually revealed evidence of viral hepatitis. However, in many cases reported as simply "no tumor cells identified," core biopsy demonstrated a variety of inflammatory and degenerative diseases of the liver. The

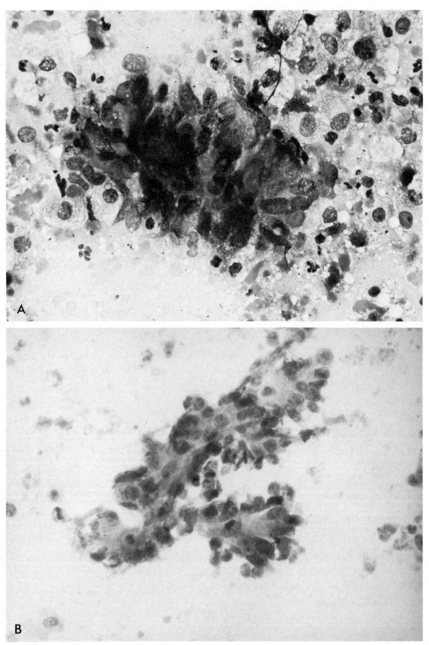

Figure 8–8   Carcinoma of the duodenum metastatic to the liver. Aspirate of liver mass obtained with CAT-scan imaging. Note the acinar arrangement of the elongated malignant cells. The pattern is similar to that of metastatic colonic carcinoma, with a large amount of necrotic debris in the background. *A*, Diff-Quik × 375. *B*, Papanicolaou × 375.

TABLE 8–2. NEEDLE BIOPSY OF THE LIVER IN MALIGNANT DISEASE: COMPARISON OF CORE BIOPSY AND CYTOLOGY FROM THE SAME SPECIMEN

	Positive for Metastatic Tumors	Hepatoma	False-Positive	False-Negative	Unsatisfactory
Cytology	29	2	1	10	1
Tissue Biopsy	24	3	0	5	0

one false-positive result is of interest and is illustrated in Figure 8–9. This patient was said to have a hepatic mass suggesting a hepatoma. The aspirate showed several atypical liver cells as demonstrated. This finding was considered indicative of hepatoma, and a positive diagnosis was reported. Additional history revealed that this patient had been receiving methotrexate for treatment of psoriasis. That drug is known to produce very atypical liver cells, as confirmed by the tissue core biopsy of the same tumor.

Other Metastatic Tumors. Other examples of metastatic tumors reported from the needle rinse specimen are depicted in Figures 8–10 to 8–12. Some of these cases are quite difficult to diagnose, particularly metastatic breast cancer (Fig. 8–10), in which the tumor cells may be extremely small and resemble those of malignant lymphoma. This is further emphasized by their somewhat scattered appearance. An example of oat cell carcinoma, a relatively easy diagnosis, is depicted in Figure 8–11. Large pleomorphic cells with abundant necrosis is usually the cytologic feature of metastatic colonic carcinoma (Fig. 8–12). An unusual case of a metastatic carcinoid tumor shows very small and uniform cells in a direct aspiration biopsy smear (Fig. 8–13).

Complications of Liver Aspirations

Complications with core needle biopsy of the liver are not unknown. In a series reported by Perrault and colleagues, 5 per cent of patients who had tissue needle biopsy on an outpatient basis required hospitalization. The overall complication rate of severe or moderate abdominal pain, hypotension, or both was 5.9 per cent in a series of 1000 cases.[39] In contrast, fine-needle aspiration biopsy of the liver has resulted in extremely few complications. Riska and Friman have reported one fatality that occurred after fine-needle aspiration biopsy of the liver. This patient had had an end-to-side portocaval anastomosis and splenectomy for cryptogenic liver cirrhosis. The patient was later admitted in hepatic coma. Blood studies showed that platelets were adequate; however, the prothrombin level was only 31 per cent. A suspected hepatoma was diagnosed. Eight hours after the fine-needle aspiration biopsy, the patient was found in shock with an intra-abdominal bleed. He died two days later. It is of interest that the needle had passed in one side and out the other side of a nodule of tumor on the dorsal surface of the liver. These two punctures may have accounted for the bleeding in a somewhat compromised patient.[40]

Schulz reported a single case of bile peritonitis complicating a fine-needle aspiration biopsy. This patient was a healthy subject with no liver disease who was undergoing fine-needle aspiration biopsy as a family screening procedure for hemochromatosis. Laporotomy was necessary 24 hours after the aspiration. There were about 1.5 liters of bile present in the abdominal cavity. At the time of needle aspiration biopsy, bile had appeared in the syringe. No traumatic defects of the biliary system were found during exploration. It has been established that it is important to avoid puncturing the gallbladder during fine-needle aspiration biopsy.[41]

Text continued on page 241

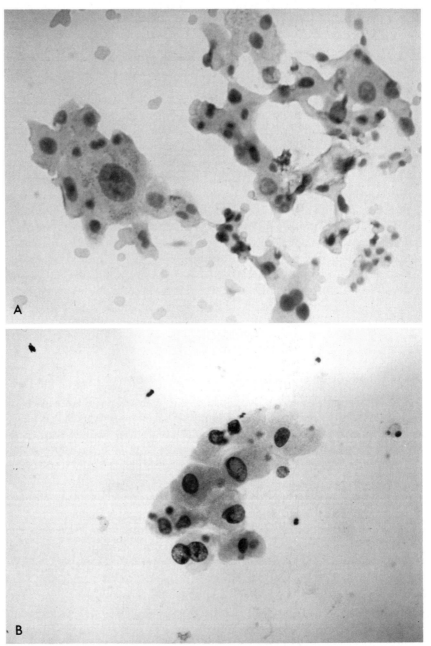

Figure 8–9   Rinse of core-needle biopsy of the liver. Note the sheets of cells with pleomorphic nuclei. Shape and cytoplasmic consistency suggest that these are liver cells. Atypical features were considered sufficient evidence for a diagnosis of hepatoma. The core biopsy revealed only atypical liver cells. Additional history revealed that this patient was taking methotrexate for psoriasis. This drug accounted for the atypia. Both *A* and *B*, Papanicolaou × 375.

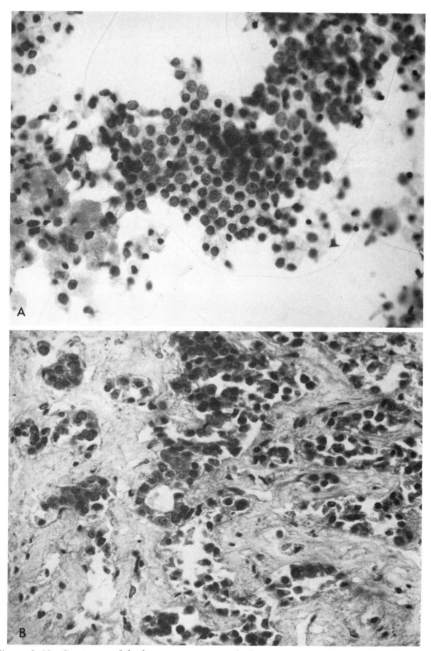

Figure 8–10 Carcinoma of the breast metastatic to the liver. *A,* Rinse of core-needle biopsy. *B,* The actual biopsy. Small uniform tumor cells visible in the cytology morphologically resemble those of lymphoma. Some cohesive groups of cells would rule out that diagnosis. *A,* Papanicolaou × 375. *B,* Hematoxylin and eosin × 375.

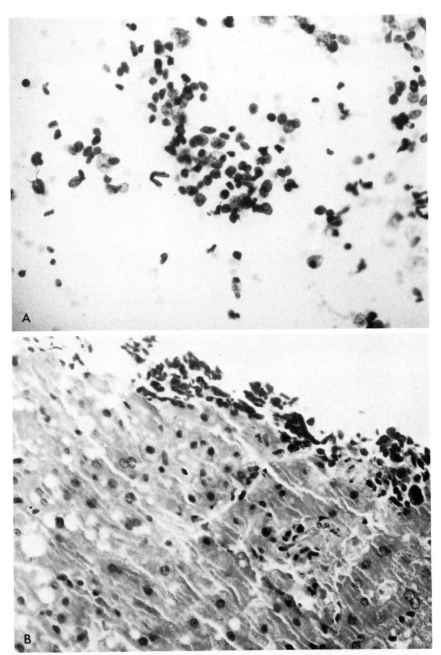

Figure 8–11   Oat cell carcinoma of the lung metastatic to the liver. *A*, Rinse of core needle biopsy. *B*, The actual biopsy. There were many small, undifferentiated tumor cells with good nuclear molding seen cytologically, while the biopsy demonstrated tumor only at the edge of the section. *A*, Papanicolaou × 375. *B*, Hematoxylin and eosin × 375.

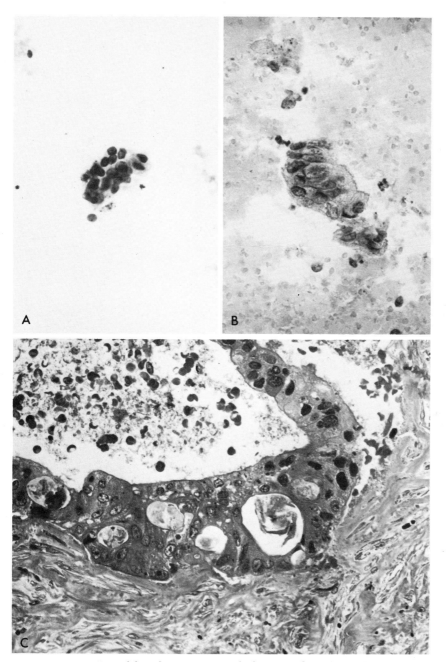

Figure 8–12   Carcinoma of the colon metastatic to the liver. *A* and *B,* Rinse of core needle biopsy. *C,* The actual core biopsy. Tumor cells are small and degenerated in the cytology specimen, but cell block section of the needle rinse demonstrates them to better advantage *(B).* A, Papanicolaou × 375. B and C, Hematoxylin and eosin × 375.

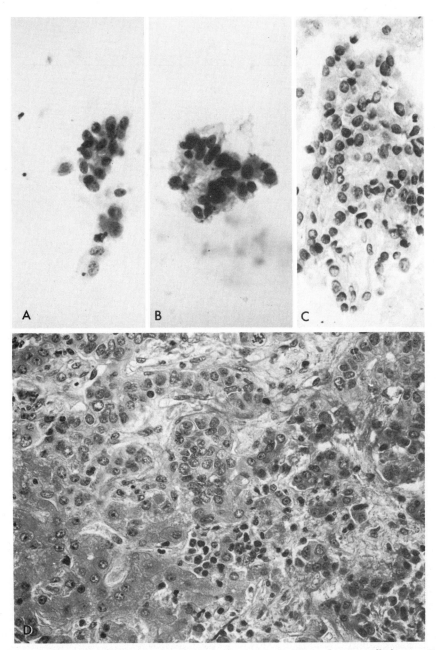

Figure 8–13 Carcinoid tumor metastatic to the liver. *A* to *C*, Rinse of core needle biopsy. *D*, The actual biopsy. Small cells in an acinar pattern are found in both the cytology (*A* and *B*) and the cell block (*C*). Note the similarity between the arrangement of the tumor cells in the tissue biopsy and that of the tumor cells in the cytologic preparations. *A* and *B*, Papanicolaou × 375. *C* and *D*, Hematoxylin and eosin × 375.

THE SPLEEN

Only Soderstrom has reported any substantial recent experience with fine-needle aspiration biopsy of the spleen.[42] Most clinicians consider this a dangerous organ to biopsy, even with a fine-needle, because of the potential for serious hemorrhage. As Soderstrom points out, a hemorrhagic diathesis is a definite contraindication for aspiration, as is a diagnosis of infectious mononucleosis with an enlarged spleen.

In Soderstrom's series, puncture was made immediately beneath the costal arch during respiratory arrest in inspiration and in the center of the palpable part of the spleen. Where the spleen was not palpable, the aspiration was made in the ninth intercostal space, slightly dorsal to the midaxillary line. It was performed during the expiratory phase of respiration. Performing an aspiration of the spleen requires less than one second.[43]

The cell types found are illustrated in both Soderstrom's monograph and a chapter written by Soderstrom in a monograph by Zajicek.[42, 43] Original extensive illustrations from an early monograph of aspiration biopsy of the spleen are found in the work by Moeschlin.[44]

OTHER INTRA-ABDOMINAL MASSES

This author's personal experience involves both palpable and nonpalpable intra-abdominal masses, usually recurrent gastrointestinal carcinoma or carcinoma of the female genital tract recurrent in the pelvis or retroperitoneal area. The majority of these aspiration biopsies have been performed to sample the palpable tumor directly, and local anesthesia has been administered through the skin, subcutaneous tissue, and muscle, down to the peritoneum. Others have been attempted in conjunction with a radiologist using both CAT scanning and ultrasonography. The same variety of methods used for the pancreas have been reported in the combined series of all intra-abdominal aspirations: ultrasonography,[45, 46] by plain fluoroscopy after radiographic contrast examination,[17, 47] during exploratory laparotomy,[48] and with a combination and variety of imaging techniques, such as angiography, radioisotope scanning, and others.[49]

Special techniques, such as intraoperative fine-needle aspiration biopsy in the differential diagnosis of colonic carcinoma and diverticular disease, have been reported.[50] Endoscopically directed biopsy of the stomach with the thorny needle of Nordenstrom has also been attempted.[51]

Colonic Adenocarcinoma.   Several examples indicate the utility of this biopsy procedure. Figure 8–14 illustrates a large mass detected in the hepatic flexure of the colon with the usual barium enema studies. This patient was not a candidate for laparotomy because of severe congestive heart failure. Aspiration was performed using the ultrasonographic image illustrated in Figure 8–15. Adenocarcinoma cells with abundant mucin production are demonstrated in the aspirate (Fig. 8–16). Their long cylindrical shape and papillary arrangement easily confirmed the diagnosis of colonic adenocarcinoma.

Embryonal Rhabdomyosarcoma.   Figure 8–17 shows sheets of undifferentiated, slightly spindle-shaped cells obtained from a direct aspiration of a recurrent abdominal mass that was embryonal rhabdomyosarcoma. The original primary tumor in this young patient was in the pelvic area. The recurrent tumor developed despite radiation and chemotherapy. It was easily confirmed by fine-needle aspiration biopsy. The cells of this aspirate have no specific morphologic features that would indicate that they are embryonal rhabdomyoblasts, but they are certainly compatible with the original diagnosis. Other small-cell sarcomas, particularly of soft parts, might produce a similar aspiration biopsy smear.

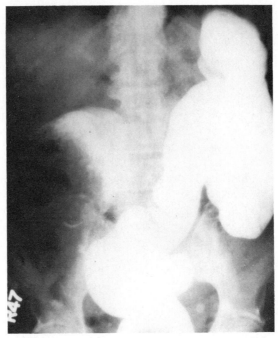

Figure 8–14   Barium enema demonstrating large obstructing mass in the hepatic flexure of the colon.

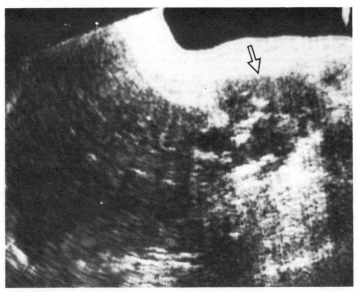

Figure 8–15   Ultrasound image of the mass depicted in Figure 8–14. The head of the patient is to the reader's left. The complex echogenic pattern of the tumor is seen to the right of the center of the illustration (arrow).

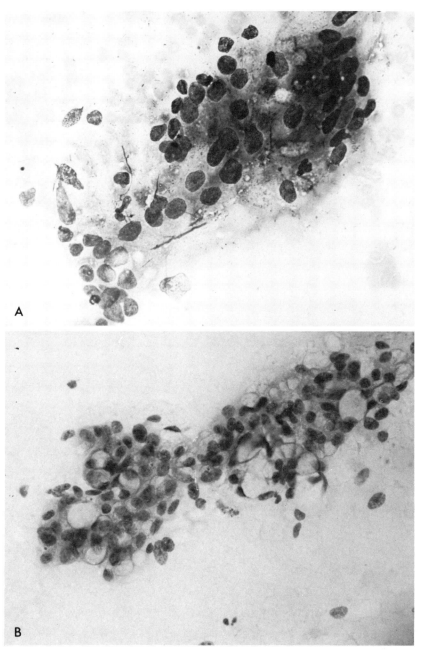

Figure 8–16   Colloid carcinoma of the colon. Aspiration performed using ultrasonic guidance (Fig. 8–15) depicts irregular clusters of malignant glandular cells in a very mucoid background that was intensely metachromatic with the Romanovsky-stained preparation. A, Diff-Quik × 375. B, Papanicolaou × 375.

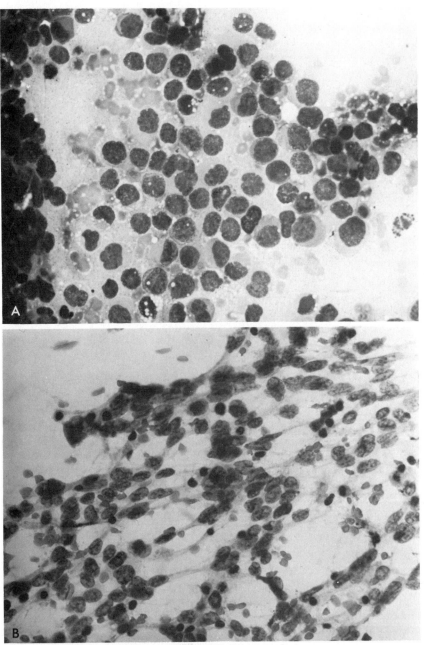

Figure 8–17 Embryonal rhabdomyosarcoma. Direct transabdominal aspiration biopsy of recurrent embryonal rhabdomyosarcoma. Cytoplasm appears light blue with the Romanovsky stains. The spindle-cell pattern of the rhabdomyoblasts is more apparent in the Papanicolaou-stained preparation. *A*, Diff-Quik × 375. *B*, Papanicolaou × 375.

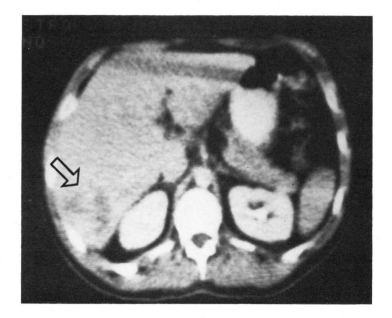

Figure 8–18 CAT-scan image of the liver, demonstrating irregular defect (arrow). Previously excised lymph node was reported as poorly differentiated lymphosarcoma. No other symptoms or physical findings were observed.

Non-Hodgkin's Lymphoma. Figure 8–18 is the CAT scan image of the liver of a 30-year-old patient from whom an enlarged groin node was removed. The tumor was diagnosed as non-Hodgkin's lymphoma. There was no other lymphadenopathy or symptoms in this patient. The scan of the liver near the kidney shows a defect. With ultrasonography, an aspiration biopsy was performed, and malignant lymphoid cells were found (Fig. 8–19*A*). A section of the original lymph node can be compared with Figure 8–19*B*. Obviously, the clinical implications of such a finding are profound, as this patient's lymphoma now must be considered stage IV instead of stage I.

Hodgkin's Disease. Recurrent Hodgkin's disease is illustrated in Figure 8–20*B*, which depicts several examples of Reed-Sternberg cells. This patient had been treated previously for Hodgkin's disease and remained well until six years later, when she noted increasing abdominal pain. CAT scan (Fig. 8–20*A*) demonstrates a mass of nodes adjacent to the aorta. Ultrasonography was used to guide the needle to its correct location.

Rectal Carcinoma. Cells of a poorly differentiated recurrent rectal carcinoma are depicted in Figure 8–21. This elderly patient had remained completely well for approximately one year after his original abdominoperineal resection for rectal cancer. He then was found to have an elevated carcinoembryonic antigen. CAT scan revealed a small mass adjacent to the urinary bladder. (Fig. 8–21*B*). Aspiration biopsy was CAT-scan directed. Compare the tumor cells of the aspirate with those of the original primary rectal carcinoma (Fig. 8–22).

SUMMARY

Result of this author's series are summarized in Table 8–3. There have been three false-negative biopsies for malignant tumors, all diagnosed correctly on a second

TABLE 8–3.   TRANSABDOMINAL ASPIRATION BIOPSIES

	Malignant Tumors		Benign Tumors	Inflammation	False-Positive	False-Negative
Carcinomas	*Sarcomas*	*Lymphomas*				
41	3	2	15	12	—	3*

*One ovarian carcinoma, one rhabdomyosarcoma, and one pancreatic carcinoma diagnosed correctly on second attempt.

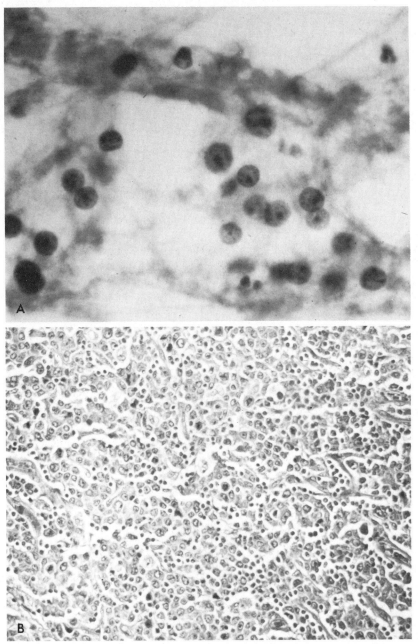

Figure 8–19   Aspirate of lesion in the liver (Fig. 8–18), revealing undifferentiated lymphoid cells that indicate liver involvement by non-Hodgkin's lymphoma. Compare with original lymph node biopsy (B). A, Papanicolaou × 900. B, Hematoxylin and eosin × 240.

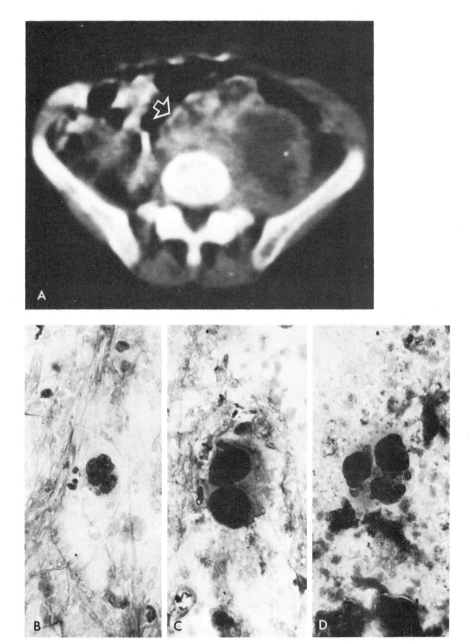

Figure 8–20   Recurrent Hodgkin's disease in the retroperitoneum. *A,* CAT-scan image of a mass of enlarged periaortic lymph nodes (arrow) detected six years after the original diagnosis and treatment of Hodgkin's disease. *B* to *D,* Aspirate illustrating several examples of pleomorphic Reed-Sternberg cells. *B, C,* and *D,* Diff-Quik × 375.

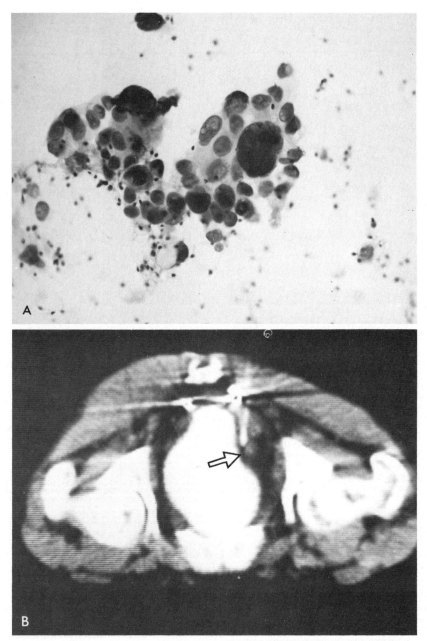

Figure 8–21 Recurrent carcinoma of the rectum. Aspiration directed by CAT-scan that revealed a mass adjacent to the bladder (*B*, arrow). Large, extremely hyperchromatic cells surrounded by smaller malignant cells form a gland-like configuration. *A*, Papanicolaou × 375.

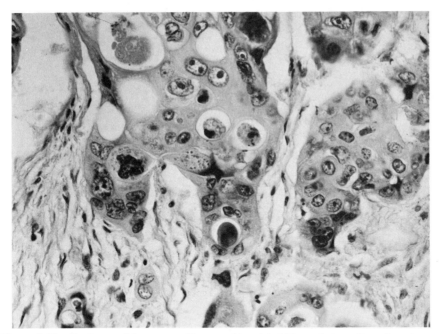

Figure 8–22 Carcinoma of the rectum. Compare this original histopathology of rectal carcinoma with the aspirate from the recurrent carcinoma depicted in Figure 8–21. Note the similarity between the large tumor cells of the two specimens. Hematoxylin and eosin × 375.

attempt. In each case, these first aspirates were not entirely satisfactory, showing only a few inflammatory cells. Skolnick and colleagues reported a series of 26 cases that included one technical failure and four false-negative results. The remaining cases were diagnosed correctly for an overall accuracy of 81 per cent. The four false-negative diagnoses occurred in two cases of carcinoma of the pancreas and two cases of carcinoma of the kidney, one primary and one metastatic. The pancreatic tumors ranged from 3.5 cm to 5 cm in diameter, while both neoplasms in the kidney were approximately 5 cm in diameter.[45] There have been no complications in this author's series of transabdominal aspirations. The procedure seems quite harmless as reported by others.[45-49]

REFERENCES

1. Holm, H. H., Pedersen, J. F., Kristensen, J. K., et al.: Ultrasonically guided percutaneous puncture. Radiol. Clin. N. Am. *12*:493–503, 1975.
2. Johansen, P., and Svendsen, K. N.: Scan-guided fine needle aspiration biopsy in malignant hepatic disease. Acta Cytol. *22*:292–296, 1978.
3. Haaga, J. R., and Alfidi, R. J.: Precise biopsy localization by computed tomography. Radiology *118*:603–607, 1976.
4. Tao, L. C., Ho, C. S., McLoughlin, M. J., et al.: Percutaneous fine-needle aspiration biopsy of the pancreas. Acta Cytol. *22*:215–220, 1978.
5. Tyler, U., Arnesjo, B., Kindberg, L. G., et al.: Percutaneous biopsy of carcinoma of the pancreas guided by angiography. Surg. Gynecol. Obstet. *142*:737–739, 1976.
6. Oscarson, J., Stormby, N., and Sundgren, R.: Selective angiography in fine needle aspiration cytodiagnosis of gastric and pancreatic tumors. Acta Radiol. Diagn. *12*:737–749, 1972.
7. Christoffersen, P., and Poll, P.: Preoperative pancreas aspiration biopsies. Acta Pathol. Microbiol. Scand. Suppl. *212*:28–32, 1970.
8. Arnesjo, B., Stormby, N., and Akerman, M.: Cytodiagnosis of pancreatic lesions by means of fine-needle biopsy during operation. Acta Chir. Scand. *139*:363–369, 1972.
9. Koiveniemi, A., Lempinen, M., and Pantzar, P.: Fine-needle aspiration biopsy of pancreas. Ann. Chir. Gynaecol. Fenn. *61*:273–280, 1972.

10. Kline, T. S., Abramson, J., Goldstein, F. et al.: Needle aspiration biopsy of the pancreas at laparotomy. Am. J. Gastroenterol. *68*:30–33, 1977.

11. Hancke, S.: Ultrasonic scanning of the pancreas. J. C. V. *4*:223–230, 1976.

12. Hancke, S., Holm, H. H., and Koch, F.: Ultrasonically guided percutaneous fine-needle biopsy of the pancreas. Surg. Gynecol. Obstet. *140*:361–364, 1975.

13. Hidvegi, D., Nieman, H. L., DeMay, R. M., et al.: Percutaneous transperitoneal aspiration of pancreas guided by ultrasound. Acta Cytol. *23*:467–470, 1979.

14. Lutz, H., and Petzoldt, R.: Ultrasonography of pancreatic diseases. Zentralbl. Chir. *101*:1369–1375, 1976.

15. Stormby, N.: Pancreas (Chapter 7); in Zajicek, J.: *Monographs in Clinical Cytology.* Vol. 7. New York, S. Karger, 1979, pp. 194–211.

16. Smith, E. H., Bartrum, R. J., Chang, Y. C., et al.: Percutaneous aspiration biopsy of the pancreas under ultrasonic guidance. N. Engl. J. Med. *292*:825–828, 1975.

17. Zornoza, J.: *Percutaneous Needle Biopsy.* Baltimore, Williams & Wilkins, 1981, pp. 102–115 (pancreas), 115–119 (liver), 119–133 (retroperitoneum).

18. McLoughlin, M. I., Ho, C, S., Langer, B., et al.: Fine needle aspiration biopsy of malignant lesions in and around the pancreas. Cancer *41*:2413–2419, 1978.

19. Ho, C. S., McLoughlin, M. J., McHattie, J. D., et al.: Percutaneous fine needle aspiration biopsy of the pancreas following endoscopic retrograde cholangiopancreatography. Radiology *125*:351–353, 1977.

20. Frederiksen, P., Thommesen, P., and Skjoldborg, H.: Fine needle aspiration biopsy of the pancreas. Scand. J. Gastroenterol. *11*:785–791, 1976.

21. Shorey, B. A.: Aspiration biopsy of carcinoma of the pancreas. Gut *16*:645–647, 1975.

22. Bartrum, R. J., Jr., and Crow, H. C.: *Gray-Scale Ultrasound: A Manual for Physicans and Technical Personnel.* Philadelphia, W. B. Saunders Co., 1977, pp. 191–202.

23. Kirstaedter, H. J., and Meyer-Burg, J.: Cytology of the pancreas and its neoplasms by means of fine needle aspiration cytology during peritoneoscopy. Verh. Dtsch. Ges. Pathol. *57*:379–383, 1973.

24. Bodner, A., Aufschnaiter, M., Mikuz, G., et al.: Cytobiopsy as the best present method of intraoperative diagnosis of tumors of the pancreas. Chir. Ital. *29*:1–11, 1977.

25. Dekker, A., and Lloyd, J. C.: Fine-needle aspiration biopsy in ampullary and pancreatic carcinoma. Arch. Surg. *114*:592–596, 1979.

26. Evander, A., Ishe, I., Lunderquist, A., et al.: Percutaneous cytodiagnosis of carcinoma of the pancreas and bile duct. Ann. Surg *188*:90–92, 1978.

27. Goldstein, H. M., Zornoza, J., Wallace, S., et al.: Percutaneous fine-needle aspiration biopsy of pancreatic and other abdominal masses. Radiology *123*:319–322, 1977.

28. Ferrucci, J. T., Jr., Wittenberg, J., Margolies, M. N., et al.: Malignant seeding of the tract after thin-needle aspiration biopsy. Radiology *130*:345–346, 1979.

29. Stormby, N., and Akerman, M.: Aspiration cytology in the diagnosis of granulomatous liver lesions. Acta Cytol. *17*:200–204, 1973.

30. Soderstrom, N.: *Fine Needle Aspiration Biopsy.* Stockholm, Almqvist and Wiksell, 1966, pp. 122–136.

31. Wasastjerna, C.: Liver; in Zajicek, J.: *Monographs in Clinical Cytology.* Vol. 7. New York, S. Karger, 1979, pp. 167–193.

32. Lundquist, A.: Fine needle aspiration biopsy of the liver. Application in clinical diagnosis and investigation. Acta Med. Scand. Suppl. *520*:5–28, 1971.

33. Dominis, M., Cerlek, S., and Crepinko, I.: Diagnosis of malignant liver tumors by thin needle aspiration biopsy. Acta Med. Iugosl. *29*:307–316, 1975.

34. Vido, I., Atay, Z., Zobl, H., et al.: Diagnostic value of cytological investigations in metastatic tumors of the liver: Comparison of laparoscopy, histology and cytology. Dtsch. Med. Wochenschr. *100*:2602–2604, 1975.

35. Tao, L. C., Donat, E. E., Ho, C. S., et al.: Percutaneous fine-needle aspiration biopsy of the liver. Cytodiagnosis of hepatic cancer. Acta Cytol. *23*:287–291, 1979.

36. Gerdes, K., Bossaert, H., and Nijs, L.: Carcinoma of the liver: Cytopathologic diagnosis. J. Am. Geriatr. Soc. *26*:411–413, 1978.

37. Ho, C. S., McLoughlin, M. J., Tao, L. C., et al.: Guided percutaneous fine needle aspiration biopsy of the liver. Cancer *47*:1781–1785, 1981.

38. Sherlock, P., Kim, Y. S., and Koss, L. G.: Cytologic diagnosis of cancer from aspirated material obtained with liver biopsies. Am. J. Dig. Dis. *12*:396–402, 1967.

39. Perrault, J., McGill, D. B., Ott, B. J., et al.: Liver biopsy: Complications in 1000 patients. Gastroenterology *74*:103–106, 1978.

40. Riska, H., Friman, C.: Fatality after fine needle aspiration biopsy of the liver (letter). Br. Med. J. *1*:517, 1975.

41. Schulz, T. B.: Fine needle aspiration biopsy of the liver complicated with bile peritonitis. Acta Med. Scand. *199*:141–142, 1976.

42. Soderstrom, N.: Spleen; in Zajicek, J.: *Monographs in Clinical Cytology*, Vol. 7, New York, S. Karger, 1979, pp. 224–247.

43. Soderstrom, N.: *Fine Needle Aspiration Biopsy.* New York, Grune and Stratton, 1966, pp. 122–136.

44. Moeschlin, S.: *Spleen Puncture.* London, Heinemann, 1951.

45. Skolnick, M. L., Dekker, A., and Weinstein, B. J.: Ultrasound guided fine-needle aspiration biopsy of abdominal masses. Gastrointest. Radiol. *3*:295–302, 1978.

46. Weidenhiller, S., Lutz, H., and Petzoldt, R.: Ultraschallgezielte Feinnadelpunktion von abdominal- und retroperitoneal Tumoren. Med. Klin. *70*:973–976, 1975.
47. Pereiras, R. V., Meiers, W., Kunhardt, B., et al.: Fluoroscopically guided thin needle aspiration biopsy of the abdomen and retroperitoneum. Am. J. Roentgenol. *131*:197–202, 1978.
48. Ihara, S., Satoh, H., Takahashi, H., et al.: Fine needle aspiration biopsy cytology in surgical field. Gan. No. Rinsho. *24*:1009–1018, 1978.
49. Ho, C. S., Tao, L. C., and McLoughlin, M. J.: Percutaneous fine needle aspiration biopsy of intraabdominal masses. Can. Med. Assoc. J. *119*:1311–1314, 1978.
50. Axelsson, C. K., and Francis, D.: Preoperative fine-needle aspiration biopsy: An aid to differential diagnosis between diverticular disease and colonic cancer? A preliminary report. Dis. Colon Rectum *21*:319–321, 1978.
51. Asaki, S., Sato, A., Wakui, K., et al.: New device for diagnosis of gastric submucosal tumor: Endoscopic direct biopsy using thorny needle. Tohoku J. Exp. Med. *127*:257–264, 1979.

Chapter Nine

Urogenital System

ASPIRATION OF THE ORGANS OF THE UROGENITAL SYSTEM

The methods and applications of fine-needle aspiration biopsy for lesions of the urogenital system are essentially similar to those for masses in the gastrointestinal tract. Specific sites in which aspiration biopsy has been used include the kidney,[1, 2, 6] the ovary,[3-5, 7] the testis,[6] and the prostate.[6, 9-13] In this system, the prostate is the organ that has been most frequently biopsied by fine-needle aspiration with a transrectal approach and the Franzen needle guide.[6] Over 30 references, most from the Scandinavian and the other European literature, were found describing the application of fine-needle aspiration biopsy to the diagnosis, prognosis, and hormonal management of prostatic carcinoma.

THE KIDNEY

Renal tumors are readily biopsied by fine-needle methods, either directly as described by Soderstrom or with a combination of techniques for imaging, including pyelography and angiography with fluoroscopic control.[2, 6, 14] More recently, ultrasonography has been added.[15] Zajicek preferred a needle 1.2 mm in outer diameter and 5 cm to 8 cm in length to penetrate the renal fascia. A fine needle, 14 cm in length and 0.6 mm in external diameter, was then threaded through the thick needle and introduced into the renal tumor. The mechanics of the actual aspiration and smear preparation are similar to those previously described in Chapter 2. A screw needle, developed by Nordenstrom, is used if the tumor is radiographically found to be extremely dense.[6] Some authors have preferred a large needle measuring 1.2 mm in outer diameter for cysts, feeling that it is easier to aspirate them completely.[13]

Soderstrom performs the puncture without imaging or fluoroscopic control immediately below the twelfth rib and one hand's-breadth lateral to the midline. He introduces the needle without an attached syringe so that he can feel the resistance of the renal capsule. He states that it may be necessary to make aspirations of upper pole tumors through the pleura during deep expiration.[1]

Renal Cysts. Most of this author's experience has been devoted to the examination of specimens aspirated from renal cysts. Only recently, with the advent of ultrasonography and computerized axial tomography, have aspiration biopsies been performed other than intraoperatively or with a needle smaller than an 18-gauge one. Examination of renal cyst fluid has been singularly unrewarding in that no cases of malignancy have been found from approximately 15 cases per year over an eight year period. These fluids either are acellular or contain only a few nonspecific cells, probably renal tubular type.

Carcinoma. Recently, solid tumors of the kidney have been aspirated using a fine needle with the use of ultrasonographic guidance. Several examples are illustrated. Figure 9–1 depicts a moderately well-differentiated renal cell carcinoma. The aspirate is abundantly cellular, with the cells having a granular, almost metachromatic cytoplasm, as seen with the Romanovsky stains. A prominent feature is the presence of large blue nucleoli. When giant nucleoli are present, they strongly suggest renal cell carcinoma. Tumor cells have been described by Soderstrom as arranged along a delicate metachromatic background substance. Phagocytosis of erythrocytes may often be observed.[1] With Papanicolaou-stained slides, the cells of moderately well- or well-differentiated renal cell carcinoma may appear relatively bland (Fig. 9–2A). The nuclear chromatin is finely granular but may not be abnormally distributed. Another example of a more pleomorphic and obviously malignant renal cell carcinoma is depicted in Figures 9–3 and 9–4. A greater degree of cell variation, most often of the nuclei, in both the air-dried smears stained with Diff-Quik and the Papanicolaou preparations, easily leads to a diagnosis of carcinoma.

This author has not performed enough aspiration biopsies of renal cell carcinoma to appreciate the differences with respect to tumor grades as described in detail by Zajicek.[6] He divides the renal cell carcinomas into well-differentiated, moderately well-differentiated, and poorly differentiated tumors. The aspirates from the well-differentiated carcinomas show cells without pleomorphism in tubular and alveolar patterns. Aspirates of moderately well-differentiated tumors contain some cells that have a pleomorphic nuclear structure as well as tubular and alveolar arrangements. Poorly differentiated tumor aspirates show neither tubular nor alveolar patterns and have marked nuclear and cellular pleomorphism. The clear cell variant of renal cell carcinoma in Zajicek's cases demonstrates a finely vacuolated tumor cell cytoplasm, best seen with the May-Grunwald-Giemsa stains. The same stain applied to the granular cell neoplasms of renal parenchyma provides a slate gray cytoplasmic color.[6]

Zajicek and his colleagues have advocated preoperative radiotherapy in those cases of renal cell carcinoma classified as poorly differentiated.[6] Correlation with treatment and survival has been good using this evaluation of the differentiation of renal cell neoplasms.[6, 17]

The differential diagnosis of renal cell carcinoma includes adrenal gland carcinoma and pheochromocytoma. Both are found to have cells with abundant cytoplasm. Pheochromocytoma also has many naked nuclei in a sea of cytoplasm. Liver cell carcinoma that is well differentiated, liver cell adenoma, or even normal liver cells may look like well-differentiated renal cell carcinoma.[6] This author believes the correct diagnosis partly depends on accurate placement of the needle in a clearly defined renal mass, for which imaging is absolutely essential.

Nephroblastoma. Nephroblastoma (Wilm's tumor) can be diagnosed from fine-needle aspiration biopsy. This tumor occurs primarily in young children and presents as a large abdominal mass. Recognition of these clinical features is important in correctly diagnosing this tumor. The mass is frequently so large that direct aspiration may be attempted if it is desirable to make a preoperative diagnosis. This is usually *not* done since a renal mass in a child is considered a surgical emergency. An aspirate from such a tumor is illustrated in Figures 9–5 and 9–6, which demonstrate loose clusters of very undifferentiated small cells. In a number of specimens described by Zajicek, the cells have round to oval nuclei and scanty cytoplasm. Differentiating between a retroperitoneal sarcoma and some other poorly differentiated tumor, including neuroblastoma, would not be possible.[6]

Text continued on page 258

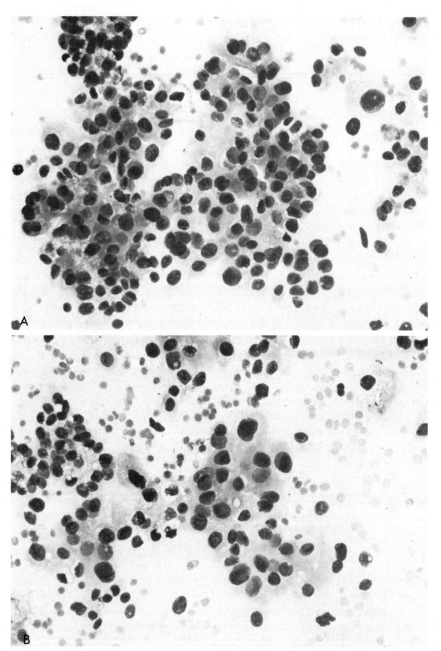

Figure 9–1 Renal cell carcinoma, moderately well differentiated. Aspirate is very cellular with some variation in size and shape of the nuclei. Cytoplasm is granular and metachromatic with Diff-Quik stain. Both *A* and *B*, Diff-Quik × 375.

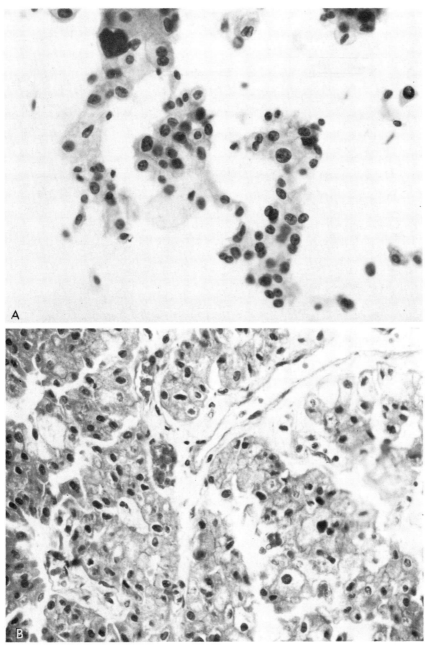

Figure 9–2   Renal cell carcinoma, moderately well differentiated. Note the nuclear chromatin pattern and some cells with prominent nucleoli (A). Compare with histologic section (B). A, Papanicolaou × 375. B, Hematoxylin and eosin × 375.

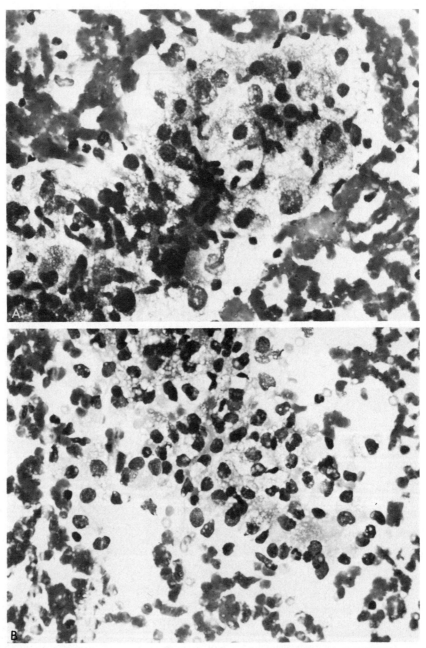

Figure 9–3   Renal cell carcinoma, poorly differentiated. Variation in cell size and shape is evident in comparison to the previous figures. Some spindle-shaped cells may suggest a sarcomatous pattern. Diff-Quik × 375.

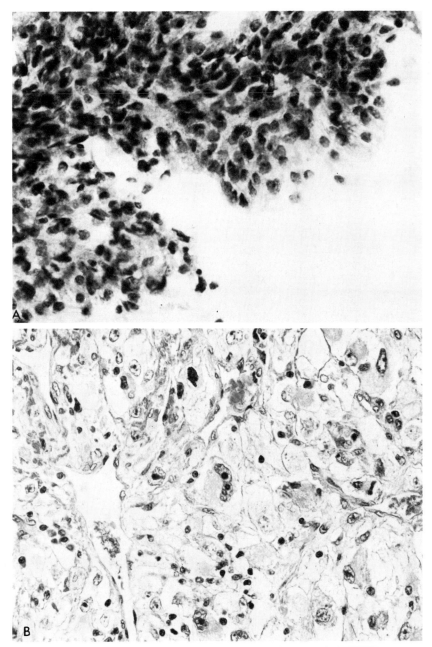

Figure 9–4 Renal cell carcinoma, poorly differentiated. Spindle-cell and pleomorphic pattern is even more obvious in the Papanicolaou-stained smear *(A)*. Compare with the pleomorphic tissue pattern *(B)*. A, Papanicolaou × 375. *B*, Hematoxylin and eosin × 375.

Normal Kidney Parenchyma.   In contrast to aspirations of neoplasms, aspirations of normal kidney parenchyma yield a variety of cell types. Renal tubular cells characteristically have a paravacuolar granulation, that is, dense dark blue granules around a central vacuole. There are also large clear cells, large granulated cells, and small basophilic cells. Actual tubular fragments may be found, and they are most characteristic of aspirates from normal renal parenchyma.[1]

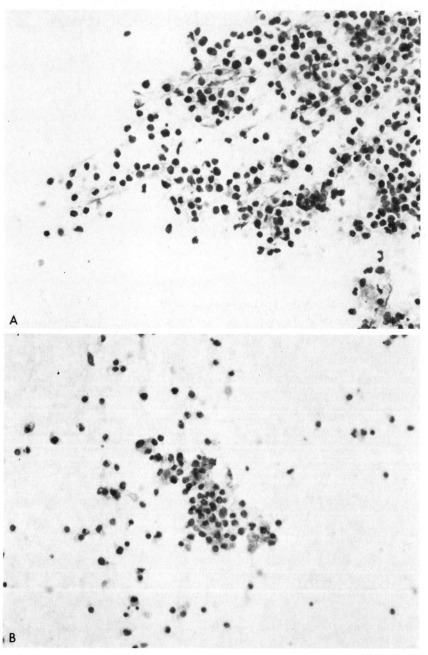

Figure 9–5   Nephroblastoma (Wilms' tumor). Sheets and loose clusters of undifferentiated small malignant cells. No identifiable tubular pattern is found. Both *A* and *B*, Papanicolaou, × 375.

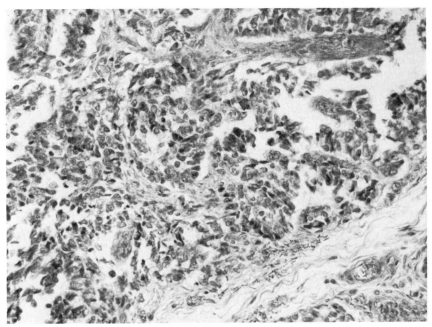

Figure 9–6 Nephroblastoma (Wilm's tumor). Histologic section from the tumor aspirate shown in Figure 9–5. Hematoxylin and eosin × 240.

Results of Kidney Aspirations

Results of several studies have provided reasonably accurate diagnoses of both cysts and solid tumors of the kidney. Edgren and colleagues reported a group of 55 cases diagnosed by aspiration combined with angiography. Malignant tumors were present in 42 of these patients. Angiography was diagnostically accurate in 94 per cent of the cases, while fine-needle aspiration was accurate in only 71 per cent of the cases. Combined accuracy for both techniques was 97 per cent. Fine-needle aspiration provided positive results in each of the four cases of renal pelvis carcinoma, while the results of angiography were negative.[14] Holm and colleagues diagnosed 43 of 49 solid renal tumors by aspiration biopsy. This group was also successful in aspirating 57 of 61 renal cysts.[15] Holm's series included aspirations of not only kidney masses but also liver, pancreas, and retroperitoneal tumors. Only one complication occurred in 1200 aspirations: a hematoma that appeared two months after aspiration of a pancreatic pseudocyst.[15]

A single false-positive diagnosis of renal cell carcinoma was reported by Thommesen and Nielsen in a series of 49 patients in whom a renal tumor had been aspirated. Of these masses, 28 were cysts, 18 were malignant tumors, and three were benign tumors. There were no false-negative reports.[2] One false-negative result has occurred in this author's limited experience. The cytologic features of this biopsy are illustrated in Figure 9–7. This rather acellular smear from a large renal mass contained a few pleomorphic cells with a finely vacuolated cytoplasm. There was also a fair amount of inflammatory cell background, suggesting the possible diagnosis of xanthogranulomatous pyelonephritis. After it was excised and carefully studied, this tumor was reported as a well-differentiated renal cell carcinoma with extensive areas of hemorrhage and necrosis (Fig. 9–8). It is probably the latter feature that falsely suggested a histiocyte-like pattern and inflammatory exudate.

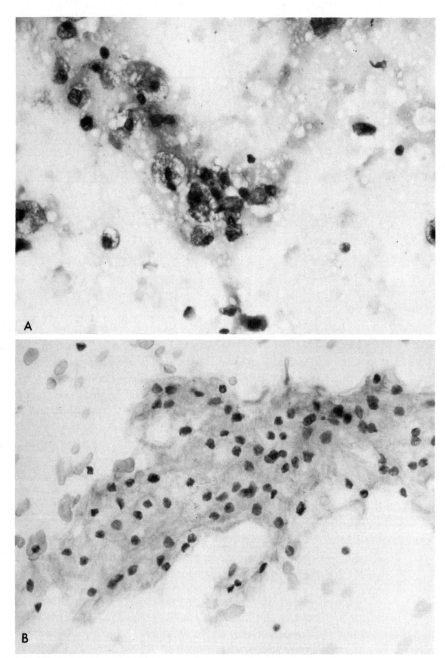

Figure 9–7 Renal cell carcinoma, well differentiated. False-negative case demonstrating scattered single cells as well as sheets and clusters of cells having a histiocytic appearance. Lack of any nuclear features suggesting malignancy prohibited a diagnosis of renal cell carcinoma, but cohesiveness of the cells in B supported a diagnosis of renal cell carcinoma rather than the original diagnosis of possible xanthogranulomatous pyelonephritis. A, Diff-Quik × 375. B, Papanicolaou × 375.

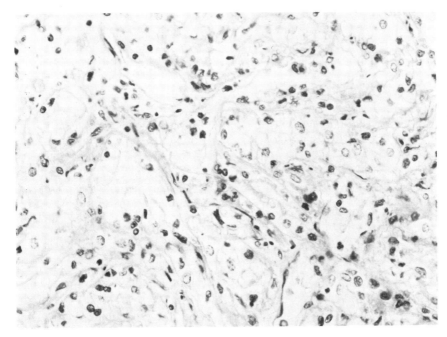

Figure 9–8   Renal cell carcinoma, well differentiated. Histologic section of the neoplasm diagnosed as possible xanthogranulomatous pyelonephritis (Fig. 9–7).

Complications of Kidney Aspirations

Few complications have been described by those reporting major series of fine-needle aspiration biopsies of the kidney. Soderstrom described some cases of micro-hematuria, whereas Zajicek reported no complications.[1, 6] Two cases of needle tract seeding following needle biopsy have been reported.[15-17] Riches, who used a tissue needle biopsy to aspirate renal cysts, cites a case reported by Hanley in which dissemination of tumor cells in the needle tract occurred. The case is poorly documented, and, since a core biopsy needle was used, it bears no relationship to the fine-needle aspiration method.[17, 18]

The case of Gibbons and colleagues appears to be an authentic example of needle tract implantation that occurred approximately 20 months after needle aspiration biopsy. Aspiration was attempted on two different occasions through a posterior approach. An 18-gauge needle was used, but no tumor cells were obtained, only blood. Despite the negative results of this essentially unsatisfactory aspiration, tumor did appear at the site of the needle tract. Interpreting the case is difficult because the patient was operated upon and the tumor resected through an anterior subcostal transperitoneal incision. Although it cannot be proved that tumor was removed intact with no violation of the capsule, we must accept the author's word for that. The exact anatomic relationship of the surgical incision to the aspiration is not described. The fact that cancer grew in the needle tract even though the aspiration did not yield any diagnostic cells is bizarre. The authors concluded from this single case that needle aspiration should be reserved for renal cysts or benign masses. This author cannot agree with that statement on the basis of the documentation provided by this single case.[19]

Von Schreeb and colleagues found no evidence of spread of tumor cells following renal puncture. Their series included a minimum of five years follow-up and a control group of patients in whom renal puncture was not performed. The external diameter of needles used varied from 0.75 mm to 1.5 mm.[20] In a small number of cases that this author has experienced to date, there have been no complications or evidence of needle tract seeding.

THE FEMALE UROGENITAL TRACT

While most of the literature devoted to fine-needle aspiration of female genital tract neoplasms discusses the ovary, the method really has general application throughout the field of gynecologic oncology. Indications are summarized in Table 9–1. They include detection of either occult or gross disease from carcinoma of the cervix, the endometrium, and the ovary.[21] The usual procedure for diagnosing a pelvic mass is the transrectal or transvaginal approach. To accomplish the biopsy easily, the Franzen needle guide is mandatory (Figs. 9–21 and 9–22).[7] Tumor involving the parametria, usually recurrence of carcinoma of the cervix or endometrium, is sampled by this method using a transvaginal route. In a series of 48 patients, fine-needle biopsy of the parametria was found to be just as accurate as Vim-Silverman needle biopsy.[22]

Special methods may also be employed. This author has performed aspirations in conjunction with the Department of Radiology using ultrasonography and computerized axial tomography to diagnose recurrent carcinoma of the female genital tract as well as prostatic and rectal cancer in which there was no palpable mass. Fine-needle aspiration biopsy of ovarian tumors through the laparoscope has been described by Kovacic and colleagues. These authors cannulated the abdominal wall to perform the actual aspiration under direct laparoscopic view. They used a needle measuring 0.8 mm in external diameter. Specifically, they recommended avoiding the hilus of the ovary because of the potential for bleeding. Descriptions of the cytologic findings for follicular cysts, corpus luteum, benign cystic teratoma, thecosis, tubular androblastoma, germinal inclusion cysts, endometriosis, and benign common epithelial tumors are all included in their paper. They admit that some of these conditions provide few cells and may be difficult to diagnose but can at least be determined to be benign.[8]

Adenoid Cystic Carcinoma.   Palpable masses involving the vulva, such as an enlarged Bartholin's gland, are readily aspirated for diagnosis. While most of these are cysts, a rare tumor may be encountered. An example is illustrated in Figure 9–9, which depicts the very uncommon adenoid cystic carcinoma.[23] The pattern of the aspirate is identical with that of the same tumor in major salivary glands: cylindrical aggregates of highly metachromatic mucopolysaccharide substance surrounded by uniform small epithelial cells. In this case, this tumor proved just as dangerous as it is in salivary glands. The patient developed bone metastases approximately two years after the original diagnosis and radical surgical treatment.

Recurrence of Pelvic Tumors

Cervical Carcinoma.   The following discussion includes brief case histories that exemplify the use of fine-needle aspiration biopsy for diagnosing pelvic tumors. Figure 9–10 illustrates an example of a pelvic recurrence of squamous cell carcinoma of the cervix in an elderly female. The sheets of malignant cells are readily recognized in both the Romanovsky-stained smear and the Papanicolaou preparation. The cytomorphologic appearance is also an excellent match for that of the original primary neoplasm (Fig. 9–11).

Endometrial Carcinoma.   Figure 9–12 illustrates an example of mixed adenosquamous carcinoma of the endometrium, also a pelvic recurrence. Cells in both sheets

TABLE 9–1.   INDICATIONS FOR FINE-NEEDLE ASPIRATION BIOPSY IN GYNECOLOGIC ONCOLOGY

1. Primary diagnosis of pelvic masses.
2. Detection of occult disease after radiation therapy for carcinoma of the cervix, endometrium, or ovary.
3. Diagnosis of enlarged lymph nodes or soft tissue masses or both associated with gynecologic malignancy.
4. Diagnosis of intra-abdominal masses before or after detection of gynecologic malignancy.

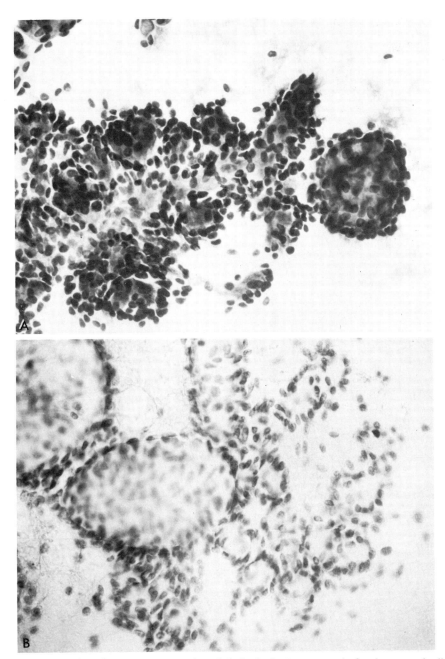

Figure 9–9   Adenoid cystic carcinoma of Bartholin's gland. Numerous cylindrical masses of cells are present with a homogeneous matrix in the center that is very metachromatic with the Diff-Quik stain (A). The epithelial cells themselves are very uniform and have little anaplasia. A, Diff-Quik × 375. B, Papanicolaou × 375.

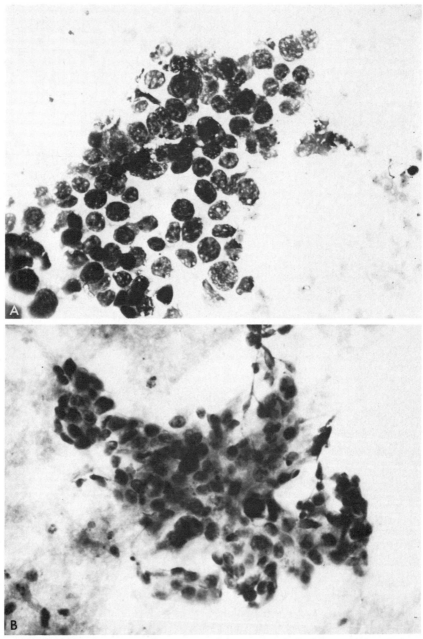

Figure 9–10 Squamous cell carcinoma of the cervix, poorly differentiated, recurrent in the pelvis. Sheets of anaplastic cells without definable cell boundaries are visible in the air-dried preparation (A). Neoplastic cells with some suggestion of cell boundaries are evident in B. A, Diff-Quik × 375. B, Papanicolaou × 375.

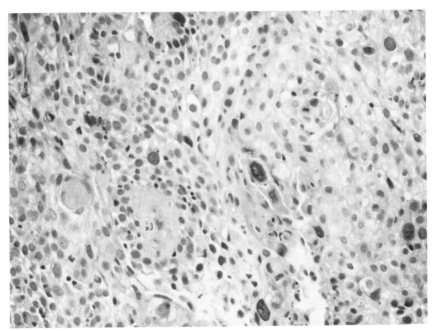

Figure 9–11   Squamous cell carcinoma of the cervix. Original cervix biopsy for comparison with the aspirate illustrated in Figure 9–10. Hematoxylin and eosin × 240.

and clusters are demonstrated. Both elements of this mixed pattern of endometrial carcinoma are found in the smear. This neoplasm is becoming an increasingly more common histologic type of endometrial carcinoma. It carries a bad prognosis.

Ovarian Carcinoma.   A pleomorphic example of the clear cell variant of recurrent ovarian carcinoma presenting in the parametria is depicted in Figures 9–13 and 9–14. The cells have a light and dark finely vacuolated cytoplasm with hobnail-like nuclei, even in the aspiration smear. Note the correlation between the morphologic features of the smear and those of the original tissue (Fig. 9–14, *B*).

Bladder Carcinoma.   Recurrent bladder cancer in the pelvis following radical cystectomy has also been diagnosed by transrectal aspiration biopsy (Fig. 9–15). The histopathologic appearance of the smear is comparable to that of the original primary (Fig. 9–16).

Primary Ovarian Carcinoma.   This author has had only limited experience with direct aspiration of ovarian tumors for a primary diagnosis. An example of a poorly differentiated ovarian carcinoma diagnosed by direct transabdominal aspiration is illustrated in Figures 9–17 and 9–18. The glandular pattern seen in the histologic sections was only focally present; the tumor otherwise grew in a completely undifferentiated manner. The original primary had been resected three years previously.

The variety of cytomorphologic patterns that may be found with primary ovarian cysts and tumors is well described by Kjellgren and Angstrom in a chapter in Zajicek's monograph.[7] This report is extremely useful for comparative purposes in the diagnosis of an original primary ovarian neoplasm. It has also been useful in situations in which the cytopathologist is dealing with a recurrent tumor but does not have the original histopathologic specimen for matching with the aspiration smear. Lack of experience can be overcome by using the regimen reported by Ramzy and colleagues, who aspirated a variety of ovarian masses either intraoperatively or postoperatively and developed a reference set of slides for diagnosis.[24]

Text continued on page 272

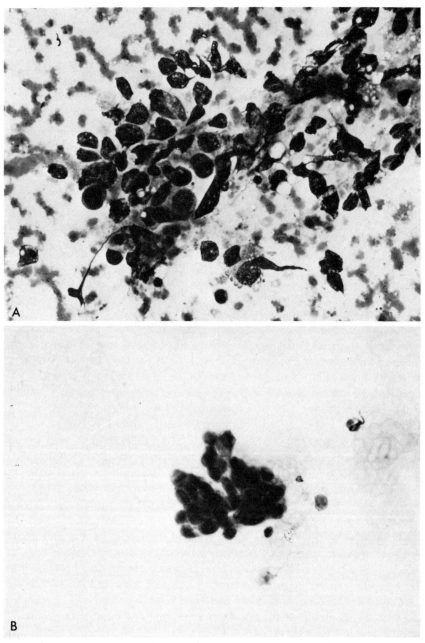

Figure 9–12 Carcinoma of the endometrium, mixed adenosquamous type, recurrent in the pelvis. Malignant features of these tumor cells are obvious. The contrasts between the sheets of cells in *A* and the clusters of cells in *B* suggest the mixed tumor pattern of adenosquamous carcinoma. *A*, Diff-Quik × 375. *B*, Papanicolaou × 375.

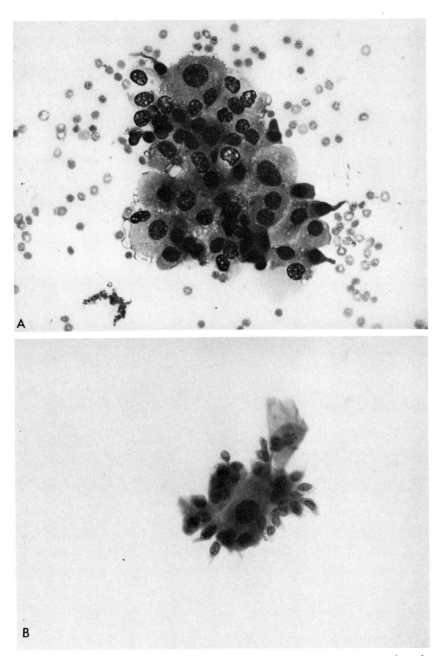

Figure 9–13 Clear cell carcinoma of the ovary recurrent in the parametria. Note the voluminous cytoplasm of these neoplastic cells and the light and dark staining that is frequently seen with the clear cell carcinomas of the female genital tract. A, Diff-Quik × 375. B, Papanicolaou × 375.

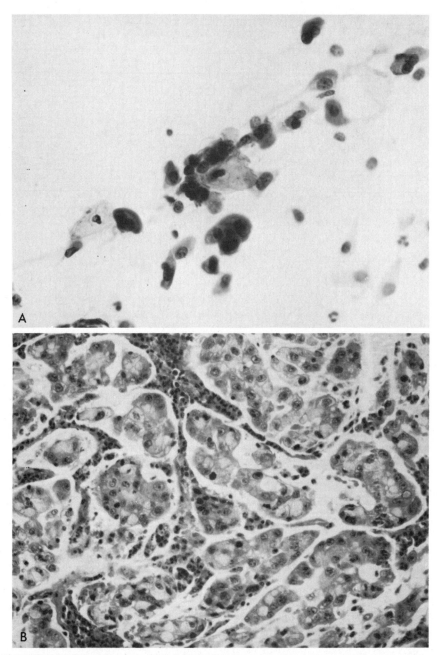

Figure 9–14 Clear cell carcinoma of the ovary, recurrent in the parametria. The clear cells are more evident than the tumor cells with dense cytoplasm in this field of the smear. Compare with the original ovarian tumor (B). A, Papanicolaou × 375. B, Hematoxylin and eosin × 240.

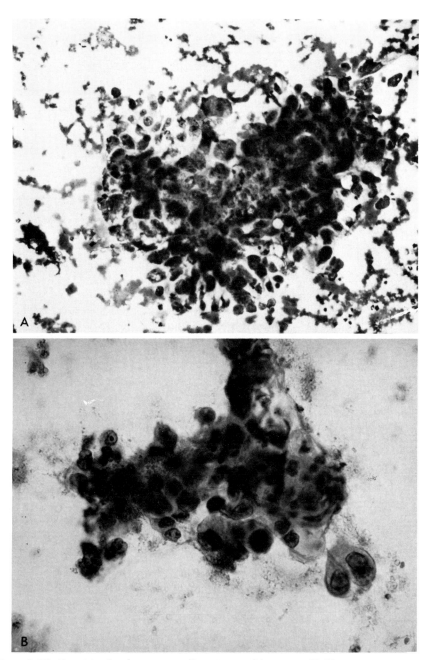

Figure 9–15   Transitional and squamous cell carcinoma of the urinary bladder, recurrent in the pelvis. Sheets of anaplastic tumor cells are quite evident, the usual pattern for poorly differentiated transitional cell carcinomas. In *B*, the very well-defined boundaries of some of the cells suggest squamous cell carcinoma. *A*, Diff-Quik × 240. *B*, Papanicolaou × 375.

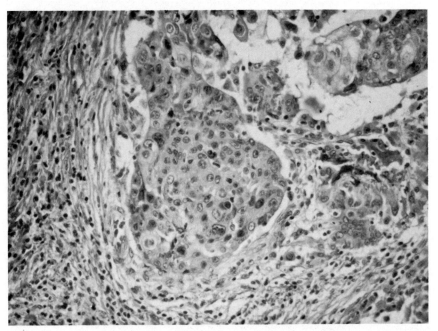

Figure 9–16   Transitional and squamous cell carcinoma of the urinary bladder, recurrent in the pelvis. Original carcinoma of the bladder can be compared with the aspiration. Squamous features are present in a small area at the top right of the illustration. Hematoxylin and eosin × 240.

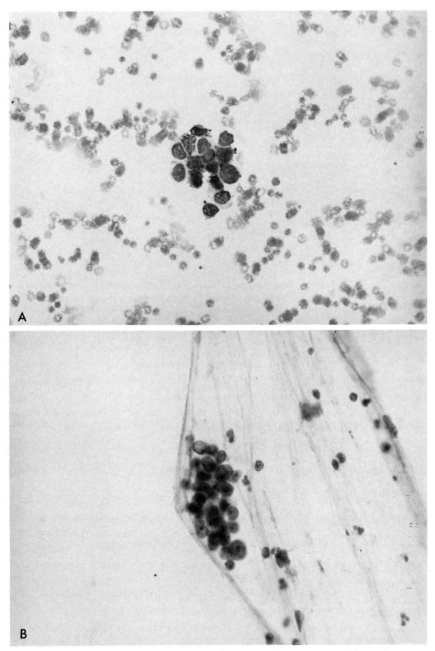

Figure 9–17 Carcinoma of the ovary, poorly differentiated. Direct transabdominal aspiration of a lower abdominal mass three years after resection of a poorly differentiated carcinoma of the ovary. A single cluster of very undifferentiated neoplastic cells is present in A and B. This neoplasm has no specific features that would support a diagnosis more definitive than carcinoma. A, Diff-Quik × 375. B, Papanicolaou × 375.

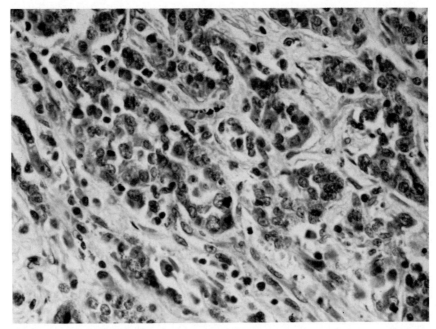

Figure 9–18   Carcinoma of the ovary, poorly differentiated. Original primary carcinoma for comparison with aspirate in Figure 9–17. Most of the tumor grows in a solid undifferentiated manner. A few foci had a tubular pattern. Note the similarity between the nuclear structure of the histologic section and that of the aspiration smear. Hematoxylin and eosin × 375.

Table 9–2 combines results from three large series in terms of both negative and positive reports for a diagnosis of malignant tumor of the ovary. The sensitivity and specificity of a positive or negative test have been calculated.[24] Except for the series of Geier and colleagues, the reports document an accuracy rate of over 90 per cent. This would support the contention that fine-needle aspiration biopsy is a very useful step toward the diagnosis of benign and malignant ovarian tumors.[3, 4, 7]

THE MALE UROGENITAL TRACT

The Testis

Testicular Tumors.   Only the Scandinavian literature yields any information concerning fine-needle aspiration biopsy of testicular masses.[6, 26, 27] Two cases are illustrated in Figures 9–19 and 9–20. These are part of a small personal series of aspiration biopsies of testicular tumors. The first shows undifferentiated sheets of tumor cells in an air-dried, Giemsa-stained smear from a seminoma. The cytoplasm is finely vacuolated, and the uniform cell pattern and the scattered lymphocytes should rather convincingly suggest the correct diagnosis. A similar pattern has been found by this author in the aspirates from both a cervical lymph node and an occipital mass in a patient with metastatic seminoma (see Fig. 10–35). Figure 9–20 illustrates a chorio-carcinoma with pleomorphic, undifferentiated cytotrophoblastic and syncytiotrophoblastic cells. The latter cells are multinucleated and have very densely staining cytoplasm.

Differential Diagnosis.   The specific classification of malignant testicular tumors by fine-needle aspiration can prove difficult, since many of them may be mixed types. The cytomorphologic features that provide a clue to a mixed pattern are often not apparent. A single cell pattern with a vesicular nuclear chromatin, a finely vacuolated cytoplasm, and cells that are evidently very fragile are the cytologic features of

TABLE 9–2.   RESULTS FROM MAJOR SERIES OF FINE-NEEDLE ASPIRATION BIOPSIES OF OVARIAN TUMORS

Reference	True-Positives	False-Positives	True-Negatives	False-Negatives	Sensitivity (%)*	Specificity (%)†
Angstrom et al.[3]	39	2	36	3	93	95
Kjellgren and Angstrom[7]	75	3	59	1	98	95
Geier et al.[4]	28	1	53	5	85	98

*Sensitivity = positive diagnosis of a malignant tumor[24] $\dfrac{TP}{TP + FN} \times 100$

†Specificity = negative aspiration for tumor or diagnosis.[24] $\dfrac{TN}{FP + TN} \times 100$

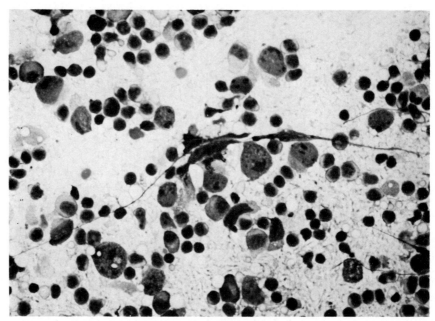

Figure 9–19 Seminoma of the testis. Direct aspiration of testicular mass. Large single undifferentiated neoplastic cells are seen in a background of lymphocytes. Giemsa × 375. (Courtesy of Dr. A. W. Handy.)

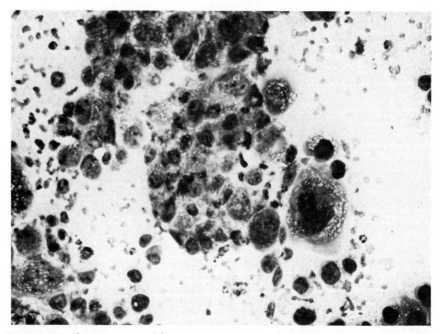

Figure 9–20 Choriocarcinoma of the testis. Aspiration revealing sheets of large cytotrophoblastic cells with vesiculated cytoplasm and multinucleated syncytial cells with very hyperchromatic nuclei. This combination of cell types supports a diagnosis of choriocarcinoma. Giemsa × 240. (Courtesy of Dr. A. W. Handy.)

seminoma. Embryonal carcinoma is made up of numerous cohesive clusters of markedly hyperchromatic cells with pronounced nuclear chromatin clumping. Each nucleus contains a very prominent nucleolus. Teratoma usually yields a scanty aspirate, and cystic areas may be entered with the aspiration of only fluid. Unless a mixed epithelial cell pattern is found, the actual diagnosis of teratoma may be quite difficult.[6]

In Zajicek's series, only a few cases of Sertoli-Leydig cell tumor were encountered. No examples are illustrated. It is stated that the crystalloids of Reinke can be seen with a Papanicolaou stain but not with a May-Grunwald-Giemsa preparation.[6]

Complications.   Urologists have always thought that any biopsy of a testicular mass, which is potentially a malignant tumor, may cause dissemination. However, in a follow-up study, averaging 2 to 18 years and including 100 cases of aspiration biopsy of malignant testicular tumors, only one patient was found to have a local recurrence that demonstrated gross extension to the scrotum. In another case, metastasis to one inguinal lymph node occurred.[6]

Spermatogenesis.   Persson and colleagues as well as Zajicek have evaluated spermatogenesis in a series of fine-needle aspiration biopsies. Persson also compared the histologic and cytologic features, finding that both were equal in evaluating spermatogenesis, but a specific histologic diagnosis was not established by aspiration biopsy unless simple spermatogenic arrest was present. Persson and colleagues also believed that normal histologic features with a cytologic appearance of azoospermia occurred only with obstruction of the epididymis or spermatic duct.[26] After studying 160 cases, Zajicek concluded that aspiration biopsy was excellent if there was normal or absent spermatogenesis. He also reported no complications with the procedure.[6]

The Prostate

Prostatic Tumors.   A transrectal fine-needle aspiration biopsy of the prostate has been the preferred method for the diagnosis of prostatic carcinoma in the Scandinavian countries as well as throughout other parts of Europe.[10, 11, 28, 29] Scant attention has been paid to this type of biopsy in the American literature. Only Rheinfrank and Nulf and Kline and coworkers have reported using this technique.[30, 31] The diagnosis of prostatic carcinoma by aspiration biopsy was first described by Ferguson in 1930. The approach was transperineal, and an 18-gauge needle measuring 15 cm in length was used. Ferguson also injected local anesthesia in the perineal area and guided the biopsy needle down to the prostatic capsule with a finger placed in the rectum. The needle was positioned to one side of the midline, and the rectal wall and the urethra were avoided. Although Ferguson at first intended to obtain a small core of tissue, he instead made smears and stained them with hematoxylin and eosin, as has been the practice at Memorial Center for Cancer since the advent of the needle aspiration biopsy at that institution.[32]

No results were given in Ferguson's paper, and the method was not practiced again until 1960, when Franzen and colleagues published a report describing their preliminary results with the transrectal biopsy.[33] The guide used by Franzen and his colleagues (Figs. 9–21 and 9–22) allowed the aspirating needle to be positioned accurately and directly into a suspicious prostatic nodule through the rectum. The fine caliber of the needle ensured a nontraumatic aspiration requiring no anesthesia. The procedure could be repeated many times. These favorable features were demonstrated in an extremely large number of aspirations performed in this manner, and they are still evident today.

To date, this author has had little opportunity to perform thin-needle aspiration biopsies for carcinoma of the prostate because his coworker, a urologist, prefers the

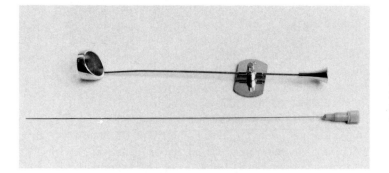

Figure 9–21 Franzen prostatic aspiration needle guide with 20.0 cm 22-gauge needle. This needle is easily threaded through the guide and will project about 5.0 cm beyond the end of the guide.

traditional transperineal Vim-Silverman needle biopsy. Three examples of aspirates from prostatic nodules are illustrated in Figures 9–23 and 9–24. Figure 9–23 depicts sheets of uniform prostatic epithelial cells with bland oval nuclei from a case of prostatic hyperplasia. In contrast, Figure 9–24 depicts an example of a well-differentiated prostatic carcinoma with an acinar pattern visible among the rather uniform cells. The presence of the microacini is the most helpful feature in diagnosing carcinoma. The tumor cells are also somewhat larger than normal prostatic cells. The uniformity of the cells suggests a well-differentiated neoplasm.

It is rare to find normal prostatic cells mixed with those arranged in an acinar pattern suggesting carcinoma. Even in well-differentiated tumors, the smears are composed of a preponderance of malignant cells. Figure 9–24 does illustrate some areas of benign prostatic epithelium (*B,* lower center) mixed with carcinoma cells, revealing the differences in nuclear size and pattern. Figures 9–25 and 9–26 illustrate the aspirate from a moderately well-differentiated prostatic carcinoma. Malignancy is easily reported based on the irregularity of the cells and the obvious malignant nuclear chromatin structure. There is also loss of cell cohesion, so more free tumor cells and naked nuclei are found. Poorly differentiated carcinoma has a pattern of limited acinar structures and more irregular clusters of tumor cells with increased pleomorphism and many dissociated tumor cells.[6, 34]

Prostatitis. A variety of other diseases of the prostate diagnosed by aspiration biopsy are described in a recent monograph by Zajicek. As expected, acute prostatitis is made up of many acute inflammatory cells and degenerated epithelial cells.[6] Clinical evidence of acute inflammation of the prostate is now considered an absolute contraindication for transrectal aspiration biopsy.

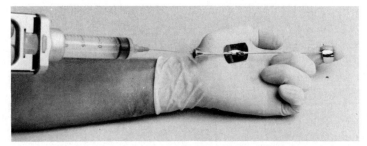

Figure 9–22 Use of Franzen needle guide for prostatic aspiration. Needle with syringe and pistol grip have been assembled. Needle is threaded into the guide with the finger in the rectum directing the tip of the guide and the needle to the prostatic nodule for aspiration. A finger cot is placed over the examining finger and needle guide. This same equipment is employed to aspirate nodules or tumors in the pelvis using a transvaginal or transrectal approach.

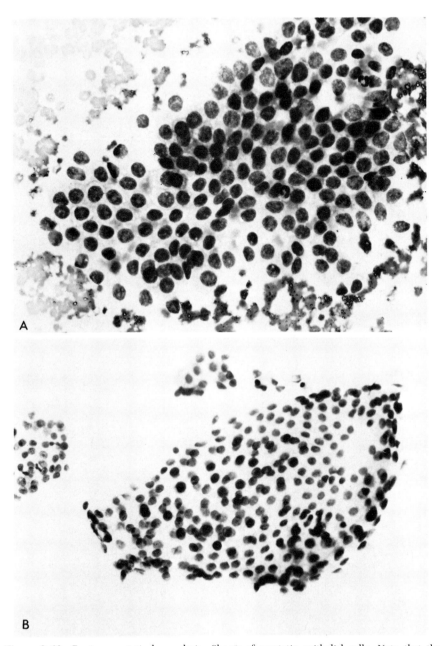

Figure 9–23 Benign prostatic hyperplasia. Sheets of prostatic epithelial cells. Note that there is neither any variation in size and shape of the cells nor any microfollicle formation. The aspirate is not specific except for the presence of prostatic epithelium that is normal in appearance. *A,* Diff-Quik × 375. *B,* Papanicolaou × 375.

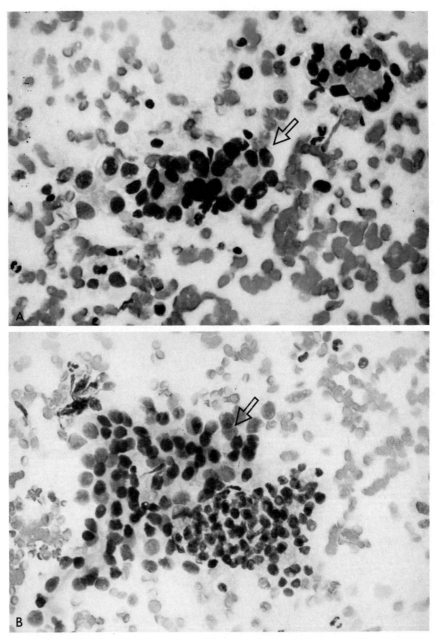

Figure 9–24 Well-differentiated carcinoma of the prostate. Sheets of prostatic cells with some variation in cell size but little alteration in shape. The most notable feature that suggests a diagnosis of carcinoma is the microfollicle pattern (*A* and *B*, arrows). There are several foci of normal prostatic cells (lower center of *B*) for comparison with the carcinoma cells. In carcinoma of the prostate, the presence of both normal and carcinoma cells in the same aspirate is unusual. *A*, Diff-Quik × 375. *B*, Papanicolaou × 375.

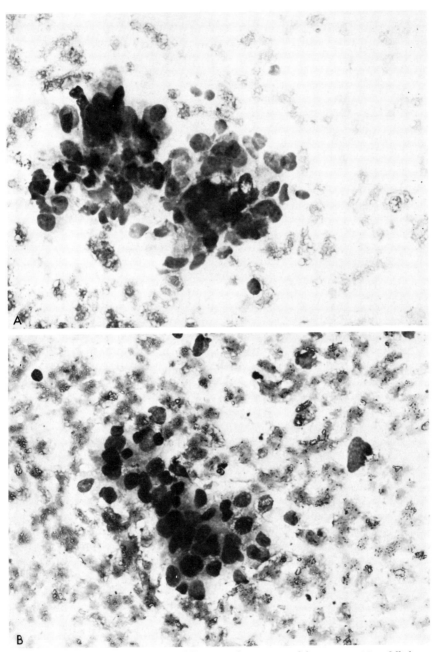

Figure 9–25 Moderately well to poorly differentiated carcinoma of the prostate. Microfollicle arrangement of cells appears with some loose neoplastic cells varying moderately in size and shape. One would expect a carcinoma of the prostate with both solid undifferentiated areas and some areas with gland formation. A, Diff-Quik × 375. B, Papanicolaou × 375.

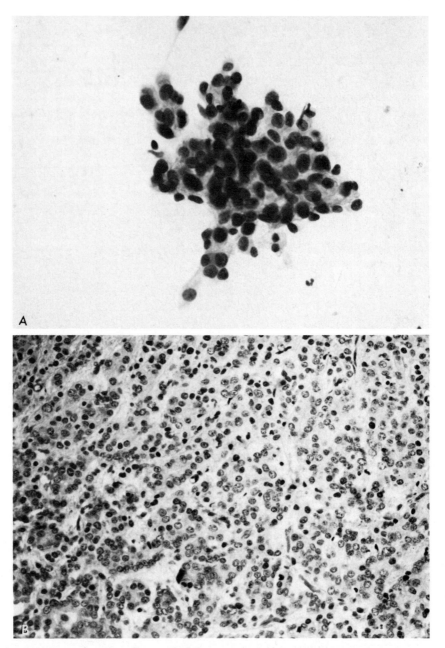

Figure 9–26   Moderately well to poorly differentiated carcinoma of the prostate. Papanicolaou-stained smear (A) shows sheets of neoplastic cells with foci suggesting a microfollicle pattern. There is slight dissociation of peripheral cells. Compare with the histology of this prostatic carcinoma, which depicts the follicle pattern of carcinoma merging with solid areas (upper right of B). A, Papanicolaou × 375. B, Hematoxylin and eosin × 240.

Chronic prostatitis demonstrates chronic inflammatory cells and some prostatic epithelium. Granulomatous prostatitis reveals epithelioid cells and a mixed inflammatory infiltrate. Zajicek believes that when the aspirate reveals a great deal of necrosis as well as epithelioid cells and a mixed inflammatory cell infiltrate, one should suspect tuberculosis of the prostate. Basophilic staining of the atypical reactive prostatic epithelial cells is also common in inflammatory conditions but extremely rare in carcinoma. This is important, since granulomatous prostatitis as well as some cases of chronic prostatitis may simulate carcinoma clinically.[6]

Hyperplasia.   Cases of atypical hyperplasia may be difficult to distinguish from well-differentiated prostatic carcinoma. One study of 31 examples in which acridine orange was applied to the smears was reviewed. This procedure seemed to distinguish atypical hyperplasia from carcinoma, the carcinomas showing many cells with strongly positive orange fluorescence.[36] This work has not been confirmed. The general application of fluorescent stains to cytologic preparations has not been considered very specific in the past.

Complications of Prostatic Aspirations

Four cases of sepsis caused by *Escherichia coli* have been reported among 1400 transrectal aspirations performed at the Karolinska Institute. One of these patients had fatal septicemia. The authors also found three additional case reports of this complication. They noted that three of their four cases were referrals from the Department of Rheumatology, accounting for nearly all the complications in that group of 63 aspirations in 51 patients.[35] The overall complication rate in a 10-year period during which 3002 transrectal aspiration biopsies were performed was 0.4 per cent and included two cases of slight transient hematuria, five cases of limited pyrexia, one case of acute epididymitis, and three cases of hemospermia.[6]

Other Diagnostic Methods

Phosphatase Studies.   Other adjuvant methods applied to aspiration biopsies of prostatic neoplasms include measurement of acid phosphatase activity, DNA studies, flow-through fluorescence cytophotometry, and electron microscopy.[37-39] Esposti and colleagues performed parallel measurements of acid phosphatase on prostatic aspiration biopsy smears from cases of benign prostatic hypertrophy and carcinoma. Using micrograms of phenol liberated per hour as the unit of measurement, the authors calculated that for cases of benign prostatic hypertrophy, values ranged from 3.9 μg/hr to 26.6 μg/hr, while in cases of carcinoma, values ranged from 0.1 μg/hr to 0.8 μg/hr.[37] Linsk and colleagues also studied acid and alkaline phosphatase, concomitant bone marrow aspiration, skeletal survey, bone scan, clinical palpation through the rectum, core biopsy, and transurethral resection compared with fine-needle aspiration biopsy of prostatic carcinoma in 27 cases. The numbers are rather small, but aspiration biopsy diagnosed 20 of the 27 tumors considered positive by clinical evaluation. Of four of those tumors that had been needled by core biopsy, only one was positive by that procedure, while all four were positive by aspiration biopsy. In contrast, 11 of 15 patients with transurethral resection were positive for carcinoma. Of these, 10 were diagnosed correctly by aspiration biopsy, while five were proved negative. Other examinations also seemed to support the accuracy of aspiration biopsy in comparison with several tests used to diagnose or document dissemination in prostatic carcinoma.[40]

DNA Analysis.   Flow-through analysis of DNA using fluorescent cytophotometry in a series of 220 fine-needle aspiration biopsies did not prove helpful in the diagnosis of carcinoma. Compared with traditional cytologic methods of diagnosis, DNA analysis provided a false-negative rate of 11.4 per cent and a false-positive rate of 29.7 per cent. Ten per cent of the aspirates were unsatisfactory for flow-through cytophotometry, whereas only 4.5 per cent of the smears were unsuitable for cytologic study. False-positive results provided by cytophotometry were attributed to proliferating cells, usually found with inflammatory conditions. It was also noted that large numbers of cells were needed for the flow-through procedure. The authors felt the results were too poor for routine use of the method.[38]

Results of Prostatic Aspirations

A number of reported series are too incomplete to make an accurate assessment of the utility of fine-needle aspiration biopsy of the prostate. For example, rates of accuracy reportedly range from 63 per cent[41] to 91 per cent.[30] Only one of the papers states a false-negative rate (17.7 per cent) in hormonally treated patients.[42] Two others report false-positive rates of 2 per cent and 28 per cent.[28] From some of these communications, one cannot even determine how many cases were actually biopsied.[28-30]

Eight studies have compared simultaneous fine-needle aspiration and tissue needle biopsy in diagnosing prostatic carcinoma.[11, 13, 31, 43-47] The rate of accuracy ranges from 85 per cent to 95 per cent, with a fair degree of concordance between core and fine-needle aspiration biopsy. Epstein reported 118 cases, 53 of which were actually carcinoma. Fine-needle aspiration diagnosed 86.6 per cent of these and core needle biopsy diagnosed 85.6 per cent. There were no false-positive results, while agreement between methods was 95.8 per cent for cases of carcinoma.[11] Kline and colleagues also had no false-positive results in a comparative series of 51 cases, 32 of which were diagnosed prostatic carcinoma by tissue needle biopsy. Aspiration diagnosed 25 of these cases positively and two others as suspicious for carcinoma.[31] Alfthan and colleagues compared a larger group of 220 patients, 82 of whom actually had prostatic carcinoma. Of these carcinomas, 84 per cent were diagnosed by aspiration biopsy with only a 5 per cent failure rate, whereas 88 per cent were diagnosed by Vim-Silverman core biopsy. Vim-Silverman biopsy failed in 12 per cent of the cases. There were five false-positive results in the original interpretation of the cytologic specimens obtained by aspiration. Three were considered to be actual false-positives. The other two patients will remain in follow-up until it can be determined whether or not they have carcinoma.[43] Ekman and colleagues also had similar results in a series of 100 patients, approximately half of whom had carcinoma of the prostate diagnosed by histopathologic studies. One interesting feature of this study was that in six of seven cases originally diagnosed as carcinoma by fine-needle aspiration rather than by core needle biopsy, repeat core biopsy identified prostatic carcinoma.[44]

Sonnenschein reported a false-positive rate of 6.5 per cent, the highest found in this series of comparative studies. There were 1700 biopsies performed with a cytologic diagnostic accuracy for prostatic carcinoma of 93.3 per cent. Less than 3 per cent of cases of carcinoma were not detected by aspiration biopsy, while 3.7 per cent were diagnosed cytologically but not confirmed histologically.[13] It would seem that an attempt to diagnose very well-differentiated tumors leads to an increase in false-positive reports, even though it raises the overall rate of accuracy of fine-needle aspiration biopsy. Some of these tumors may be occult carcinomas that cannot be detected histologically with core biopsy alone. A longer follow-up period and complete autopsies might verify that contention.

All the authors agree that the ease and utility of fine-needle aspiration make it the preferred initial biopsy method for the diagnosis of a prostatic nodule. If clinical suspicion of tumor remains after a negative needle aspiration, then either a repeat aspiration or a tissue needle biopsy should be recommended. Several authors also note that performing multiple aspirations not only of the nodule but also of other areas of the prostate at the same examination probably contributes to diagnostic accuracy.[44, 46]

Table 9–3 summarizes four selected series in which the data is sufficient to calculate both sensitivity and specificity.

TABLE 9–3.   RESULTS OF SELECTED SERIES OF FINE-NEEDLE ASPIRATION BIOPSIES OF PROSTATE

Reference	True-Positive	False-Positive	True-Negative	False-Negative	Sensitivity (%)	Specificity (%)	Unsatisfactory
Faul et al.[12]	24	1	81	4	86	99	16
Eposti[10]	60	4	101	5	92	96	4
Bishop and Oliver[9]	37	1	113	1	97	99	30
Williams et al.[48]	33	0	15	3	91	100	12

Sensitivity for the diagnosis of carcinoma of the prostate ranged from 86 per cent to 97 per cent, while specificity was better than 96 per cent in all reports. Specificity tended to be higher when there were a greater number of unsatisfactory smears, suggesting in several of these studies very strict criteria for making an initial interpretation.[9, 10, 12, 48] Esposti also emphasized that 10 per cent of carcinomas of the prostate are not diagnosed at the first aspiration, and he therefore strongly recommended multiple repeat aspirations. This tends to reduce the false-negative results to nearly zero.[10]

Esposti also tried to grade prostatic carcinomas on the basis of the morphologic features of the cells in the aspirate. In a series of 469 patients with prostatic carcinoma, correlation was good in separating low-grade or well-differentiated tumors from poorly differentiated neoplasms with respect to survival. Moderately well-differentiated cancers fell somewhere in the middle of the survival curve, with a shift toward survival approximating that of well-differentiated cases. The cytologic basis for this grading has been described and illustrated previously (Figs. 9–24 and 9–25).[10]

REFERENCES

1. Soderstrom, N.: *Fine Needle Aspiration Biopsy.* Stockholm, Almqvist and Wiksell, 1966, pp. 137–147.
2. Thommesen, P., and Nielsen, B.: The value of fine needle aspiration biopsy and intravenous pyelography in the diagnosis of renal masses. Fortschr. Geb. Roentgenstr. Nuklearmed. *122*:248–251, 1975.
3. Angstrom, T., Kjellgren, O., and Bergman, F.: The cytologic diagnosis of ovarian tumors by means of aspiration biopsy. Acta Cytol. *26*:336–341, 1972.
4. Geier, G., Kraus, H., and Schuhmann, R.: Fine needle aspiration biopsy in ovarian tumors; in DeWatteville, H., et al. (Eds.): *Diagnosis and Treatment of Ovarian Neoplastic Alterations.* Amsterdam, Excerpta Medica, 1975, pp. 73–76.
5. Kjellgren, O., Angstrom, T., Bergman, F., et al.: Fine needle aspiration biopsy in diagnosis and classification of ovarian carcinoma. Cancer *28*:967–976, 1971.
6. Zajicek, J.: *Aspiration Biopsy Cytology. Part 2. Cytology of Infradiaphragmatic Organs.* Monographs in Clinical Cytology. Vol. 7. New York, S. Karger, 1979, pp. 1–37, 104–128, 129–166.
7. Kjellgren, O., and Angstrom, T.: Transvaginal and Transrectal Aspiration Biopsy in Diagnosis and Classification of Ovarian Tumours; in Zajicek, J.: *Monographs in Clinical Cytology.* Vol. 7. New York, S. Karger, 1979, pp. 80–103.
8. Kovacic, J., Rainer, S., Levicnik, A., et al.: Cytology of Benign Ovarian Lesions in Connection with Laparoscopy; in Zajicek, J.: *Monographs in Clinical Cytology.* Vol. 7. New York, S. Karger, 1979, pp. 57–79.
9. Bishop, D., and Oliver, J. A.: A study of transrectal aspiration biopsies of the prostate with particular regard to prognostic evaluation. J. Urol. *117*:313–315, 1977.
10. Esposti, P.: Cytologic diagnosis of prostatic tumors with the aid of transrectal aspiration biopsy. A critical review of 1,110 cases and a report of morphologic and cytochemical studies. Acta Cytol. *10*:182–186, 1966.
11. Epstein, N. A.: Prostatic biopsy: A morphological correlation of aspiration cytology with needle biopsy histology. Cancer *38*:2078–2087, 1976.
12. Faul, P., Klosterhalfen, H., and Schmiedt, E.: Erfahrungen mit der Feinnadebiopsie (Saug-bzw. Aspirationsbiopsie nach Franzen) der Prostata. Urologe *10*:120–126, 1971.
13. Sonnenschein, R.: The effectiveness of transrectal aspiration cytology in the diagnosis of prostatic cancer. Eur. Urol. *1*:189–192, 1975.
14. Edgren, J., Taskinen, E., Alfthan, O., et al.: Radiology and fine needle aspiration biopsy in the diagnosis of tumours of the kidney. Ann. Chir. Gynaecol. Fenn. *64*:209–216, 1975.
15. Holm, H. H., Pederson, J. F., Kristensen, J. K., et al.: Ultrasonically guided percutaneous puncture. Radiol. Clin. N. Am. *13*:493–503, 1975.
16. von Schreeb, T., Franzen, S., and Ljungqvist, A.: Renal adenocarcinoma. Scand. J. Nephrol. *1*:265–269, 1967.
17. Riches, E.: Endoscopic and laboratory investigations; in Riches E. (Ed.): *Tumours of the Kidney and Ureter.* Edinburgh, E. & S. Livingstone Ltd., 1964, p. 157.
18. Hanley, H. G.: Discussion on cyst and tumor occurring in the same kidney. Trans. Am. Assoc. Gen. Urin. Surg. *55*:126–128, 1963.
19. Gibbons, R. P., Bush, W. H., and Burnett, L. L.: Needle tract seeding following aspiration of renal cell carcinoma. J. Urol. *118*:865–867, 1977.
20. von Schreeb, T., Abner, O., Skovsted, G., et al.: Renal carcinoma. Is there a risk of spreading tumor cells in diagnostic puncture? Scand. J. Urol. Nephrol. *1*:270–276, 1967.
21. Sevin, B., Greening, S. E., and Nadji, M.: Fine needle aspiration cytology in gynecologic oncology. Acta Cytol. (Abstr.) *22*:602, 1978.

22. Geier, G.: Aspirationszytologie am Parametrium. Geburtsch. u. Frauenheilk. *37*:423–428, 1977.
23. Frable, W. J., and Goplerud, D. R.: Adenoid cystic carcinoma of Bartholin's gland. Diagnosis by aspiration biopsy. Acta Cytol. *19*:152–153, 1975.
24. Ramzy, I., Delaney, M., and Rose, P.: Fine needle aspiration of ovarian masses. II. Correlative cytologic and histologic study of nonneoplastic cysts and noncelomic epithelial neoplasms. Acta Cytol. *23*:97–104, 1979.
25. Galen, R. S., and Gambino, S. R.: *Beyond Normality: The Predictive Value and Efficiency of Medical Diagnosis.* New York, John Wiley and Sons, 1975.
26. Persson, P. S., Ahren, C., and Obrant, K. S.: Aspiration biopsy smear of testis in azoospermia. Scand. J. Urol. Nephrol. *5*:22–26, 1971.
27. Ekelung, L., and Gothlin, J.: Fine needle biopsy of metastases at retrograde pyelography, directed by fluoroscopy. Report of a case with malignant teratoma of the testis. Scand. J. Urol. Nephrol. *10*:261–262, 1976.
28. Ventura, M., Barasolo, E., Morano, E., et al.: Franzen needle transrectal prostatic biopsy in the cytologic diagnosis of prostatic cancer. J. Urol. Nephrol. (Paris) *83*:858–862, 1977.
29. Sparwasser, H., and Luchtrath, H.: Die transrectale Saugbiopsie der Prostata. Urologe *9*:281–285, 1970.
30. Rheinfrank, R. E., and Nulf, T. H.: Fine needle aspiration biopsy of the prostate. Endoscopy *1*:27–32, 1969.
31. Kline, T. S., Kelsey, D. M., and Kohler, F. P.: Prostatic carcinoma and needle aspiration biopsy. Am. J. Clin. Pathol. *67*:131–133, 1977.
32. Ferguson, R. S.: Prostatic neoplasms, their diagnosis by needle puncture and aspiration. Am. J. Surg. *9*:507–511, 1930.
33. Franzen, S., Giertz, G., and Zajicek, J.: Cytological diagnosis of prostatic tumours by transrectal aspiration biopsy: A preliminary report. Br. J. Urol. *32*:193–196, 1960.
34. Esposti, P. L.: Cytologic malignancy grading of prostatic carcinoma by transrectal aspiration biopsy. Scand. J. Urol. Nephrol. *5*:199–209, 1971.
35. Esposti, P. L., Elman, A., and Norlen, H.: Complications of transrectal aspiration biopsy of the prostate. Scand. J. Urol. Nephrol. *9*:208–213, 1975.
36. De Gaetani, C. F., and Trentini, G. P.: Atypical hyperplasia of the prostate. A pitfall in the cytologic diagnosis of carcinoma. Acta Cytol. *22*:483–486, 1978.
37. Esposti, P. L., Estborn, B., and Zajicek, J.: Determination of acid phosphatase activity in cells of prostatic tumours. Nature *188*:663–664, 1960.
38. Sprenger, E., Michaelis, W. E., Vogt-Schaden, M., et al.: The significance of DNA flow-through fluorescence cytophotometry for the diagnosis of prostate carcinoma. Beitr. Pathol. *159*:292–298, 1976.
39. Epstein, N. A.: Primary papillary carcinoma of the prostate: Report of a histopathologic, cytologic and electron microscopic study on one case. Acta Cytol. *21*:543–546, 1977.
40. Linsk, J. A., Axilrod, H. D., Solyn, R., et al.: Transrectal cytologic aspiration in the diagnosis of prostatic carcinoma. J. Urol. *108*:455–459, 1972.
41. Sunderland, H., and Lederer, H.: Prostatic aspiration biopsy. Br. J. Urol. *43*:603–607, 1971.
42. Schulte-Wissermann, H., and Luchtrath, H.: Aspirationsbiopsie und Cytologie beim Prostatacarcinom. Virchows Arch. Pathol. Anat. Physiol. *352*:122–129, 1971.
43. Alfthan, O., Klintrup, H. E., Koivuniemi, A., et al.: Cytological aspiration biopsy and Vim-Silverman biopsy in the diagnosis of prostatic carcinoma. Ann. Chir. Gynaecol. Fenn. *59*:226–229, 1970.
44. Ekman, H., Hedberg, K., and Persson, P. S.: Cytological versus histological examination of needle biopsy specimens in the diagnosis of prostatic cancer. Br. J. Urol. *39*:544–548, 1967.
45. Schnürer, L. B., Fritjofsson, A., Lindgren, A., et al.: Fine needle versus coarse needle in punction diagnosis of prostatic carcinoma. Acta Pathol. Microbiol. Scand. *76*:150–160, 1969.
46. Staehler, W., Ziegler, H., Volter, D., et al.: *Zytodiagnostik der Prostata.* Stuttgart, Schattauer, 1975.
47. Alfthan, O., Klintrup, H. E., Koivuniemi, A., et al.: Comparison of thin-needle and Vim-Silverman needle biopsy in the diagnosis of prostatic cancer. Duodecim *84*:506–511, 1968.
48. Williams, J. P., Still, B. M., and Pugh, R. C. B.: The diagnosis of prostatic cancer: Cytological and biochemical studies using the Franzen biopsy needle. Br. J. Urol. *39*:549–554, 1967.

Chapter Ten

Bone and Soft Tissue

TECHNIQUE

The original studies of needle aspiration biopsy, by Martin and Ellis and later by Stewart, contained a few cases of soft tissue sarcomas.[1, 2] It was Coley and colleagues, however, who first reported a definitive series of 35 consecutive cases of needle aspiration of bone tumors. The data are somewhat scanty in that study, but three errors occurred: one metastatic carcinoma diagnosed as osteosarcoma; one neurogenic sarcoma diagnosed as an osteosarcoma; and one case in which the pathologist was unable to make a diagnosis. In 18 cases there was no open biopsy, but confirmation of the diagnosis was obtained by a clinical follow-up and radiographic studies.[3] This series was subsequently expanded and again reported in 1945 by Snyder and Coley, who performed 567 aspirations in 474 patients. The three major sites were the femur (146 cases), the pelvis (111 cases), and the ribs (72 cases). The authors concluded that aspiration biopsy was most valuable in true neoplasms. They also stated that there was no dissemination of tumor cells by this biopsy method and no cases of needle tract implantation.[4]

Few other clinicians or pathologists have developed an interest in performing aspiration biopsy of the bone. In fact, there has been considerable negative feeling among surgical pathologists primarily interested in bone tumors. A few have advocated core needle biopsy, while others favor combining aspiration with preparation of histologic sections using a cell block.[5, 6] Several large series have been reported, however, by Valls and colleagues as well as by Ottolenghi and by Schajowiez and coworkers.[7, 8, 9, 10] Valls and Ottolenghi, in two separate papers, illustrate their approach in detail and the results from 86 and 1061 cases, respectively. The latter series includes aspirations of vertebral bodies. They both stress the necessity of correct placement of the needle. This has been facilitated in recent years by better imaging methods, including fluoroscopy and CAT scanning.[7, 9, 11, 12]

BONE

Osteogenic Sarcoma. This author's experience has been quite limited with primary malignant bone tumors. It includes the aspiration of three osteogenic sarcomas and one case each of plasma cell myeloma, chondrosarcoma, chordoma, and Ewing's sarcoma. Figure 10–1 illustrates the aspiration smear from an osteosarcoma of the proximal end of the tibia in an 11-year-old girl. The typical radiographic features are illustrated in Figure 10–2. The smear is quite cellular and the cells are pleomorphic.

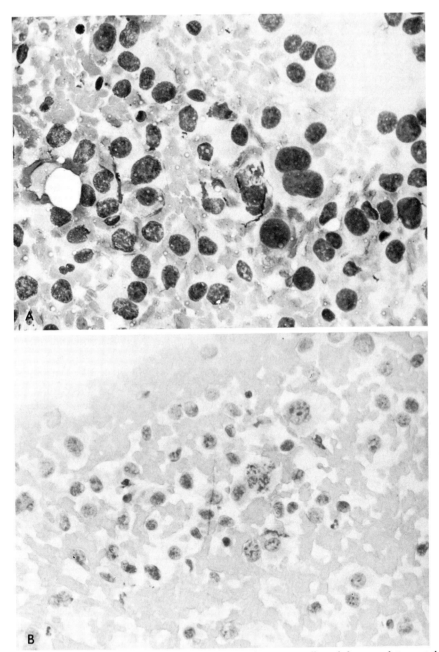

Figure 10–1 Ostogenic sarcoma of the tibia. Pleomorphic tumor cells with large nuclei are visible in both *A* and *B*. The stromal pattern, which is a combination of osteoid and blood, interdigitates between the cells. *A*, Diff-Quik × 375. *B*, Papanicolaou × 375.

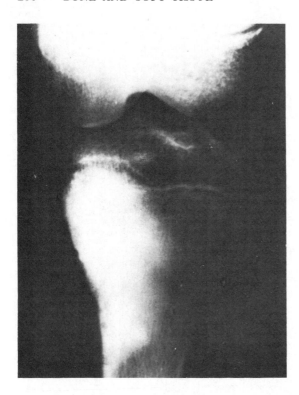

Figure 10–2 Radiograph of the osteogenic sarcoma diagnosed from the biopsy depicted in Figure 10–1.

Their relatively large size and abundant cytoplasm are particularly well demonstrated in the Romanovsky-stained preparations. The nuclear structure and the nucleoli are seen better in the wet-fixed, Papanicolaou-stained aspirate. If stained by hematoxylin and eosin, these tumor cells will have a very eosinophilic cytoplasm resembling in some respects a keratinizing squamous cell carcinoma. Occasionally, multinucleated tumor giant cells are found, but they are not useful as a specific diagnostic feature for any of the bone diseases having giant cells.[10]

In an aspirate from an osteogenic sarcoma, there is a scant amount of blue homogeneous background staining, which may represent osteoid and is best seen in the Romanovsky-stained smears. With the Papanicolaou stain, this "stroma" may appear pinkish-red and homogeneous, containing entrapped cells. The pattern is analogous to what has been described as malignant osteoid. From this author's experience with the aspiration of a few primary bone sarcomas, it can not be determined whether this cell stromal interface is in any way specific.

Figure 10–3 illustrates the same patient whose aspirates are shown in Figure 10–1, a child who was treated by primary amputation after osteogenic sarcoma was diagnosed by aspiration biopsy. The gross tumor was highly sclerotic, except in the area of perforation of the periosteum, from which the aspirate had been obtained (Fig. 10–4). The histopathologic specimen is typical of osteogenic sarcoma (Fig. 10–5).

Figure 10–6 illustrates another osteosarcoma in a 16-year-old child, a destructive lesion of the proximal tibia. The tumor cells in this case are more spindle-shaped, and the apparent osteoid matrix is brightly eosinophilic. With metachrome B staining, which was performed on an air-dried aspirate in this case, the background stroma representing possible osteoid is slightly metachromatic (Fig. 10–6).

Chondrosarcoma.   A chondrosarcoma occurred in an 11-year-old child and radiographically presented as a destructive but much less sclerotic mass (Fig. 10–7) that was actually palpable over the anterior aspect of the proximal tibia. An abundant aspirate was obtained with a strikingly metachromatic background surrounding enlarged,

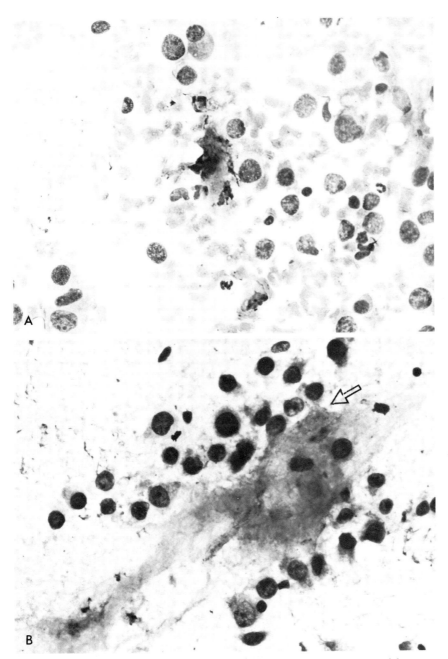

Figure 10–3 Osteogenic sarcoma of the tibia. Two fields demonstrate the proximity of the tumor cells to the osteoid matrix (*B*, arrow). This matrix is very metachromatic with the Romanovsky stains. Both *A* and *B*, Diff-Quik × 375.

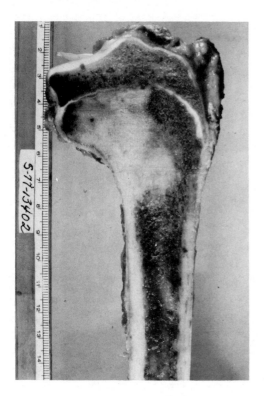

Figure 10–4 Gross specimen of osteogenic sarcoma diagnosed from the aspiration biopsy illustrated in Figures 10–1 and 10–3.

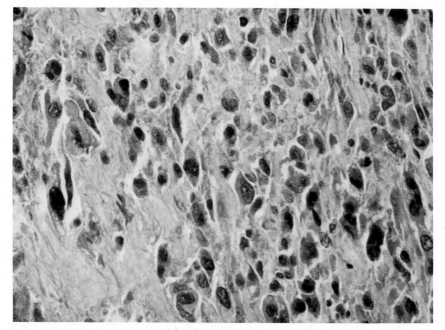

Figure 10–5   Osteogenic sarcoma of the tibia. Typical malignant cells of this bone tumor are found in an osteoid matrix. Hematoxylin and eosin × 240.

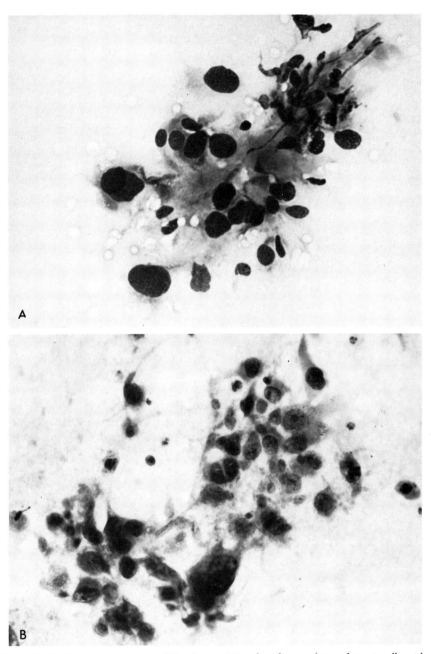

Figure 10–6 Osteogenic sarcoma of the femur. Note the pleomorphic malignant cells with some metachromatic stroma, more apparent in A. Good chromatin detail with large nucleoli is found in the Papanicolaou-stained preparation (B). A, Diff-Quik × 375. B, Papanicolaou × 375.

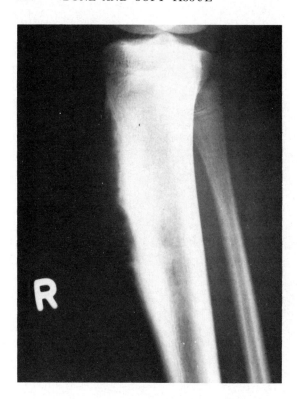

Figure 10–7 Radiograph of chondrosarcoma of the tibia. There was a large palpable mass over the anterior aspect of the tibia. Aspiration was taken from that area.

multinucleated cartilaginous cells (Fig. 10–8). A few foci that are better demonstrated on the alcohol-fixed, Papanicolaou-stained smear reveal cells with a spindle configuration and a greater degree of nuclear abnormality. This part of the smear does not differ significantly from the aspirate of an osteosarcoma; however, the radiograph is not diagnostic of that neoplasm. The bone destruction evident on the radiograph confirms that one is dealing with a malignant bone tumor. Hence, all of the evidence leads one to suspect a chondrosarcoma that is probably in part poorly differentiated. Primary amputation confirmed this diagnosis. The histopathologic features of less differentiated areas are illustrated in Figure 10–9.

Ewing's Sarcoma. The case of Ewing's sarcoma studied by this author was detected during a follow-up in a 15-year-old patient who was treated for two and one half years by radiation and maintenance chemotherapy for primary Ewing's sarcoma of the scapula. Six months prior to the aspiration, chemotherapy was discontinued. Approximately three months later, pain occurred in the right arm. Radiographs did not reveal any changes at first, but two months later there was evidence of periosteal elevation over the distal humerus (Fig. 10–10). While no mass was palpable, an aspiration performed in the area of the periosteal elevation revealed many small undifferentiated tumor cells in sheets and clusters. In Figure 10–11, the two types of aspiration smears are compared: an air-dried smear stained with metachrome B and a Papanicolaou-stained, wet-fixed preparation. In the latter smear, there is some clustering of neoplastic cells in a rosette-like pattern. Malignant features of these small cells, such as increased nuclear cytoplasmic ratio, granular nuclear chromatin, and nucleoli, are easily found. The background is bloody and necrotic. A follow-up bone survey of this child revealed other metastatic sites. Chemotherapy and radiation were reinstituted.

Paget's Disease. Only three benign bone tumors have been examined by aspiration biopsy in this author's personal series, no doubt a reflection of the reluctance of his colleague, an orthopedic surgeon, to use this diagnostic procedure and the

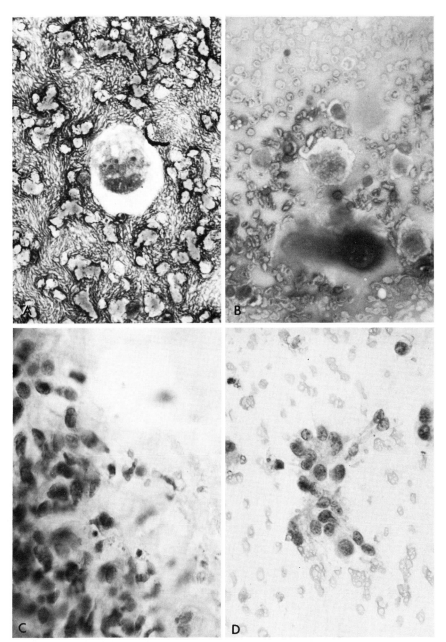

Figure 10–8   Chondrosarcoma of the tibia. Both *A* and *B* show abundant highly metachromatic stroma with large pleomorphic double-nucleated cartilaginous cells. Note the large nucleolus in the tumor cell in the lower half of *B*. More spindle-shaped cells with some chromatin clumping and a much less obvious chondromatous matrix are found in the Papanicolaou preparation *(C and D)*. *A* and *B*, Diff-Quik × 375. *C* and *D*, Papanicolaou × 375.

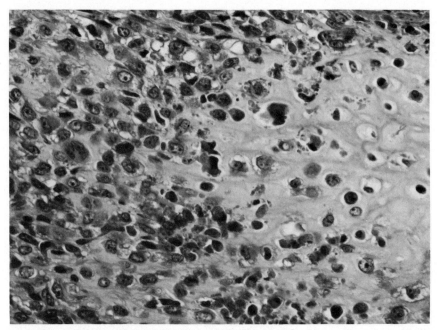

Figure 10–9   Chondrosarcoma of the tibia. Histopathology shows both moderately well and poorly differentiated areas in this field. Hematoxylin and eosin × 375.

relative rarity of such neoplasms. Figure 10–12 illustrates the radiographs of a patient with known Paget's disease of the skull who developed several lumps over the mandible. Aspiration of one of these masses (Fig. 10–13) revealed many tumor giant cells and small stromal cells with active nuclei, findings that are entirely consistent with giant cell tumor as seen in Paget's disease. Certainly, the aspiration pattern would not be specific. Only the clinical features of this case and the rare but well-known development of giant cell tumors with Paget's disease suggest the diagnosis. Later, a surgical excision performed for cosmetic purposes confirmed the aspiration report.

   Enchondroma.   An aspiration of an enchondroma of the metacarpal was the result of a follow-up in a nine-year-old girl who had been treated by curettage for an eosinophilic granuloma of the cervical spine. A bone survey was performed to determine whether there were other lesions. An expanded smooth-bordered radiolucent area was found in the second metacarpal (Fig. 10–14). This tumor radiographically appeared to be an enchondroma rather than an eosinophilic granuloma. An aspirate,

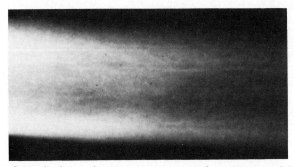

Figure 10–10   Radiograph of Ewing's sarcoma metastatic to the periosteum of the humerus. Note the fuzzy elevated appearance of the periosteum. Differential diagnosis would be osteomyelitis.

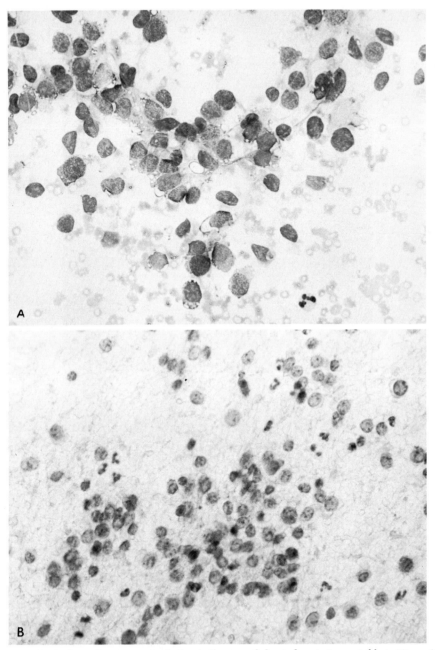

Figure 10–11 Ewing's sarcoma. Aspiration in the area of elevated periosteum visible in Figure 10–10 reveals small undifferentiated malignant cells. Note the fine fibrillar background and rosette-like pattern in the Papanicolaou preparation (B). A, Diff-Quik × 375. B, Papanicolaou × 375.

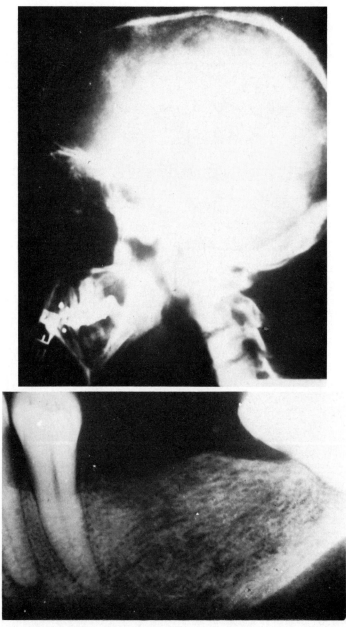

Figure 10–12 Paget's disease of the skull, with giant cell tumor of both sides of the mandible. Radiographs show the marked thickening of the skull bones consistent with a diagnosis of Paget's disease. Alkaline phosphatase was also extremely elevated. Both views of the mandible show areas of rarefaction beneath the palpable masses that were present bilaterally over the body of the mandible in this patient.

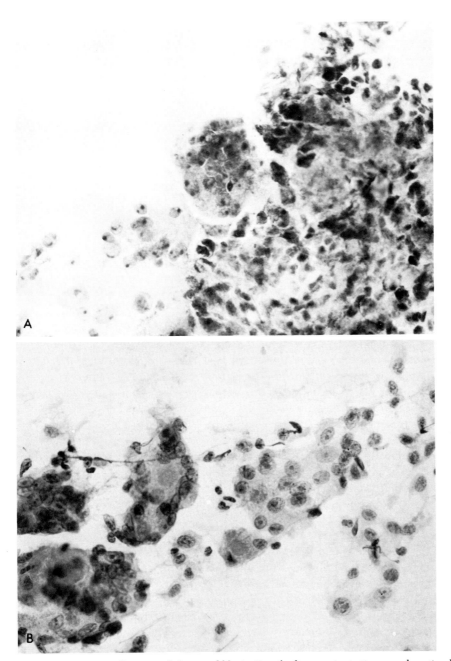

Figure 10–13 Giant cell tumor of the mandible in Paget's disease. Aspiration reveals active but morphologically uniform spindle cells mixed with many large multinucleated giant cells. The pattern is typical of what would be expected from an aspirate of a giant cell tumor of bone. Both lesions were excised from this patient without recurrence to date. A, Papanicolaou × 375. B, Diff-Quik × 375.

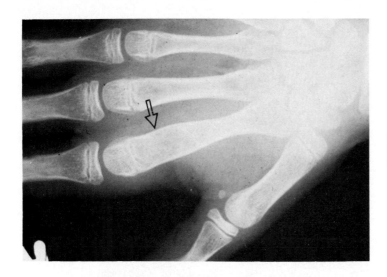

Figure 10–14 Radiograph of enchondroma of metacarpal (arrow) in a young girl with eosinophilic granuloma of the cervical spine.

obtained with a 22-gauge, 3.75 cm (1.5 in) spinal needle with a stylus, also documented the diagnosis. The thin cortex of the metacarpal was easily penetrated. An abundant specimen that was highly metachromatic with scant cellularity made up the smear (Fig. 10–15). The uniformity of the few cartilaginous cells and the extensive background matrix confirmed the diagnosis of enchondroma. This tumor was later curetted.

Metastatic Tumors. In several series in the literature as well as in this author's experience, it is in cases of carcinoma metastatic to bone that the needle aspiration biopsy is most useful. This is particularly true because aspiration can be performed on an outpatient basis with only local anesthesia administered through the skin to the periosteum. The fine-needle method can not be used unless either the cortex has been broken by the metastatic tumor or it is extremely thin. Otherwise, a stiff and larger bore needle is necessary for biopsy.[13] Several examples of aspirates from tumors metastatic to bone are illustrated in Figures 10–16 to 10–18. The cells of most of these biopsies appear to be highly undifferentiated. Care must be taken in matching them with the original primary cancer. Histologic sections of the primary tumor are usually available for study and comparison. The use of special stains as previously described for lymph node aspirates is also helpful. The undifferentiated nature of secondary cancers in bone often precludes determining the primary site when metastasis is the original presentation.

Inflammatory Lesions. When destructive, inflammatory bone disease is present, specimens can be obtained for culture, by needle aspiration. The aspirates themselves are often not specific, showing only an acute inflammatory exudate or a relatively limited sample with chronic inflammatory cells and some fibroblasts. Rarely, a definite organism may be recognized, as in the case of a patient with a soft tissue mass in the back that showed destruction of the eighth thoracic vertebra. An aspirate from this area revealed acute inflammatory exudate and *Actinomyces israelii* organisms (Fig. 10–19). This case also emphasizes the use of the cell blocks when a large volume of biopsy material is obtained. The organisms in this case were more easily seen in the agar-embedded cell block stained with hematoxylin and eosin (Fig. 10–19*B*).

SUMMARY OF BONE ASPIRATIONS

This author's experience with aspiration biopsy of bone is summarized in Table 10–1. While the results substantiate a high rate of accuracy, it should be remembered that there are only a handful of primary malignant bone tumors in this series, and

Text continued on page 304

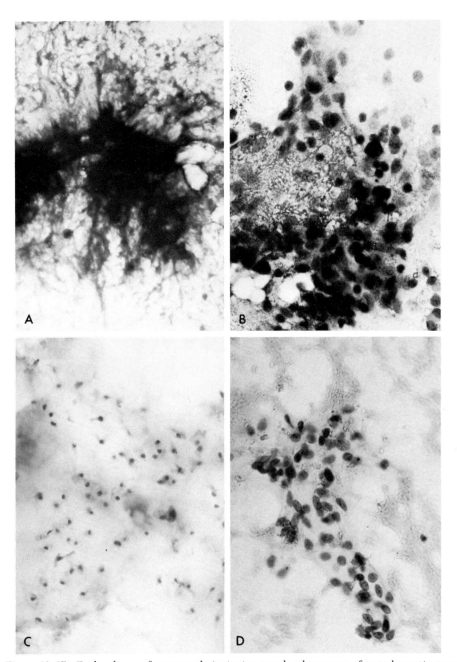

Figure 10–15 Enchondroma of metacarpal. Aspiration reveals a large mass of metachromatic stroma (A) nearly devoid of cells. Focal cellular areas were visible in some areas, but the tumor cells are quite uniform (B and D). Benign and typical cartilaginous tissue is evident in C, which illustrates Papanicolaou-stained aspirate. A and B, Diff-Quik × 375. C and D, Papanicolaou × 375.

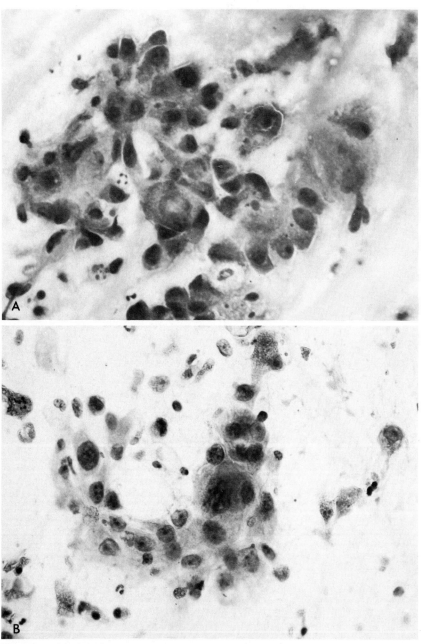

Figure 10–16   Mixed adenosquamous cell carcinoma of the lung, metastatic to the scapula. Aspiration is highly cellular, reflecting the undifferentiated nature as well as the pleomorphism of this metastatic lung carcinoma. Some cells have loosely textured cytoplasm; others have well-defined cell borders. *A*, Diff-Quik × 375. *B*, Papanicolaou × 375.

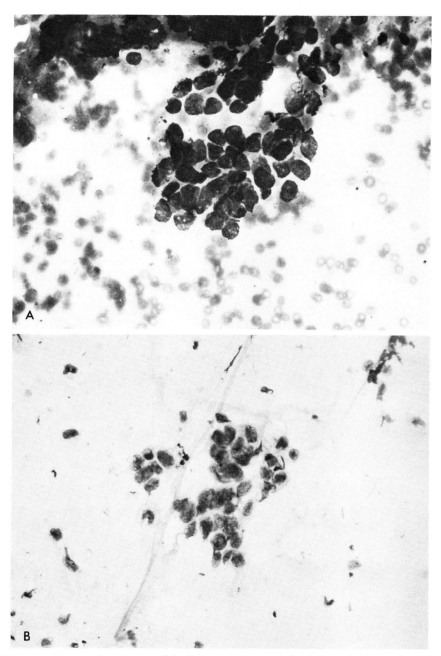

Figure 10–17 Oat cell carcinoma of the lung, metastatic to a rib. This morphology in the aspirate of small undifferentiated cells certainly suggests an oat cell carcinoma. There is good nuclear molding, more prominent in A. A, Diff-Quik × 375. B, Papanicolaou × 375.

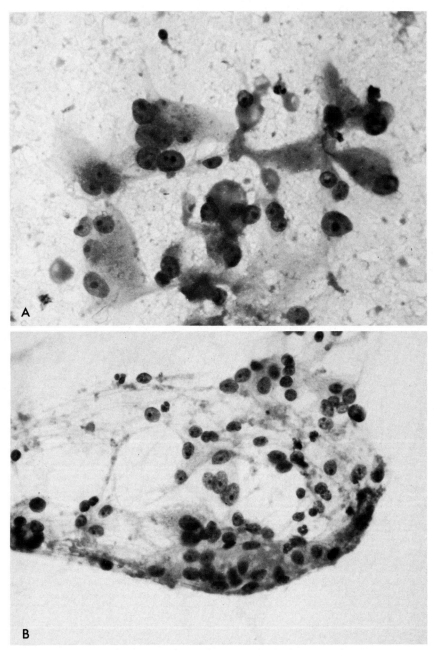

Figure 10–18 Pheochromocytoma of the adrenal gland, metastatic to the femur. This metastasis appeared several years after successful removal of a pheochromocytoma. The nuclear pattern with prominent nucleoli and the abundant cell cytoplasm are both features that correspond well with the features of the original primary tumor in this case. *A*, Diff-Quik × 375. *B*, Papanicolaou × 375.

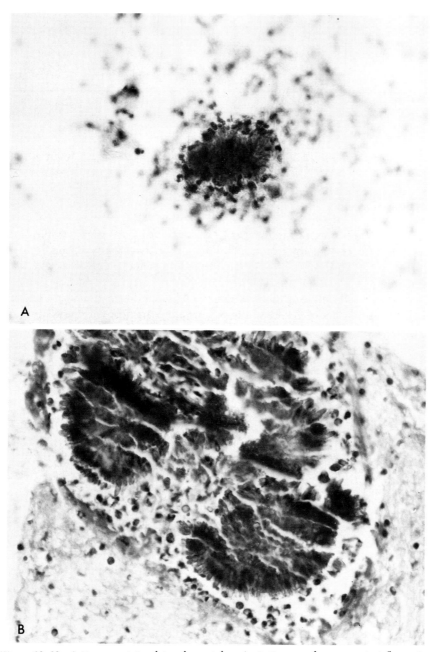

Figure 10–19 Actinomycosis involving the vertebra. Aspiration reveals many acute inflammatory cells and clusters of organisms with a club-like border. A very large organism is pictured in the cell block section (*B*). Immunofluorescent staining of a section of the cell block identified the organism as *Actinomyces israelii*. *A*, Papanicolaou × 375. *B*, Hematoxylin and eosin × 375.

TABLE 10–1.   THIN-NEEDLE ASPIRATION BIOPSY OF BONE

Primary Malignant Tumors	Metastatic Tumors	Primary Benign Tumors	Benign Tumors	False-Positive	False-Negative
8	26	3	22	—	(3)*

Total bone aspirations	59
Unsatisfactory aspirations	2
Sensitivity for tumor	92%
Specificity for the *absence* of tumor	100%

*Misssed one case of osteosarcoma, one case of eosinophilic granuloma, and one case of metastatic carcinoma.

even fewer primary benign bone neoplasms. Several more extensive reports from the literature document that the rate of accuracy for the diagnosis of primary malignant bone tumors is approximately 75 per cent.[14-18] Accuracy for metastatic tumors seems to be somewhat better.[16] Several of the authors emphasize the need to vary the technique depending upon the type of neoplasm, most often in cases of primary bone tumors, in which the smear alone may not be sufficient for an exact classification. An example would be making the differential diagnosis between chondromas and chondrosarcomas.[13, 14, 15] Only the report of Hadju and Melamed tabulates the actual cell types and other cytologic features for several different primary bone sarcomas. The cytologic patterns fall between those of large-cell tumors (osteosarcoma, chondrosarcoma, chordoma, malignant giant-cell tumor, and fibrosarcoma) and those of small-cell tumors (Ewing's sarcoma, malignant lymphoma, and plasma cell myeloma). Osteoid was seen in all the osteosarcomas and in two of the chondrosarcomas but in none of the other tumors. This report does not discuss the results of their diagnoses, but presumably there were no false-positive or false-negative results in a series of 86 aspirations.[19]

The report of deSantos and colleagues confirms that diagnostic accuracy may be improved with the experience of the cytopathologist. These authors compiled the results of aspiration biopsies in 34 cases of suspected primary bone tumors. In 31 cases, an adequate sample was obtained. There was an overall accuracy rate of 93 per cent. However, in almost all these cases core biopsies were performed, except in those in which a lytic lesion was clearly present or the tumor was in the spine.[20]

SOFT TISSUE

A review of the literature reveals no substantial series of fine-needle aspiration biopsies of soft part tumors. Even Hadju's exhaustive work on the cytopathologic features of sarcomas contains only a few examples of aspiration biopsy of these neoplasms. Most of the cytologic findings are based either on imprints or on the appearance of sarcomas in pleural and peritoneal fluids.[21] Other recent reports have included examples of benign schwannoma that demonstrate Verocay bodies on the aspiration smear, malignant hemangiopericytoma, synovial sarcoma, malignant fibrous histiocytoma, myxofibrosarcoma, and nodular fasciitis.[22-27]

The aspirations of soft tissue masses performed at the Medical College of Virginia are documented in Table 10–2. As in bone tumors, there are only a small number of primary malignant soft part sarcomas, and the majority of these are diagnosed by needle aspiration biopsy as recurrent neoplasms. This illustrates the greatest utility,

TABLE 10–2.   THIN-NEEDLE ASPIRATION BIOPSY OF SOFT TISSUE

Primary Malignant Tumors	Metastatic Tumors	Benign Tumors	Negative NOS*	False-Positive	False-Negative
26	139	17	98	(2)†	(8)

Total soft tissue aspirations	281
Unsatisfactory aspirations	12
Sensitivity for tumor	95%
Specificity for the *absence* of tumor	98%

*NOS = not otherwise specified.

†One case of fat necrosis interpreted as metastatic renal cell carcinoma. One case of aspiration of a pelvic mass that was diverticulitis with abcess formation reported as recurrent carcinoma of the cervix.

other than the diagnosis of metastatic carcinomas to soft tissue, of fine-needle aspiration biopsy.

It has not been difficult to identify a sarcoma on the basis of the cytologic pattern of the aspiration biopsy, but usually it is a problem to classify the neoplasm precisely. The following cases illustrate the variety of aspiration smears from soft part sarcomas and some of the complexities involved in their interpretation.

Fibrosarcoma.   Figure 10–20 illustrates the aspirate from a forearm mass in a 54-year-old man who had previously had a soft part resection of that area for a low-grade fibrosarcoma. There are many pleomorphic cells with a somewhat spindle-shaped configuration. Some of the cells are multinucleated and have an almost histiocytic appearance. The nuclear shape and size conform to the original primary tumor as seen in Figure 10–21. Hence, a diagnosis of recurrent fibrosarcoma is easily made. Because of the pleomorphic and multinucleated appearance, this neoplasm might have been classified as a malignant fibrous histiocytoma. But in either case, the cytomorphologic pattern of the aspirate corresponds quite well with that of the original lesion. An amputation was required in order to control the recurrent tumor, which had invaded the radius.

Liposarcoma.   Figures 10–22 and 10–23 illustrate aspirates from liposarcomas. The patterns are variable, with sheets of spindle-shaped cells and a very delicate cytoplasm that is metachromatic with the Romanovsky stains. This is best appreciated in the aspirate of an axillary mass that was a moderately well- to poorly differentiated liposarcoma (Fig. 10–22). A mass in the abdominal wall had a round cell undifferentiated pattern, also with a metachromatic stroma (Fig. 10–23). As expected, this tumor histologically showed a round cell undifferentiated pattern of liposarcoma (Fig. 10–24).

Embryonal Rhabdomyosarcoma.   An example of embryonal rhabdomyosarcoma is illustrated in Figures 10–25 and 10–26. The cells are round and completely undifferentiated, varying in size and shape. A few of them exhibit a small, relatively dense, blue cytoplasmic tag that suggests the histopathologic pattern of embryonal rhabdomyosarcoma (Fig. 10–26). There are no specific features identifying this tumor as a rhabdomyosarcoma on the wet-fixed, Papanicolaou-stained smear. A few mitotic figures were visible throughout the sheets of tumor cells.

Differentiation from Fibrosarcoma.   The difficulty of exactly diagnosing sarcoma when confronted with a primary rather than a recurrent tumor is illustrated in Figures 10–27 and 10–28, which depict the aspirate from a painless mass in the left occipital and cervical area of a nine-year-old child. The undifferentiated round cell composition of the tumor is obvious and quite similar to the pattern of the embryonal rhabdomyosarcoma that was previously illustrated. The same undifferentiated and

Text continued on page 312

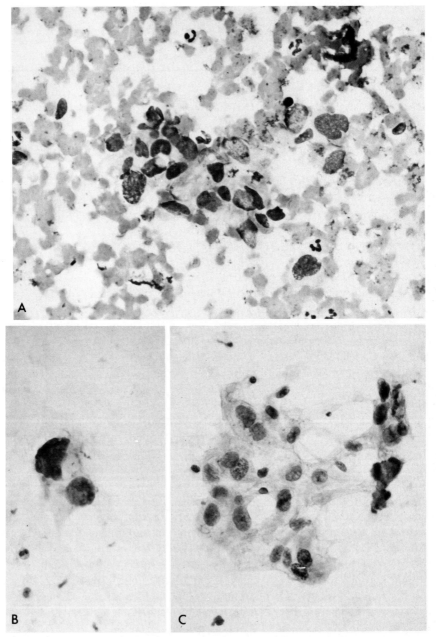

Figure 10–20   Fibrosarcoma of the forearm, recurrent. Aspiration shows pleomorphic spindle-shaped cells without other specific identifying features. The nuclear shapes are very similar to those in the original tissue, depicted in Figure 10–21. *A*, Diff-Quik × 375. *B* and *C*, Papanicolaou × 375.

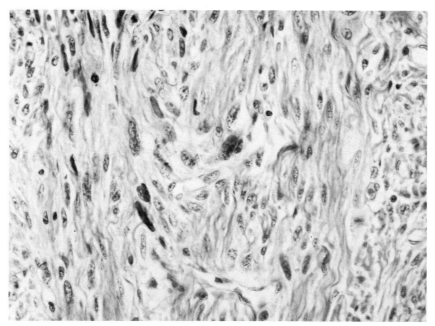

Figure 10–21   Fibrosarcoma of the forearm, recurrent. Original histopathology. Compare the spindle-shaped pleomorphic cells with those in the aspiration smear (Fig. 10–20). Hematoxylin and eosin × 375.

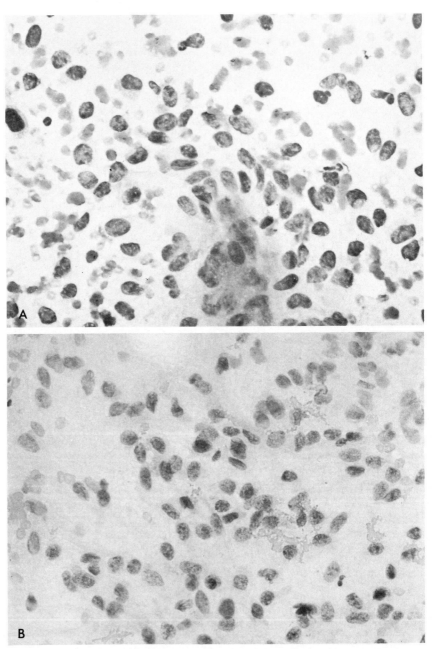

Figure 10–22   Liposarcoma, myxoid type, of axillary area. Malignant spindle-shaped cells in a myxoid background that is metachromatic with the Romanovsky stains. *A*, Diff-Quik × 375. *B*, Papanicolaou × 375.

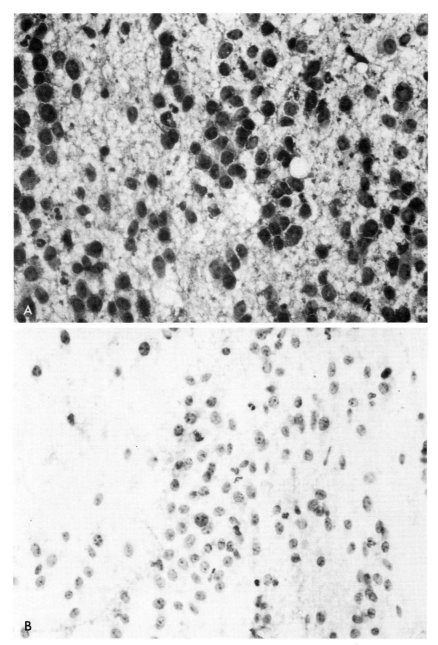

Figure 10–23 Liposarcoma, round cell type, poorly differentiated. Very undifferentiated small round cells with an epithelium-like pattern. Primary diagnosis of liposarcoma and differentiation of this tumor from a metastatic carcinoma could be difficult. A, Diff-Quik × 375. B, Papanicolaou × 375.

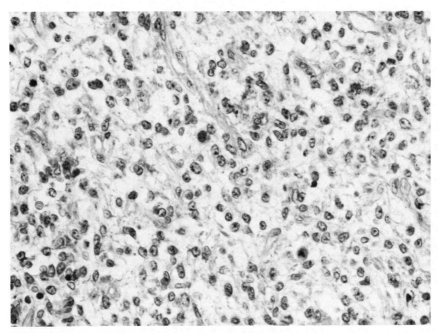

Figure 10–24   Liposarcoma, round cell type, poorly differentiated. Compare the histopathology of this recurrent tumor of the abdominal wall with the aspiration smear (Fig. 10–23). Hematoxylin and eosin × 375.

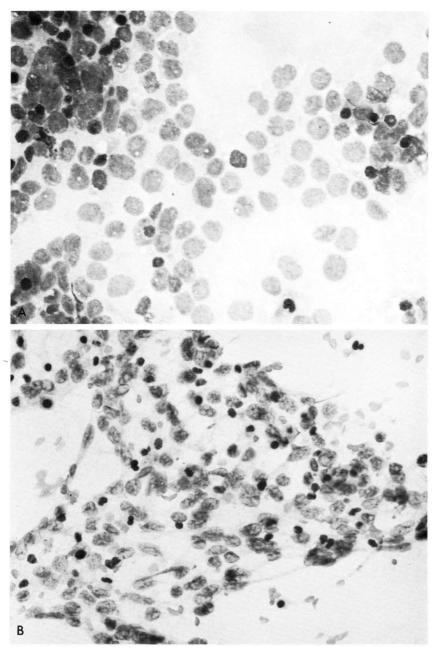

Figure 10–25   Embryonal rhabdomyosarcoma. Rounded undifferentiated cells are evident in the air-dried smear *(A)*. Some of the cells have a faint cytoplasmic tag on one side. This stains light blue in the actual smear. The fixed, Papanicolaou-stained preparation has more of a spindle-cell pattern and clumping of the nuclear chromatin. Distinguishing this tumor from other undifferentiated sarcomas can be a problem. *A*, Diff-Quik × 375. *B*, Papanicolaou × 375.

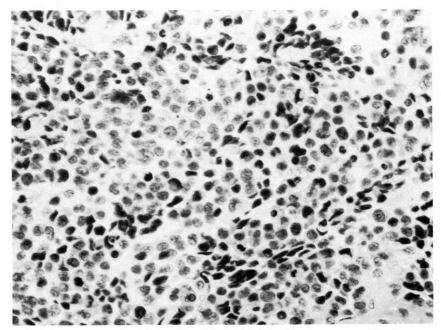

Figure 10–26   Embryonal rhabdomyosarcoma. Original histopathology of a tumor that recurred in the abdominal wall; the aspirate of the recurrent tumor is depicted in Figure 10–25. Hematoxylin and eosin × 375.

nonspecific features are also seen in the wet-fixed aspiration smear. Certainly in a child, the most likely diagnosis would be embryonal rhabdomyosarcoma if this smear pattern and clinical setting were present. Histologically, this mass revealed a poorly differentiated fibrosarcoma (Fig. 10–28*B*).

Chordoma.   Two chordomas have provided challenging aspiration biopsy smears, particularly one that presented in the cervical area. The first tumor, illustrated in Figure 10–29, occurred in a 55-year-old male who presented with pain in the perineum and a mass in the buttock. An open biopsy of the buttock tumor was diagnosed as a liposarcoma, and the patient was referred for evaluation and possible hemipelvectomy. An aspiration was also performed, revealing large bubbly cells with abundant cytoplasm, a morphologic appearance unlike that of several previously aspirated liposarcomas. Radiographs of the pelvis demonstrated destruction of the sacrum with a soft tissue mass projecting anteriorly. That finding coupled with the aspirate strongly suggested the diagnosis of chordoma. This was confirmed at the time of radical surgical excision of the tumor (Fig. 10–30).

The second tumor (Fig. 10–31) contained cells in a more sheet-like configuration, and only a few of them had definite vacuoles. The position of this mass in the high cervical area was consistent with a clinical diagnosis of salivary gland tumor, perhaps acinar cell carcinoma. Preoperative films of the neck showed an irregular lytic process along the anterior surface of several cervical vertebral bodies. At surgery, the mass appeared to arise from this area. A diagnosis of chordoma was histologically confirmed.

Schwannoma.   The aspiration smear may not always portray the malignant features of a soft part sarcoma while at the same time demonstrating other criteria for a specific diagnosis. Such was the case in the diagnosis of a mass in the low cervical area of a 26-year-old woman (Fig. 10–32). This mass was painful when palpated, and there was extension along the distribution of the radial nerve. The patient had been treated for a dysgerminoma of the ovary 12 years before. A diagnosis of metastatic

Text continued on page 319

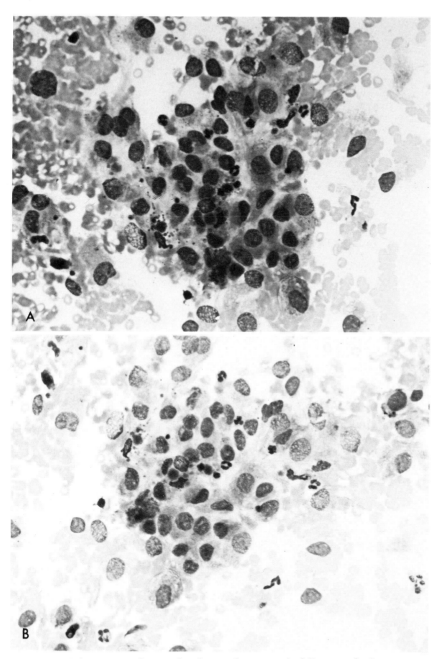

Figure 10-27   Fibrosarcoma of occipital and cervical area, poorly differentiated. This tumor appeared in a child and was clinically thought to be a rhabdomyosarcoma. The aspirate is not inconsistent with that diagnosis (compare with Fig. 10–25). The cells have a more abundant and definable cytoplasm. Both A and B, Diff-Quik × 375.

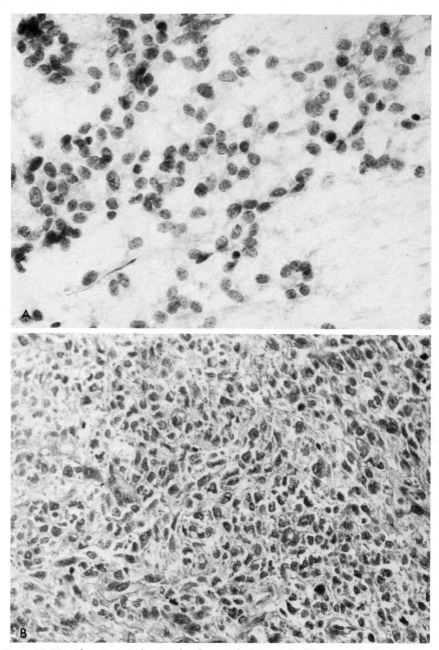

Figure 10–28   Fibrosarcoma of occipital and cervical area, poorly differentiated. The fixed smear (A) has a much rounder cell pattern that is essentially identical with that in the aspiration smear of the embryonal rhabdomyosarcoma (Fig. 10–25). The pathology of the excised tumor (B) reveals a spindle cell sarcoma that was classified as a fibrosarcoma. A, Papanicolaou × 375. B, Hematoxylin and eosin × 375.

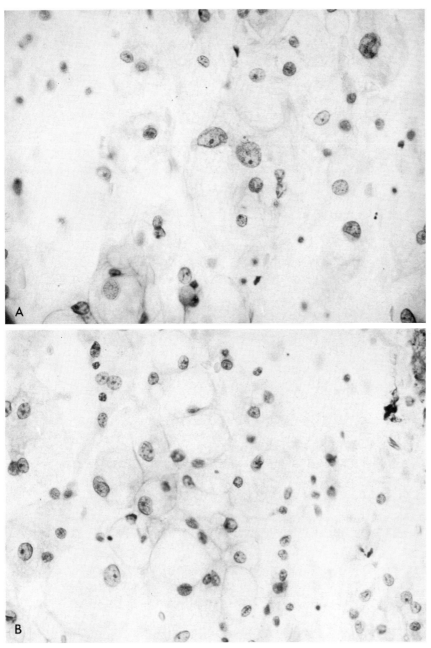

Figure 10–29 Chordoma of sacral area presenting in the buttock. Aspiration shows many large vacuolated cells with a bubble-like appearance. Nuclear chromatin is rather bland with a small but prominent nucleolus. Original surgical biopsy of this mass was reported as liposarcoma. Although the smear pattern did not suggest that diagnosis, roentgenograms revealed destruction of the sacrum and a mass pushing the rectum forward, findings that strongly supported a diagnosis of chordoma. Both A and B, Papanicolaou × 375.

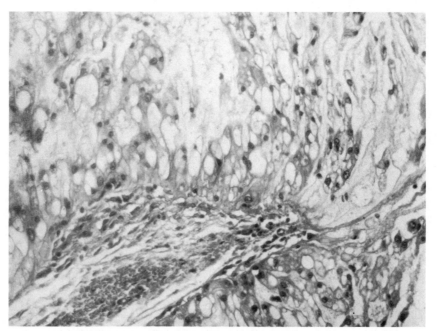

Figure 10–30   Chordoma of sacral area. Histopathology of the excised tumor whose aspirate is illustrated in Figure 10–29. Hematoxylin and eosin × 240.

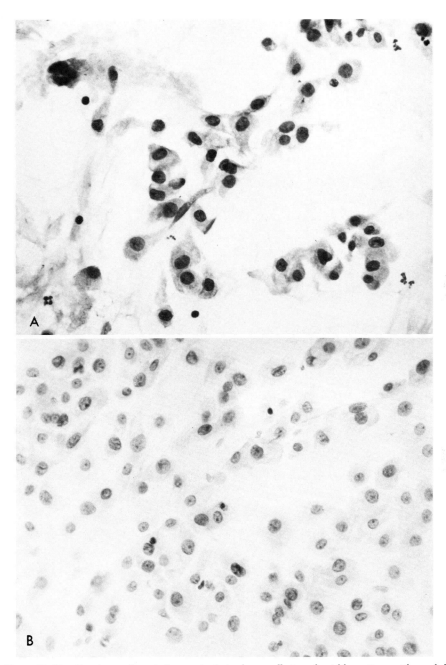

Figure 10–31   Chordoma of cervical area. Aspirate shows cells in a sheet-like pattern with much less evidence of vacuolization than in the prior case (Fig. 10–29). The bubble-like appearance of the cells is more evident in *B*. The lateral cervical presentation of this neoplasm and the aspiration pattern suggested a salivary gland tumor, possibly acinar cell carcinoma. Roentgenograms demonstrated some destruction of several cervical vertebral bodies. Exploration revealed this area as the origin of the mass. This tumor proved to be a chordoma. Both *A* and *B*, Papanicolaou × 375.

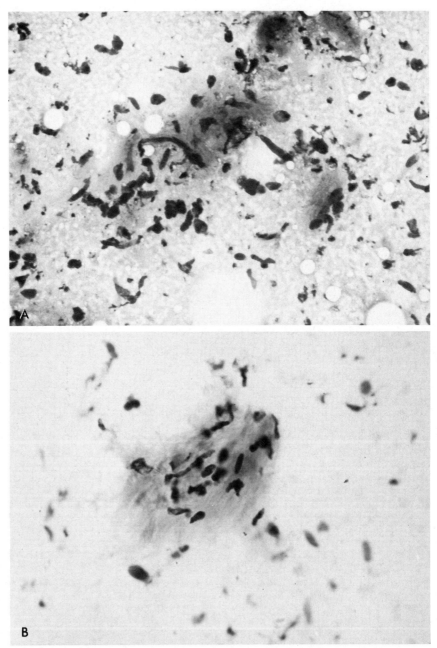

Figure 10–32 Schwannoma of brachial area. Aspiration depicts the spindle-shaped cells with peculiar twisted nuclei. Note the Verocay body in *B. A*, Diff-Quik × 375. *B*, Papanicolaou × 375.

tumor was the major consideration. The aspirate contained spindle-shaped cells with peculiar twisted nuclei and Verocay bodies. A diagnosis of schwannoma, probably benign, was reported. Histologically, this neoplasm appeared at first to be a benign schwannoma, but small foci within it of high mitotic activity and anaplasia indicated that it was malignant (Fig. 10–33).

Granular Cell Myoblastoma. The majority of benign soft tissue tumors have been lipomas, whose aspirates are composed only of fat. An identical smear pattern

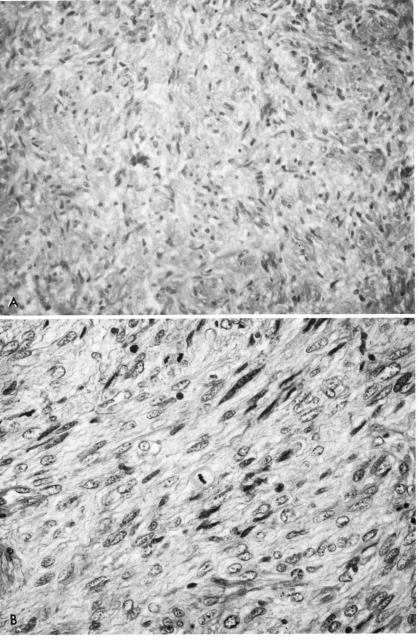

Figure 10–33 Malignant schwannoma. Excision of the mass whose aspirate is illustrated in Figure 10–32 proved to be typical benign schwannoma in most sections (A). B, however, reveals a cellular area in which the nuclei are extremely mitotic. Aspiration had failed to detect this malignant area. A, Hematoxylin and eosin × 240. B, Hematoxylin and eosin × 375.

could easily be obtained simply by aspiration of subcutaneous adipose tissue without the presence of a clinical mass. One example of a granular cell myoblastoma occurring in the thigh is depicted in Figure 10–34. The periodic acid–Schiff (PAS) stain confirmed the positive bright red granularity of the cytoplasm. This tumor was intimately associated with nerves and probably represents the so-called granular cell schwannoma. If this neoplasm were to appear in the breast, it could be easily diagnosed with aspiration biopsy on the basis of the uniformity of the cells, their granular cytoplasm, and the metachromasia of that granularity seen with the Romanovsky dyes.

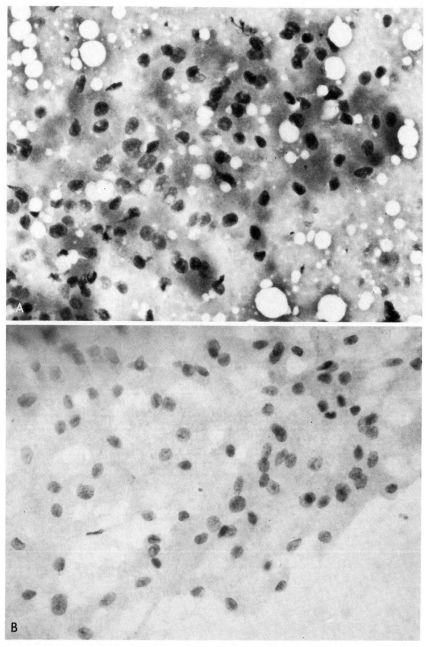

Figure 10–34   Granular cell myoblastoma of the thigh. The smears show a uniform population of cells with eccentric nuclei and a granular cytoplasmic texture. This granular and somewhat metachromatic cytoplasm is much more apparent in the smear stained with Diff-Quik. A periodic acid–Schiff (PAS) stain demonstrated a bright positive granularity. *A*, Diff-Quik × 375. *B*, Papanicolaou × 375.

Metastatic Tumors. It can be appreciated from Table 10–2 that most of the aspirates of soft tissue "lumps and bumps" are metastatic cancers, and the vast majority are the squamous cell type, usually from the lung or oral cavity. Carcinoma of the breast, recurring on the chest wall, is also common. The aspiration biopsy merely confirms what is clinically obvious, and the cytopathologist needs only to match the aspiration smear pattern and the original primary tumor. This is easily done, even with breast cancers that are undifferentiated. Figures 10–35 to 10–37 illustrate some unusual aspirates from tumors metastatic to the subcutaneous tissue. Figure 10–35

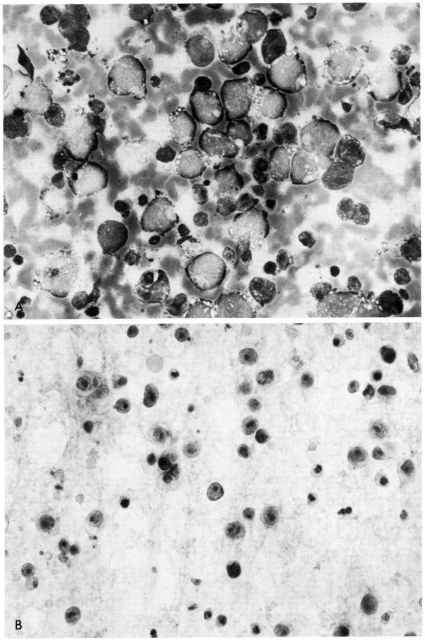

Figure 10–35 Seminoma of the testis, metastatic to the occipital area. Many round undifferentiated cells are present with a few associated lymphocytes. Cell detail with prominent nucleoli is more evident in the fixed smear *(B)*. A, Diff-Quik × 375. B, Papanicolaou × 375.

depicts an example of seminoma metastatic to the occipital area. The cells have a round to oval shape with moderate pleomorphism. There are single cells in many fields of the aspirate, suggesting the possibility of a malignant lymphoma. The nuclei have large, irregular nucleoli. The primary diagnosis of a specific tumor type in this case without the clinical history would be virtually impossible. Figure 10–36 also illustrates an undifferentiated carcinoma metastatic to the area of the inner thigh. Similarity of the nuclear and cellular structures can be seen when the aspirate is compared with the original primary ovarian carcinoma (Fig. 10–37).

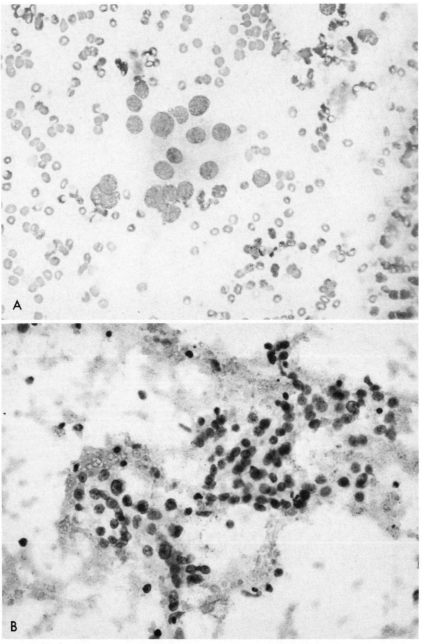

Figure 10–36 Carcinoma of the ovary, metastatic to soft tissue ᴏf the thigh. Another aspirate with round undifferentiated cells. The nuclear chromatin has a very delicate texture. *A*, Diff-Quik × 375. *B*, Papanicolaou × 375.

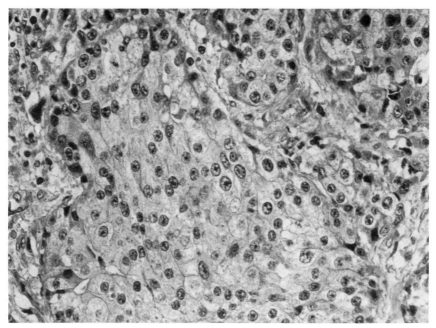

Figure 10–37 Carcinoma of the ovary, original histopathology. Compare the texture, shape, and size of these nuclei with the corresponding features of the nuclei in the aspiration smear (Fig. 10–36). Although the tumor is undifferentiated, one can detect a strong resemblance between the nuclear features of the original specimen and those of the smear. Hematoxylin and eosin × 375.

SUMMARY OF SOFT TISSUE ASPIRATIONS

All the cases described, both for primary soft part sarcomas and metastatic tumors, support most convincingly the theory that the clinical story is extremely important for success with this type of aspiration biopsy. Many of the tumors, metastatic carcinomas in particular, appear undifferentiated. The cytopathologist must have the original primary neoplasm to make an accurate comparison so that there will be a reasonable chance of ruling out a second primary malignancy.

REFERENCES

1. Martin, H. E., and Ellis, E. B.: Biopsy by needle puncture and aspiration. Ann. Surg. 92:169–181, 1930.
2. Stewart, F. W.: The diagnosis of tumors by aspiration biopsy. Am. J. Pathol. 9:801–812, 1933.
3. Coley, B. L., Sharp, G. S., and Ellis, E. B.: Diagnosis of bone tumors by aspiration. Am. J. Surg. 13:215–224, 1931.
4. Snyder, R. E., and Coley, B. L.: Further studies on the diagnosis of bone tumors by aspiration biopsy. Surg. Gynecol. Obstet. 80:517–522, 1945.
5. Norderstrom, B.: Percutaneous biopsy of vertebra and ribs. Acta Radiol. 11:114–121, 1971.
6. Schagjowicz, R.: Aspiration biopsy in bone lesions. J. Bone Joint Surg. 37A:465–477, 1955.
7. Valls, J., Ottolenghi, C. E., and Schajowicz, F.: Aspiration biopsy in diagnosis of lesions of vertebral bodies. J.A.M.A. 136:376–383, 1948.
8. Ottolenghi, C. E.: Diagnosis of orthopedic lesions by aspiration biopsy. Results of 1061 punctures. J. Bone Joint Surg. 37A:443–464, 1955.
9. Ottolenghi, C. E.: Aspiration biopsy of the spine: Techniques for thoracic spine and results of twenty-eight biopsies in this region and overall results of 1050 biopsies of other spinal segments. J. Bone Joint Surg. 51A:1531–1544, 1969.
10. Schajowicz, R., and Derqui, J. C.: Puncture biopsy in lesions of the locomotor system: Review of results of 4050 cases, including 941 vertebral punctures. Cancer 21:531–548, 1968.
11. Lalli, A. F.: Roentgen-guided aspiration biopsies of skeletal lesions. J. Can. Assoc. Radiol. 21:71–73, 1970.

12. Robinov, K., Goldman, H., Robash, H., et al.: The role of aspiration biopsy of focal lesions in lung and bone by simple needle and fluoroscopy. Am. J. Roentgenol. *101*:932–938, 1967.

13. deSantos, L. A., Lukeman, J. M., Wallace, S., et al.: Percutaneous needle biopsy of bone in the cancer patient. Am. J. Radiol. *130*:641–649, 1978.

14. Schajowicz, R., and Hokama, J.: Aspiration (puncture or needle) biopsy of bone lesions. Recent Results Cancer Res. *54*:139–144, 1976.

15. Akerman, M., Berg, N. O., and Persson, B. M.: Fine needle aspiration biopsy in the evaluation of tumor-like lesions of bone. Acta Orthop. Scand. *47*:129–136, 1976.

16. Olszewski, W., Woyke, S., and Domanski, Z.: Aspiration cytodiagnosis of neoplastic metastases to bones. Nowotwory 27:239–247, 1977.

17. Thommesen, P., and Frederiksen, P.: Fine needle aspiration biopsy of bone lesions: Clinical value. Acta Orthop. Scand. *47*:137–143, 1976.

18. Stormby, N., and Akerman, M.: Cytodiagnosis of bone lesions by means of fine-needle aspiration biopsy. Acta Cytol. *17*:166–172, 1973.

19. Hadju, S. I., and Melamed, M. R.: Needle biopsy of primary malignant bone tumors. Surg. Gynecol. Obstet. *133*:829–832, 1971.

20. deSantos, L. A., Murray, J. A., and Ayala, A.: The value of percutaneous needle biopsy in the management of primary bone tumors. Cancer *43*:735–744, 1979.

21. Hadju, S. I., and Hadju, E. O.: *Cytopathology of Sarcomas and Other Nonepithelial Malignant Tumors.* Philadelphia, W. B. Saunders Co., 1976, pp. 37, 78, 83, 99, 113, 138, 150, 158, 224, 226, 232, 235, 247, 252, 267–268, 273, 277, and 280.

22. Ramzy, I.: Benign schwannoma: Demonstration of Verocay bodies using fine needle aspiration. Acta Cytol. *21*:316–319, 1977.

23. Nickels, J., and Koivuniemi, A.: Cytology of malignant hemangiopericytoma. Acta Cytol. *23*:119–125, 1979.

24. Koivuniemi, A., and Nickels, J.: Synovial sarcoma diagnosed by fine-needle aspiration biopsy. A case report. Acta Cytol. *22*:515–518, 1978.

25. Soon-Hong, I.: Cytologic findings in a case of malignant fibrous histiocytoma. Acta Cytol. *22*:519–522, 1978.

26. Merck, C., and Hagmar, B.: Myxofibrosarcoma: A correlative cytologic and histologic study of 13 cases examined by fine needle aspiration cytology. Acta Cytol. *24*:137–144, 1980.

27. Dahl, I., and Akerman, M.: Nodular fasciitis: A correlative cytologic and histologic study of 13 cases. Acta Cytol. *25*:215–223, 1981.

Chapter Eleven

Research and Special Applications

TECHNIQUES

Fine-needle aspiration biopsy has become a powerful clinical tool in the diagnosis of tumors. Its potential in research has yet to be fully realized, but it seems promising in several areas. In this chapter, a brief review of special applications and research will be presented. The voluminous literature describing immunologic methods with which aspiration biopsy may be of use can only be superficially scanned.

The fundamental principle underlying the application of aspiration biopsy to experimental studies is its ability to procure viable tumor cells with little or no disturbance of the neoplasm itself and with excellent preservation of those cells. Some of the techniques that may then be applied to those cells are as follows: tissue culture and immunologic studies, planimetric measurements, enzyme quantitation and identification of specific tumor markers, study and measurement of hormone receptors, ultrastructural studies, monitoring of therapy and its effects on cells, and measurement of DNA and cell ploidy.

No papers concerning the direct application of tissue culture methods to aspiration biopsy were found in the literature. Availability of suspension media for the transport of aspirated cells, studies of cell viability, and the lymph node barrier to injected tumor cells during lymphography in the experimental animal all suggest that aspirated tumor cells could probably be preserved and grown in tissue culture.[1, 2, 3] Scherwin has described the juxtanuclear position of lymphocytes to breast cancer cells in tissue culture. Biopsy material was obtained in 1.0 mm cubes.[4] It seems possible that adequate cells for similar studies could be obtained by aspiration biopsy. Aspirated cells would have the added advantage of being free of most of the extraneous stromal elements present in conventional tissue biopsies.

PLANIMETRY AND IMAGING PROCESSING

Breast Tumors. Several planimetric and image analysis studies have been conducted on cells from different tissues obtained by aspiration biopsy or imprints. These studies are summarized in Table 11–1. Wallgren and Zajicek suggested the value of more precise cellular and nuclear analysis when they reviewed the observational data from a multifaceted analysis of several cytologic features seen in aspiration smears of breast carcinoma, correlating these features with prognosis. Large nuclei and nucleoli, small cell clusters, and many free single cells were associated with a poor prognosis.[5]

Text continued on page 330   **325**

TABLE 11–1.   PLANIMETRIC STUDIES AND IMAGE PROCESSING

Reference	Methods	Tumor Types Examined	Results and Comments
Cornelisse et al.[6]	Imprint from fresh tissue, air-dried and MGG-stained,* with camera lucida tracing of nuclear border	Mastopathy Fibroadenoma Breast cancer	Mean nuclear area, maximum nuclear area, percentage nuclei larger than 200 μ^2 discriminated in 60% of breast cancers and 95% of benign lesions. Carcinomas with nuclei less than 110 μ^2 were found more often in patients with negative lymph nodes.
Dziura and Bonfiglio[7]	Nordenstrom screw needle biopsy. Smears immediately fixed in alcohol. Pap stain used. Planimetric camera lucida tracings of 150 cells in each case.	Intraductal hyperplasia, slight, moderate, and marked, 5 cases each. Intraductal carcinoma, 2 cases. Infiltrating duct carcinoma, 10 cases.	Planimetric data negative. Qualitative features of nuclear overlap increased with spectrum hyperplasia to carcinoma. True syncytia seen only with carcinoma.
Zajdela et al.[8]	Air-dried aspiration smear stained with MGG. Nuclei measured with ocular micrometer at 1000×. In each case, 100 cells measured.	Infiltrating duct, breast cancer, 245 cases. Benign breast diseases, fibrocystic and fibroadenoma, 50 cases.	Those nuclei greater than 12μ in diameter classified as large nuclei; those less than 12μ classified as small nuclei. Significant overlap of benign disease (small nuclei) and stage I breast cancer. Five year survival rate with breast cancer: 90% with tumors with small nuclei; 58% with those with large nuclei.
Zajicek et al.[9]	Aspirate collected in Hank's solution, sedimented, centrifuged, and resuspended in methanol. H & E† stain of spread of cell suspension performed. Scanning microscopy with TICAS programs used.	Breast cancer, 3 cases before and after radiation doses of 800 and 1600 rads.	Differences in radiosensitive and radioresistant cases found. No long follow-up.

Reference	Material	Method	Results
Bocking[10]	Prostate cancer	85,000 data points from 1200 photographs of 50 cases recorded with Digiplan planimeter interfaced with Hewlett Packard 9815A calculator. 10,000 data points of nuclear DNA from 50 cytologic smears; Vickers M86 scanning used.	Analysis of variance used to rank diagnostic criteria. Linear discriminant analysis of image data identified 18 of 20 noncancerous tumors and 27 of 30 cancers. 10% false-positive and 10% false-negative rates.
Spaander et al.[11]	Prostatic cancer histologically diagnosed and graded.	Air-dried MGG-stained aspiration smears examined by Leitz A.S.M. image analysis system.	Differences found between observations of operators taking measurements in grade III carcinomas owing to nonselection of large, free, atypical nuclei. Repeat observations improved prognostic correlation over cytologic grading alone.
Boon et al.[12]	Thyroid tumors: 21 adenoma, 13 follicular carcinomas, 7 nontoxic goiters.	50 cells with intact nuclei and well-defined cytoplasm from air-dried, MGG-stained aspiration smears examined by Leitz A.S.M. image analysis system at 1200 ×.	Significant differences for mean nuclear area found between benign and malignant follicular neoplasms and between neoplastic cells and cells of nontoxic goiter.

*MGG = May-Grunwald-Giemsa.
†H & E = Hematoxylin and eosin.

TABLE 11–2.   DNA STUDIES

Reference	Methods	Tissue Type Examined	Results and Comments
Thommessen et al.[14]	Flow cytophotometry on fine-needle aspirates.	47 benign tissues, 58 malignant tumors.	DNA histograms are reproducible for individual patients. DNA is normal diploid in benign conditions. DNA in tumors is generally increased and dependent on differentiation. Qualitative DNA changes are sometimes observed during treatment.
Moubayed[15]	Microspectrophotometry on single cells in aspiration smears.	Breast: 23 lesions including fibroadenoma, intraductal hyperplasia, and carcinoma.	DNA histograms could not distinguish these lesions. False-negative histograms are frequent with well-differentiated breast carcinoma.
Zajicek et al.[16]	Determination of dry cell mass by microinterferometer. DNA measured by scanning microspectrophotometer at 265 nm.	3 fibroadenomas and 3 breast cancers.	Complete differentiation not possible by these methods. Cancers tend to have higher DNA values.
Auer[17]	Fuelgen-stained, air-dried aspiration smears. Rapid-scanning microspectro-photometer at 546 nm.	144 breast cancers, clinical stages I to III. 100 cancer cells plus 20 to 30 control cells detected in each case.	DNA values grouped into 4 types: I (minimal deviation from normal) through IV (marked aneuploidy). Groups correlated with survival.
Nordenskjold et al.[18]	DNA synthesis by incorporation of 3H-thymidine into tumor cells obtained by aspiration before or during endocrine therapy. Measured by autoradiography.	Breast cancers	Regression of tumor preceded by decrease in S-phase cells. Proportion of S-phase cells did not predict responders prior to endocrine therapy.
Bedrossian et al.[19]	Flow cytophotometry. Assay for estrogen receptors from imprint smears or pepsinized cell samples	Breast cancers, clinically resectable and clinically advanced	Used DNA index (G_1/G_0 tumor:G_1/G_0 normal). 72% of tumors aneuploid. Ploidy did not correlate well with clinical menopause, metastases, percentage of cells in S-phase, estrogen receptor status, histologic invasiveness, or cytologic grade. High percentage of S-phase cells associated with estrogen receptor proved negative.

Author	Material	Method	Results
Auer et al.[20]	Breast cancers, 56 patients.	Feulgen-stained nuclei on aspiration smears fixed in 4% buffered formaldehyde at 25°C. Rapid-scanning integrated microspectrophotometer off peak at 610 nm. Estrogen receptors measured by isoelectric focusing on quick-frozen tissue.	When DNA did not deviate much from diploid or tetraploid values, then estrogen receptors were high. When DNA synthesis was normal or highly aneuploid, then estrogen receptors were low or not measurable.
Patek et al.[21]	24 breast tumors, 7 benign and 17 malignant.	Imprint smears from excised tissue. Microfluorometry of individual nuclei stained by fluorochrome BAO 2.5 bis [4'-aminophenyl-(1')]1,3,4-oxydiazole.	Benign tissues all diploid. DNA values for in situ and well-differentiated invasive cancers differ. Grade II and III tumors shifted to tetraploid or total aneuploid values. Results suggest DNA values can be used to grade mammary carcinomas.
Sprenger et al.[22]	12 benign mammary dysplasias, 23 fibroadenomas, 51 invasive breast cancers, 6 noninvasive breast cancers, 2 cases of Paget's disease.	Air-dried, MGG-stained aspiration smears. Post fixed in absolute ethanol; stained with acriflavine. Fluorescence cytophotometry after Feulgen hydrolysis and removal of the MGG stain.	Invasive cancers often show DNA distribution found in benign breast diseases. DNA of noninvasive breast cancers is usually normal. Aneuploidy and increased nuclear DNA are least pronounced in small (early clinical stage) cancers.
Preece and Zippel[23]	Breast cancers. 11 lobular in situ carcinomas, 5 invasive lobular carcinomas.	Feulgen-stained 4μ tissue sections. Scanning cytophotometer to measure DNA. X-chromatin body in cells of lobular neoplasia and lobular carcinoma counted.	DNA in 8 cases of lobular neoplasia is diploid; in 3 cases, diploid to tetraploid. Five cases of invasive lobular carcinoma are diploid and tetraploid. No correlation of any kind with presence of X-chromatin body.
Kreicbergs et al.[24]	5 chondrosarcomas 7 osteosarcomas	Tissue sections and imprints fixed in buffered formalin. Feulgen staining. Rapid-scanning microspectrophotometer at 546 nm. Flow cytophotometry on cell suspension of tumor and normal tissue stained with ethidium bromide. Measured at 455 to 490 nm, 590 nm, and 630 nm, sorted on 256 multichannel analyzer.	Good correlation of modal DNA among 3 different methods. Flow proved better for aneuploid modal DNA. Presence of aneuploidy similar in all 3 methods. Single-cell analysis is time-consuming, but better for determining percentage of hyperdiploid cells. Flow is rapid.
Adams and Dahlgren[25]	Lung carcinoma	Air-dried aspiration smears fixed in Carnoy's solution. Modified Feulgen stain. Measured specimen absorbance on controlled photographs using monochromatic light at 560 nm.	Mean value of total DNA higher for tumor cells. Heteroploidy most evident in adenocarcinoma and squamous cell carcinoma. Oat cell carcinomas have narrow DNA distribution curves.

Four studies conducted on breast cancers comparing them with benign breast tumors have had variable results (Table 11–1).

Methods have varied from simple camera lucida tracings to sophisticated Taxonomic Intracellular Analytic System (TICAS) programs for image analysis. Dziura and Bonfiglio found that planimetric data were of no value in distinguishing among intraductal hyperplasia with variable degrees of atypia, intraductal carcinoma, and invasive duct carcinoma.[7] The TICAS programs were able to distinguish the cellular composition of three different breast carcinomas as well as note differences in radiosensitivity of these tumors.[9] The obvious problems with the TICAS study are the small number of cases and the lack of follow-up information or other subsequent reports in the literature. These types of studies have been limited, and the results have been difficult to interpret because of lack of standardization of methods.

Prostate Tumors.   Two planimetric studies have been performed on prostatic aspiration biopsies. One method uses data points obtained from black and white photographs of the smears combined with scanning microdensitometer measurement of samples of nuclear DNA from the cells; the other directly employs the Leitz A.S.M. image analysis system on air-dried smears stained with May-Grunwald-Giemsa.[10, 11] The rates of false-negative and false-positive results were both 10 per cent, and they were discovered during an attempt to differentiate prostatic carcinoma from benign hyperplasia and prostatitis in the combined image analysis and DNA evaluation.[10] Results were somewhat better for grading of prostatic carcinoma by image analysis of cell nuclei, but findings discovered during the initial phases of the study varied greatly among the observers. This observational discrepancy required the establishment of criteria concerning which cells to measure so that good correlative results could be obtained.[11]

Thyroid Tumors.   The single study of the planimetric analysis of thyroid cells obtained from aspiration of follicular adenomas and carcinomas showed good discrimination between these two neoplasms. This is a finding of great potential value in separating a benign lesion from a malignant tumor, and it can not be duplicated by conventional cytologic methods.[12] At present, though, this author and several colleagues have been unable to confirm these planimetric findings after studying cases of follicular adenoma and carcinoma, papillary carcinoma, and adenomatous goiter of the thyroid. The cell measurements were made using the Videoplan image analysis system on air-dried aspiration biopsy smears stained with Diff-Quik. Mean values of nuclear area, maximum and minimum nuclear diameter, and approximation to a circle were not significantly different for these four thyroid diseases. Data were nearly identical for follicular adenoma and carcinoma.[13]

MEASUREMENTS OF DNA

As an outgrowth of research in automated cytology, determination of DNA content of single cells and the degree of heteroploidy as one additional criterion for diagnosis and prognosis of tumors has been studied. Table 11–2 summarizes a number of these investigations.[14-15] Measurements of DNA have been easier to conduct on aspiration biopsy smears, touch imprints, or even tissue sections than on samples from the cervix and vagina because of the more homogeneous nature of the cell population and the absence of large numbers of inflammatory cells and debris. Tumor cell samples can be disaggregated for flow cytophotometry, or single-cell measurements of DNA can be obtained from smears, imprints, or thin tissue sections.

In several of the reports, a combination of measurements of dry cell mass, estrogen receptor, and sex chromatin have been correlated with cell ploidy to study their relationships and any prognostic implications.[16, 19, 23] Rather than measure total DNA,

Nordenstrom and colleagues studied DNA synthesis by incorporating 3H-thymidine in needle aspirates of breast carcinoma before and during endocrine therapy. These investigators found that tumor regression was preceded by a decrease in S-phase cells but that the proportion of cells in S-phase prior to therapy did not predict a response.[18]

The most commonly employed staining technique has been the Feulgen method, performed after destaining on a smear or touch imprint that has been previously air-dried and stained with May-Grunwald-Giemsa or on a smear fixed in buffered formaldehyde or absolute methanol.[17, 20, 22] Other fluorochromes that have been employed are BAO 2.5 bis[4'-aminophenyl-(1')]1,3,4-oxydiazole, acriflavine, and ethidium bromide.[21, 22, 24] Perhaps it is the differences in methods, including use of absorbance on photographic film to determine total DNA, that acounts for variation and inconsistency in results.[25]

Breast Tumors.   Breast cancers alone or in combination with benign breast disease have been evaluated most commonly by DNA determinations (eight reports). Moubayed found that DNA histograms could not be used to distinguish intraductal hyperplasia from well-differentiated duct carcinoma of the breast. Zajicek and colleagues also found considerable overlap of DNA values comparing breast carcinomas with fibroadenomas.[15, 16] This latter study included only three cases of each type. Auer reported a much larger series of 144 breast cancers (clinical stages I, II, and III) and found that DNA values could be divided into four groups. These ranged from group I with minimal deviation from the normal diploid cell population to group IV with marked aneuploidy. The degree of aneuploidy correlated directly with patient survival in each clinical stage.[17] Bedrossian and colleagues calculated a DNA index, the ratio of tumor cells to normal cells (G_1/G_0). These investigators attempted to correlate this index with clinical menopause, presence of metastases, percentage of cells in S-phase, estrogen receptor status, cytologic grade, and histologic degree of invasiveness. No correlations were found. The high percentage of cells in S-phase was associated with breast cancers with negative estrogen receptor values.[19] Auer and colleagues also studied cell ploidy with respect to estrogen receptors. DNA values that deviated only minimally from the diploid or tetraploid values were usually from tumors with high estrogen receptor values.[20] Patek and colleagues found a general correlation between histologic grade and cell ploidy of breast cancers.[21] Like Patek's group, Sprenger and colleagues found that DNA values were not useful for diagnosing well-differentiated, non-invasive breast cancers.[22]

IMMUNOPEROXIDASE AND IMMUNOFLUORESCENCE

A large number of reagents have been applied to tissue sections, fixed or fresh-frozen, to detect specific substances for cell identification. Recent reviews by Taylor and Kledzik as well as by DeLellis and colleagues list over 50 different antigens, including enzymes, polypeptide and steroid hormones, oncodevelopmental antigens, viral antigens, immunoglobulins, and other specific cell proteins, that are being identified by immunology.[26, 27] All the authors stress the careful performance of the techniques and the absolute essential use of adequate positive and negative controls.

No systematic study has been performed using the immunoperoxidase or immunofluorescence methodology upon aspiration biopsy smears. Singh and colleagues cultured human peritoneal and pleural fluid and prepared an anti–mesothelial-cell serum in rabbits. This reagent was used to study both effusions from patients to identify malignant mesothelioma and formalin-fixed tissue sections from mesothelioma. Preliminary results indicated some success with the reagent in distinguishing undifferentiated malignant tumors metastatic to the pleura or peritoneum from malignant mesothelioma.[28]

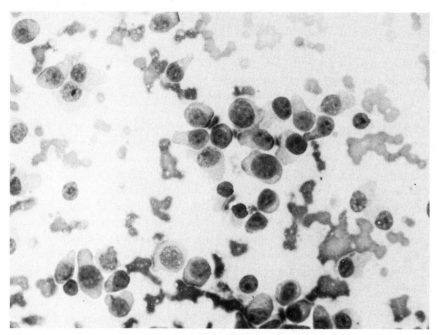

Figure 11–1 Multiple myeloma. Aspirate of neck mass in patient with known multiple myeloma demonstrates numerous atypical and frankly malignant plasma cells. Diff-Quik × 375.

Nadji has examined a number of conditions using imprints, cell blocks, and filter and cytocentrifuge preparations with an immunoperoxidase method. He found that the best fixative was either 95 per cent ethanol or buffered formol acetone. Filters did not work, which is not surprising since they are sensitive to a number of solvents. Destained cytologic slides were also found to be suitable for this study. Immunoglobulins occurred as a monoclonal pattern in two myelomas and three large-cell lymphomas. Eleven non-neoplastic lymphoid proliferations were found to be polyclonal. Small lymphocytes in smears were not suitable for study, since staining was not visible within these cells. Muramidase was found to be positive in histiocytes and macrophages as well as in reactive mesothelial cells. The latter may in fact be macrophages and not true mesothelial cells. Gastrin was positive in a functional islet cell tumor, and in two clinical non-functional islet tumors, gastrin, insulin, and glucagon were all positive in the cytologic preparations. Positive results were also obtained with (1) calcitonin in a medullary carcinoma of the thyroid and (2) carcinoembryonic antigen in liver aspirates from metastatic carcinoma of the stomach, in mucinous carcinoma of the ovary, and in cells from adenocarcinoma of the lung in peritoneal and pleural fluid. The beta subunit of human chorionic gonadotropin could be detected in syncytiotrophoblast cells in cervical vaginal smears from two pregnant women, and alphafetoprotein was positive in the cells from an endodermal sinus tumor found in peritoneal fluid. This study is the first to demonstrate the wide spectrum of applications of the immunoperoxidase methods to cytologic material.[29]

One of the difficulties with the immunoperoxidase technology is that the presence of endogenous peroxidase in tissue produces a false-positive staining. This is particularly true of red blood cells, an obvious potential source of staining with aspiration biopsies. Coleman and colleagues have employed a different reagent using an indirect immunoalkaline phosphatase to study the presence of an epithelial membrane antigen in cells from serous effusion. Their study is directed toward more sensitive identification of epithelial cells present in effusions and is concerned with distinguishing their presence from reactive mesothelial cells. Results from a preliminary communication showed some promise.[30]

Multiple Myeloma.   This author has used the immunoperoxidase methods in several cases. Figures 11–1 and 11–2 illustrate an aspirate from a metastatic nodule of multiple myeloma in the cervical area that demonstrates monoclonal staining with only alpha globulin. There is background staining by the endogenous peroxidase in the red blood cells, but the intensity is greater and definitely within the cytoplasm of the tumor cells. The brown granules are also much more sharply defined than the homogeneously stained background provided by the red blood cells. The background staining may be reduced by fixing the smears in Carnoy's solution or by pretreating the smears with very dilute hydrogen peroxide to eliminate peroxidase in the red blood cells.

Non-Hodgkin's Lymphoma.   A nodular lymphoma provided positive staining with antibodies to kappa light chains (Fig. 11–3). This lymphoma had been first diagnosed eight years prior to the present aspiration biopsy of a recurrence in a groin node. Although the lesion had originally been diagnosed as a clinical stage II tumor, the patient had done well with radiation and chemotherapy and had not required any treatment during the two years prior to the development of this present recurrence. The histologic picture still shows a nodular lymphoma with poorly differentiated cells (Figs. 11–4 and 11–5).

Carcinoma.   Figures 11–6 and 11–7 illustrate the application of Battifora's anti-keratin antibody to two aspiration biopsy smears: the first from a squamous cell carcinoma of the lung metastatic to the soft tissue of the right calf, and the second from a mixed adenosquamous cell carcinoma of the lung.[31] The staining with the keratinized squamous cell carcinoma is positive in some cells, but it is localized to peripheral areas of the cytoplasm and is present in only some of the tumor cells. The lung tumor demonstrates only a few positive cells among clusters of columnar cells as well as background staining that tends to obscure the positive cells. It is necessary to

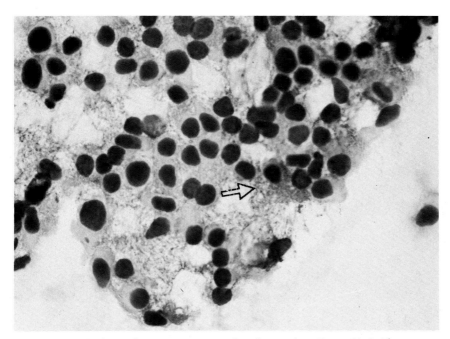

Figure 11–2   Multiple myeloma. Same case as that illustrated in Figure 11–1. This smear stains postively (arrow) with immunoperoxidase method using anti–alpha globulin reagent. Immunoperoxidase × 600.

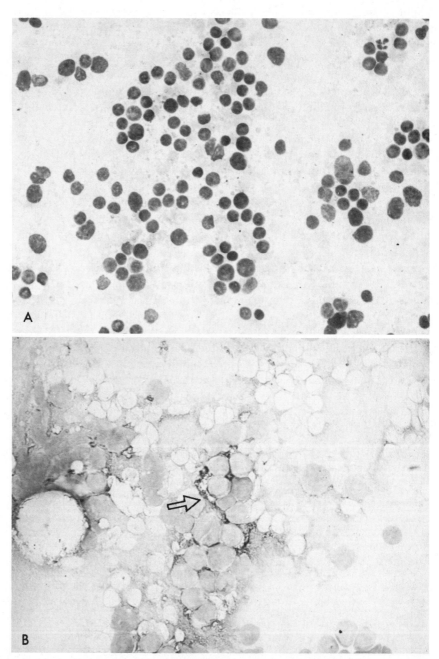

Figure 11–3 Non-Hodgkin's lymphoma, nodular, poorly differentiated. Aspirate of groin node diagnosed as nodular non-Hodgkin's lymphoma. The monomorphic pattern of poorly differentiated lymphoid cells is present. Immunoperoxidase stain was positive in this case only with anti–kappa light chain reagent (*B*, arrow). *A*, Diff-Quik × 375. *B*, Immunoperoxidase × 600.

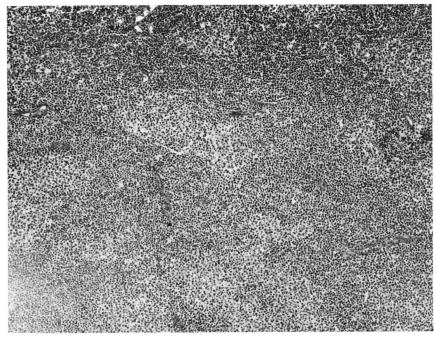

Figure 11–4 Non-Hodgkin's lymphoma, nodular, poorly differentiated. Excised node after aspiration diagnosis (Fig. 11–3) reveals nodular pattern with poorly differentiated cells. Hematoxylin and eosin × 240.

interpret the results cautiously. This antibody does not appear to be specific for keratinized cells per se but seems to stain epithelial cells and to differentiate them from lymphoid cells, as originally proposed for differentiating lymphoma from thymoma.[31] The antibody will also stain the cells of breast cancer.[32]

There has been intense interest in immunologic methods for detection of steroid hormone receptors in tumors, most importantly breast cancers. Applications have usually been made to tissue sections. They include the use of fluorescein isothiocyanate bovine serum albumin conjugated with the steroid receptor tracer applied to fresh-frozen sections according to the method of Lee and others. In one study, isoelectric focusing was performed in polyacrylamide gel from specimens obtained by fine-needle aspiration biopsy.[33-36] This author has used some of the receptor tracer material of Lee on fine-needle aspirates but has found the results inconsistent and difficult to interpret. When one views the individual cells with fluorescent microscopy, it is difficult to tell the exact type of cell that is staining. It has also been time-consuming to obtain suitable controls unless one uses tissue sections with the aspiration smears. A reliable immunoperoxidase method for identification of the receptor sites in breast cancers has not yet been developed, but a suitable reagent would have the advantage of allowing more precise identification of the cells that are actually positive.

Ultrastructural Studies

Most if not all ultrastructural features useful in diagnostic surgical pathology can be seen in aspiration biopsy specimens processed by standard methods for transmission and scanning electron microscopy. Domagala and colleagues have tested two methods with fluids: (1) fixation of the cells in glutaraldehyde followed by centrifugation of them onto glass slides, and (2) sedimentation of the cells onto the slides followed by fixation. The cells are then stained by the Giemsa method for light microscopic examination

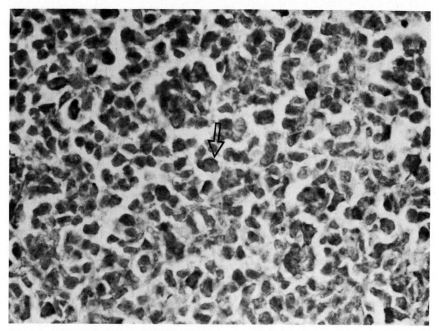

Figure 11–5   Non-Hodgkin's lymphoma, nodular, poorly differentiated. Same case as that illustrated in Figure 11–4. Presence of immunoglobulins is indicated by positive staining (dark areas of the cytoplasm) with methyl green–pyronine (arrow). Methyl green–pyronine × 600.

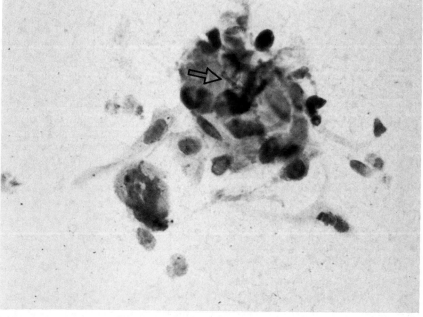

Figure 11–6   Squamous cell carcinoma of the lung, metastatic to the right calf. Malignant tumor cells are present. They show granular positive staining at the periphery of the cytoplasm with the antikeratin antibody immunoperoxidase method (arrow). Immunoperoxidase × 600.

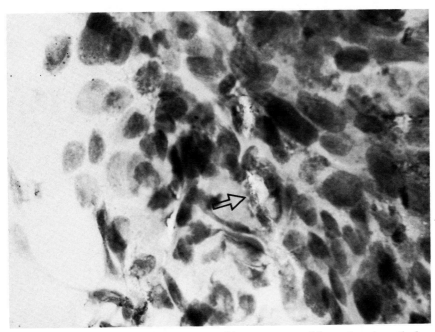

Figure 11–7   Carcinoma of the lung. Aspirate of lung mass stained by antikeratin antibody reveals some positive staining (arrow), suggesting that this carcinoma has a squamous component. However, light microscopic features of the aspirate indicate only adenocarcinoma. Immunoperoxidase × 600.

and photography. A special coverglass with etched lines is used to facilitate locating cells for subsequent ultrastructural study.[37, 38] Coleman and colleagues have described a similar method for electron microscopy of single cells in smears of urinary sediment, detecting the papova virus.[39] While studies of single cells have been valuable, the techniques are tedious and time-consuming.

For aspiration biopsies, this author has preferred either to rinse out the needle directly into buffered glutaraldehyde after preparation of direct smears for light microscopy or to take a second aspiration from the mass, placing all of that specimen in the glutaraldehyde fixative. This specimen is then centrifuged and handled in the manner of a cell block, using the same protocol that is customary for the small tissue fragments processed for electron microscopy. Some examples of aspiration biopsies studied by transmission electron microscopy are described in the following discussion.

Solitary Plasmacytoma.   Figure 11–8 illustrates the aspirate from a sternal mass in a 59-year-old man. While the configuration of the cells suggested a plasma cell tumor, there was no evident bone involvement. The ultrastructure (Fig. 11–9) demonstrates a clock-faced heterochromatin distribution without prominent nucleoli. There is abundant rough endoplasmic reticulum. Mitochondria are well developed and preserved but not giant or atypical. These features are those of well-differentiated plasma cells.[40] So far, the follow-up supports a diagnosis of solitary plasmacytoma.

Metastatic Gastrinoma.   Figure 11–10 illustrates the light microscopic features of an aspirate from a mass in the tail of the breast and axillary area of a 63-year-old woman. Previous history of this patient significantly revealed that she had had a documented gastrinoma of the duodenum with metastases to the liver and the Zollinger-Ellison syndrome three years before the appearance of the present tumor. The differential diagnosis, based on both the clinical history and the undifferentiated pattern of the cells seen on the aspirate, is metastatic gastrinoma versus a possible primary breast carcinoma. Immunoperoxidase staining with an antigastrin antibody on one of the smears was negative. Pasqual staining, also performed on an aspiration smear, was questionably positive. Figure 11–11 depicts a cell with evident neurosecre-

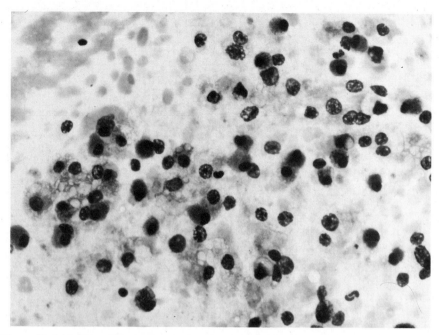

Figure 11–8 Solitary plasmacytoma. Aspirate of soft tissue mass over the sternum. Tumor is composed of well-differentiated plasma cells. Diff-Quik × 375.

tory granules and many elongated mitochondria. The granules measure up to 270 nm in diameter. While neither feature is specific for gastrinoma, the abundant and prominent mitochondria suggest a hormone-producing cell. The granules also suggest the production of some hormone, although they do not identify it specifically. The large size of the granules also supports the diagnosis. This has been true of all of the gastrinomas studied to date.[40, 41]

Metastatic Ovarian Carcinoma. A third specimen studied ultrastructurally was an aspirate from a supraclavicular lymph node in an elderly woman who had had a hysterectomy for a pelvic tumor that was originally diagnosed as an endometrioid carcinoma of the ovary. The light microscopic features of the aspirate (Fig. 11–12) support that diagnosis, demonstrating clusters and sheets of cells, the latter with squamous features. Ultrastructurally, however (Fig. 11–13), the tumor lacks the definitive characteristics of an endometrioid carcinoma. The mitochondria are neither large nor pleomorphic, and bundles of characteristic cytoplasmic microfilaments are lacking.[42]

Other Tumors. Other examples of fine-needle aspirates examined ultrastructurally include an oncocytic adenoma of the thyroid, a single cell from papillary carcinoma of the thyroid, and cells from a poorly differentiated adenocarcinoma of the lung (Figs. 11–14 to 11–16). The oncocytes have cytoplasm packed with mitochondria, and the preservation is so good that the cristae are not easily seen (Fig. 11–14). The cell from the papillary carcinoma of the thyroid (Fig. 11–15) reveals an area of cytoplasm seen through the nucleus (arrow), which perhaps represents the early formation of the optically clear nucleus that is so characteristic of this tumor. The lung carcinoma (Fig. 11–16) shows cells with many microvilli and zonula occludens. There are some cells with virus-like particles in the cytoplasm (arrow). The meaning of these particles is unknown, but they have been seen in one other aspirate of an adenocarcinoma of the lung.

Text continued on page 344

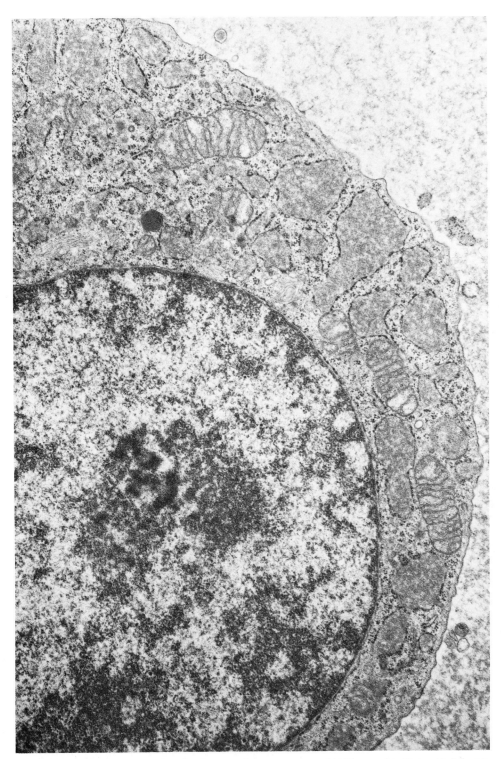

Figure 11–9 Ultrastructural study of aspirate from same case as that illustrated in Figure 11–8 depicts clock-faced heterochromatin pattern but no prominent nucleolus. There is abundant rough endoplasmic reticulum. Mitochondria are well developed, as in well-differentiated plasma cells, but they are not atypical or of giant type. × 17,000.

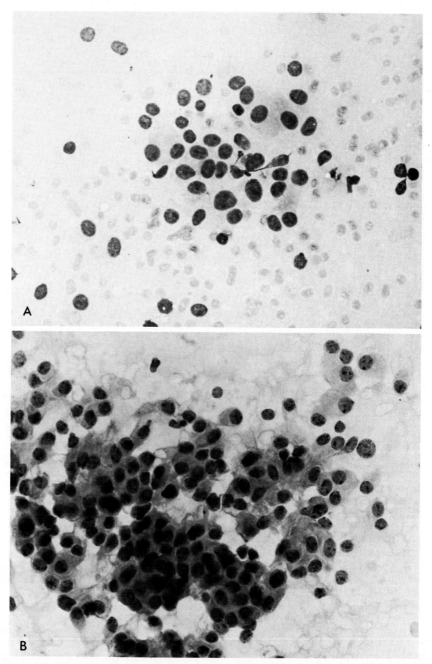

Figure 11–10 Metastatic gastrinoma. Aspirate of axillary mass revealing undifferentiated malignant cells with eccentric nuclei. Note the resemblance to aspirates of some breast cancers. *A*, Diff-Quik × 375. *B*, Papanicolaou × 375.

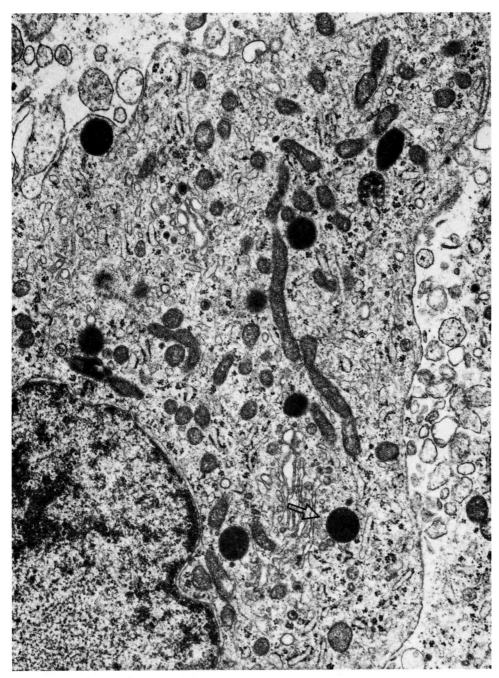

Figure 11–11 Ultrastructural study of aspirate from the same case as that illustrated in Figure 11–10. Cells have abundant elongated mitochondria and neurosecretory granules (arrow). The latter are large, some measuring over 250 nm. These features confirm the diagnosis of metastatic gastrinoma from previous primary site in the duodenum. × 27,500.

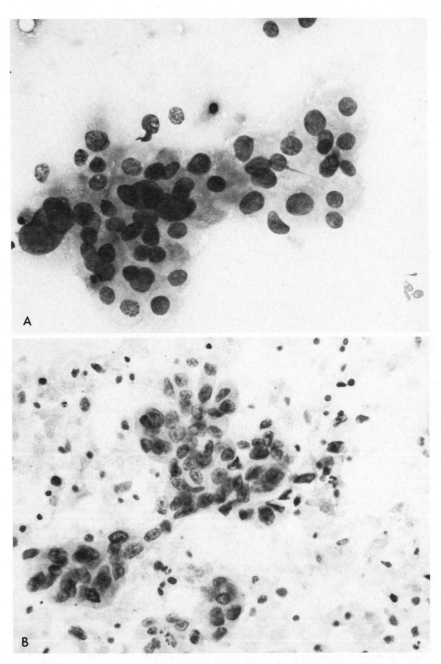

Figure 11–12   Metastatic carcinoma of the ovary. Aspirate of supraclavicular lymph node from patient in whom ovarian carcinoma, endometrioid type, was previously diagnosed. Malignant tumor cells occur in sheets and clusters, consistent with prior diagnosis of endometrioid carcinoma. A, Diff-Quik × 375. B, Papanicolaou × 375.

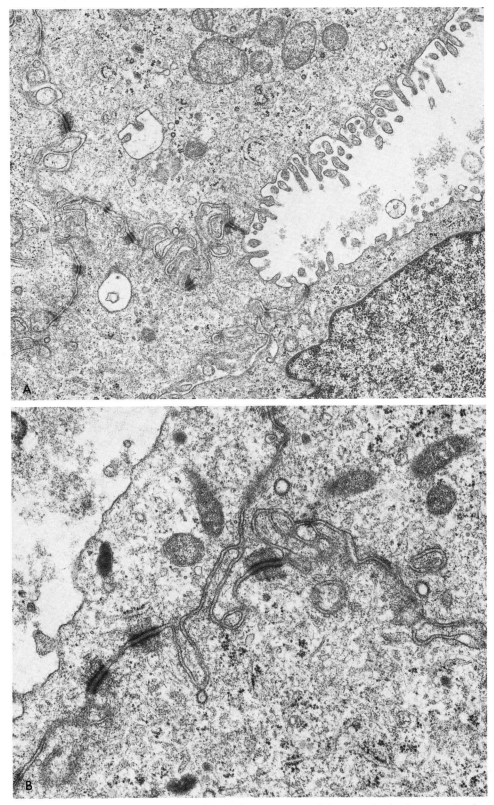

Figure 11–13 Ultrastructure of case illustrated in Figure 11–12 fails to reveal either large mitochondria or diagnostic bundles of microfilaments seen with endometrioid carcinomas. Note the well-developed desmosomes and prominent microvilli. Studies of the original tumor failed to reveal endometrioid characteristics. *A,* × 15,100. *B* × 30,000.

Only Domagala and Koss have reported any studies of cells from fine-needle aspiration biopsies examined by both scanning and transmission electron microscopy. They examined malignant lymphomas, melanomas, oat cell carcinomas, and breast cancers, concluding that the surface configuration of these tumor cells obtained directly from tissue was variable, depending on the histologic pattern. This finding contrasted with observations of the same types of tumor in fluids in which surface characteristics of malignant cells appeared to be quite similar.[43, 44]

SUMMARY

In summary, many currently popular investigative methods may be applied to cells obtained by fine-needle aspiration biopsy. The findings have clinical relevance and open new avenues for the study of human tumors within the dynamic environment of the host.

REFERENCES

1. Boon, M. E., and Lykles, C.: Imaginative approach to fine needle aspiration cytology. Lancet 2:1031–1032, 1980.
2. Engzell, U., Rubio, C., Tjernberg, B., et al.: The lymph node barrier against V × 2 cancer cells before, during and after lymphography. Eur. J. Cancer 4:305–312, 1968.
3. Johansson, B., and Zajicek, J.: Sampling of cell material from human tumours by aspiration biopsy. Nature (Lond.) 200:1333–1334, 1963.

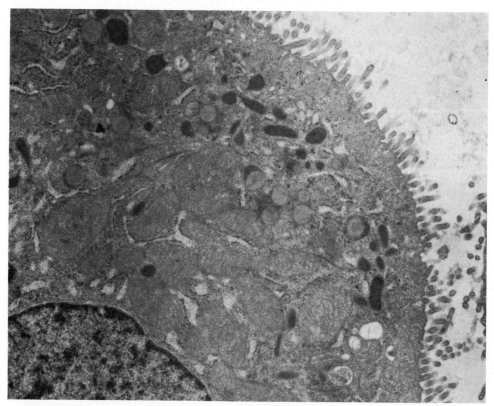

Figure 11–14 Oncocytic adenoma of the thyroid. The cells have closely packed mitochondria that are so well preserved that many of them do not reveal cristae. Aspirate was placed in buffered glutaraldehyde within less than five seconds after it was taken from the patient. × 11,250.

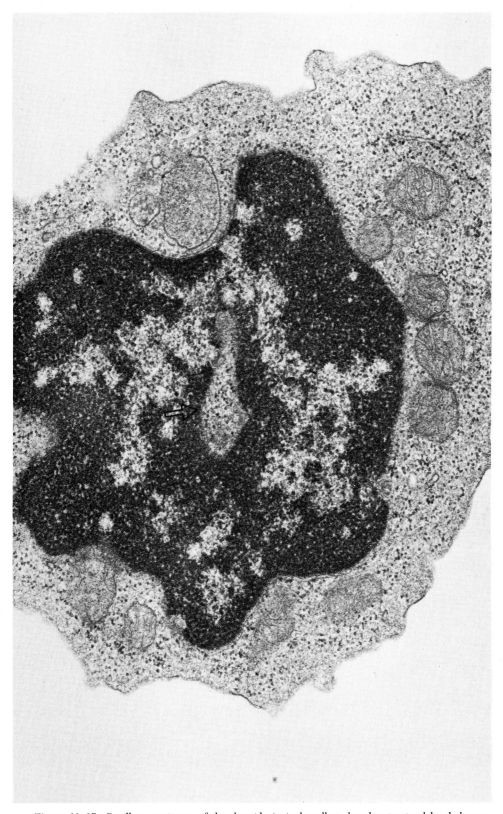

Figure 11–15 Papillary carcinoma of the thyroid. A single cell at the ultrastructural level shows a central area of cytoplasm (arrow) visible through the nucleus. Perhaps this is the beginning of the optically clear nucleus characteristic of this tumor. × 33,000.

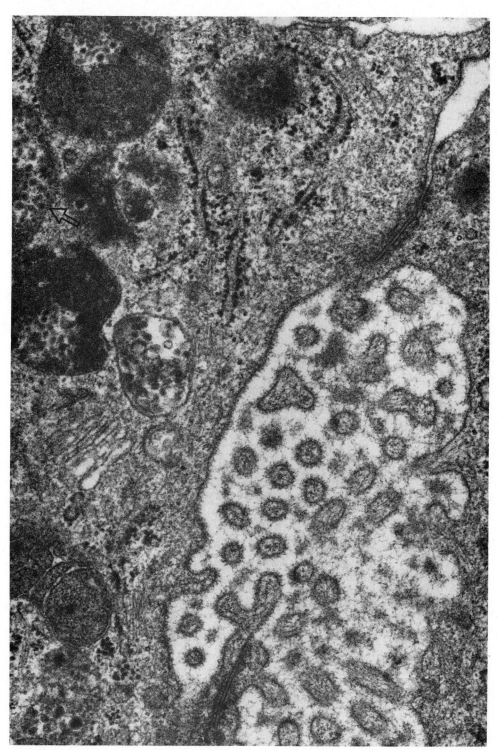

Figure 11–16 Carcinoma of lung. Tumor cells with many microvilli and zonula occludens. Note presence of virus-like particles (arrow, upper left). The significance of these particles is unknown. × 49,500.

4. Scherwin, R. P.: Juxtanuclear lymphocytes in histocultures of mammary cancer. Am. J. Clin. Pathol. 71:64–71, 1978.

5. Wallgren, A., and Zajicek, J.: The prognostic value of aspiration biopsy smear in mammary carcinoma. Acta Cytol. 20:479–485, 1976.

6. Cornelisse, C. J., de Koning, H. R., Arentz, P. W., et al.: Quantitative analysis of nuclear area variation in benign and malignant breast cytology specimens. Anal. Quant. Cytol. 3:128–134, 1981.

7. Dziura, B. R., and Bonfiglio, T. A.: Needle cytology of the breast. A quantitative and qualitative study of the cells of benign and malignant ductal neoplasia. Acta Cytol. 23:332–340, 1979.

8. Zajdela, A., De LaRiva, L. S., and Ghossein, N. A.: The relation of prognosis to the nuclear diameter of breast cancer cells obtained by cytologic aspiration. Acta Cytol. 23:75–80, 1979.

9. Zajicek, J., Bartles, P. H., Bahr, G. F., et al.: Computer analysis of needle aspirates from breast carcinomas during radiotherapy. Acta Cytol. 17:179–187, 1973.

10. Bocking, A.: Validation of diagnostic criteria in prostatic cytology by semiautomated image analysis (abstract). Anal. Quant. Cytol. 2:293, 1980.

11. Spaander, P. J., Ruiter, D. J., de Voogt, H. J., et al.: The implication of subjective recognition of malignant cells in aspiration for the grading of prostatic cancer using cell image analysis (abstract). Anal. Quant. Cytol. 2:305, 1980.

12. Boon, M. E., Lowhagen, T., and Willems, J. S.: Planimetric studies on fine needle aspirates from follicular adenoma and follicular carcinoma of the thyroid. Acta Cytol. 24:145–148, 1980.

13. Luck, J. B., Mumaw, U. R., and Frable, W. J.: Fine needle aspiration biopsy of the thyroid. Differential diagnosis by "Videoplan" image analysis. Acta Cytol. In press.

14. Thommesen, P., Frederiksen, P., Bichel, P., et al.: Flow-cytometric analysis of human tumour tissue obtained by fine needle aspiration biopsy. Ugeskr. Laeger 140:155–158, 1978.

15. Moubayed, A. P.: Zytomorphologische, zytophotometrische und histologische diagnostik an mamma-biopsien. Geburtshilfe Frauenheilkd. 36:905–911, 1976.

16. Zajicek, J., Caspersson, T., Jakobsson, P., et al.: Cytologic diagnosis of mammary tumors from aspiration biopsy smears. Comparison of cytologic and histologic findings in 2,111 lesions and diagnostic use of cytophotometry. Acta Cytol. 14:370–376, 1970.

17. Auer, G. U., Caspersson, T. O., and Wallgren, A. S.: DNA content and survival in mammary carcinoma. Anal. Quant. Cytol. 2:161–165, 1980.

18. Nordenskjold, B., Lowhagen, T., Westerberg, H., et al.: 3H-thymidine incorporation into mammary carcinoma cells obtained by needle aspiration before and during endocrine therapy. Acta Cytol. 20:137–143, 1976.

19. Bedrossian, C. W. M., Raber, M., and Barlogie, B.: Flow cytometry and cytomorphology in primary resectable breast cancer. Anal. Quant. Cytol. 3:112–116, 1981.

20. Auer, G. U., Caspersson, T. O., Gustafsson, S. A., et al.: Relationship between nuclear DNA distribution and estrogen receptors in human mammary carcinomas. Anal. Quant. Cytol. 2:280–284, 1980.

21. Patek, E., Johannisson, E., Krauer, F., et al.: Microfluorometric grading of mammary tumors. A pilot study. Anal. Quant. Cytol. 2:264–271, 1980.

22. Sprenger, E., Ulrich, H., and Schondorf, H.: The diagnostic value of DNA determination aspiration cytology of benign and malignant lesions of the breast. Anal. Quant. Cytol. 1:29–36, 1979.

23. Preece, P. E., and Zippel, H. H.: X-chromatin (Barr Bodies) correlated with DNA content of lobular neoplasia and invasive lobular carcinoma in the female breast. Acta Cytol. 23:163–168, 1979.

24. Kreicbergs, A., Cewrien, G., Tribukait, B., et al.: Comparative single-cell and flow DNA analysis of bone sarcoma. Anal. Quant. Cytol. 3:121–127, 1981.

25. Adams, L. R., and Dahlgren, S. E.: Cytophotometric measurements of the DNA content of lung tumours. Acta Pathol. Microbiol. Scand. 72:561–574, 1968.

26. Taylor, C. R., and Kledzik, G.: Immunohistologic techniques in surgical pathology—a spectrum of "new" special stains. Human Pathol. 12:590–596, 1981.

27. DeLellis, R. A., Sternberger, L. A., Mann, R. B., et al.: Immunoperoxidase technics in diagnostic pathology. Report of a workshop sponsored by the National Cancer Institute. Am. J. Clin. Pathol. 71:483–488, 1979.

28. Singh, G., Dekker, A., and Whiteside, T. L.: Anti–mesothelial cell serum: A diagnostic reagent for malignant mesothelioma (meeting abstract). Fed. Proc. 38:912, 1979.

29. Nadji, M.: The potential value of immunoperoxidase techniques in diagnostic cytology. Acta Cytol. 24:442–447, 1980.

30. Coleman, D. V., To, A., Ormerod, M. G., et al.: Immunoperoxidase staining in tumor marker distribution studies in cytologic specimens (letter). Acta Cytol. 25:205, 1981.

31. Battifora, H., Sun, T., Bahu, R. M., et al.: The use of antikeratin antiserum as a diagnostic tool: Thymoma versus lymphoma. Human Pathol. 11:635–640, 1980.

32. Battifora, H.: Significance of new and special methods in human tumor diagnosis in surgical pathology. Presentation, Specialty Conference. International Academy of Pathology, Annual Meeting, March 5, 1981.

33. Lee, S. H.: Cellular estrogen and progesterone receptors in mammary carcinoma. Am. J. Clin. Pathol. 73:323–329, 1980.

34. Brigati, D. J., Bloom, N. D., Tobin, E. H., Kim, D. S., et al.: Morphologic methods of steroid hormone receptor analysis in human breast cancer: A review. Breast 5:27–33, 1979.

35. Pertschuk, L. P., Gaetjens, E., Carter, A. C., et al.: Histochemistry of steroid receptors in breast cancer: An overview. Ann. Clin. Lab. Sci. 9:219–224, 1979.

36. Silfversward, C., and Humla, S.: Estrogen receptor analysis on needle aspirates from human mammary carcinoma. Acta Cytol. *24*:54–57, 1980.

37. Domagala, W., Kahan, A., and Koss, L. G.: A simple method of preparation and identification of cells for scanning electron microscopy. Acta Cytol. *23*:140–146, 1979.

38. Ruiter, D. J., Mauaw, B. J., and Beyer-Boon, M. E.: Ultrastructure of normal epithelial cells in Papanicolaou stained cervical smears. An application of a modified open-faced embedding technique for transmission electron microscopy. Acta Cytol. *23*:507–515, 1979.

39. Coleman, D. V., Russell, W. J. I., Hodgson, J., et al.: Human papova virus in Papanicolaou smear of urinary sediment detected by transmission electron microscopy. J. Clin. Pathol. *30*:1015–1020, 1977.

40. Ghadially, F. N.: *Diagnostic Electron Microscopy of Tumours.* Boston, Butterworths & Co., Ltd., 1980, pp. 190–197.

41. Trump, B. F., and Jones, R. T.: *Diagnostic Electron Microscopy.* Vol. 3. New York, John Wiley & Sons, 1980, p. 473.

42. Trump, B. F., and Jones, R. T.: *Diagnostic Electron Microscopy.* Vol. 2. New York, John Wiley & Sons, 1979, pp. 292–293.

43. Domagala, W., and Koss, L. G.: Configuration of surfaces of human cancer cells obtained by fine needle aspiration biopsy. A comparative light microscopic and scanning electron microscopic study. Acta Cytol. *24*:427–434, 1980.

44. Domagala, W., and Koss, L. G.: Configuration of surfaces of human cancer cells in effusions: A scanning electron microscropic study of microvilli. Virchows Arch. Abt. B. Zellpathol. *26*:27–42, 1977.

INDEX